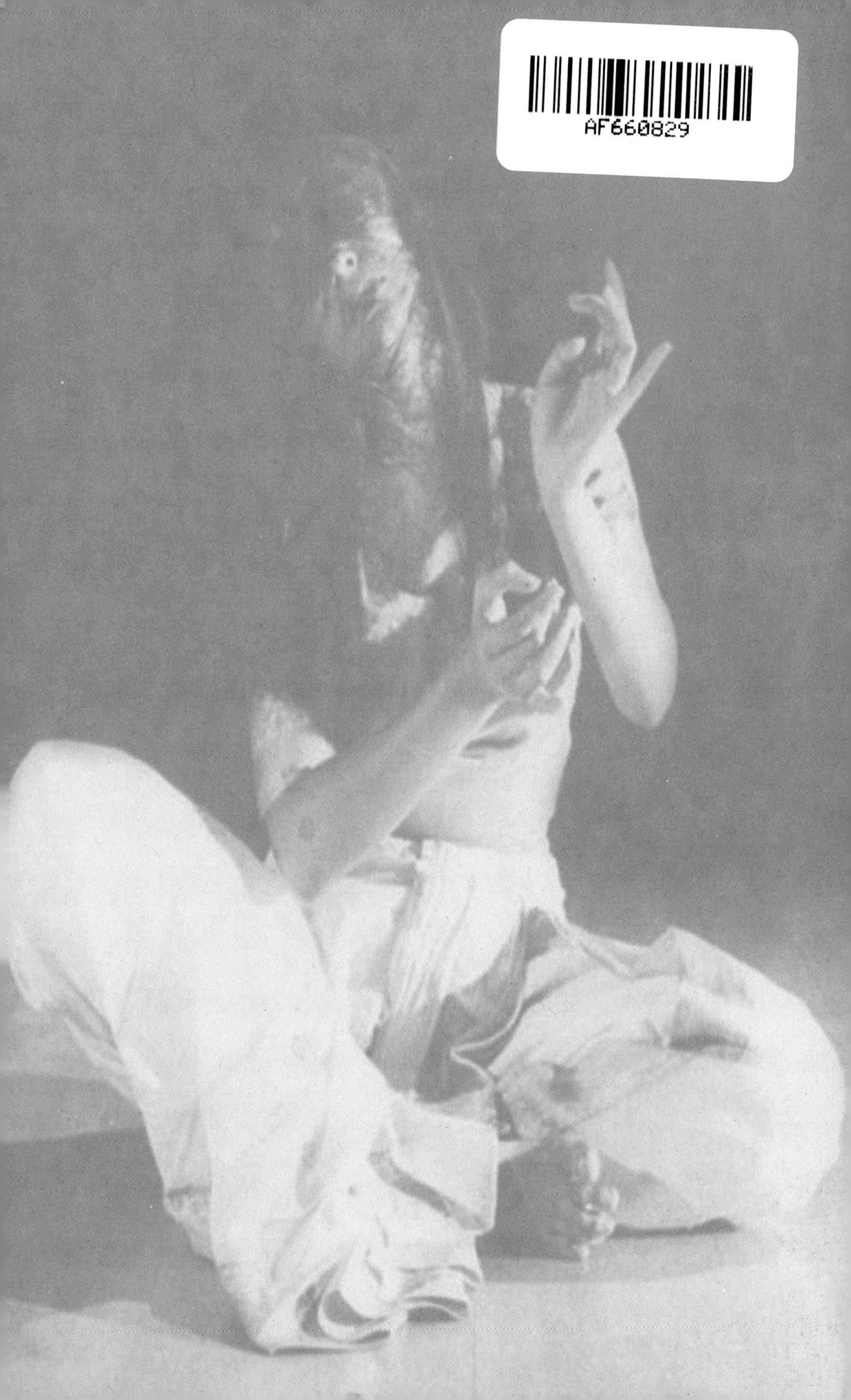

THE MOVING SPACE

The Moving Space
WOMEN IN DANCE

edited by

URMIMALA SARKAR MUNSI
AISHIKA CHAKRABORTY

PRIMUS BOOKS

PRIMUS BOOKS
An imprint of Ratna Sagar P. Ltd.
Virat Bhavan
Mukherjee Nagar Commercial Complex
Delhi 110 009

Offices at
CHENNAI LUCKNOW
AGRA AHMEDABAD BENGALURU COIMBATORE DEHRADUN GUWAHATI
HYDERABAD JAIPUR JALANDHAR KANPUR KOCHI KOLKATA MADURAI
MUMBAI PATNA RANCHI VARANASI

First published 2018

ISBN: 978-93-86552-50-1 (hardback)
ISBN: 978-93-86552-51-8 (POD)

Published by Primus Books

Laser typeset by Mithu Karmakar
mithu.karma@gmail.com

Printed and bound in India by
Replika Press Pvt. Ltd.

To

SREEMATI AMALA SHANKAR

and

LATE DR MANJUSRI CHAKI-SIRCAR

who have shaped our lives and scholarship

Contents

Part III: Choreographing the Space: Identity and Creativity

Part IV: Transformative Space: Empathy and Activism

Acknowledgements

This book is dedicated to two women dancers, Sreemati Amala Shankar and Late Dr Manjusri Chaki-Sircar, who have taught us the magic of moving as dancers, and also have been instrumental in helping us think of the dance space as a constantly moving and evolving dynamic entity that controls the dancer as much as the dancer controls it. Years spent as a student, performer, troupe member, teacher and eventually also a senior administrator at Uday Shankar India Culture Centre (for Urmimala) was not only a training in dance but also of moving through life and the world with dance. Dancers' Guild (for Aishika) brings back memories of wonderfully exciting and back-breaking work associated with classes, rehearsals, movements and choreographies, and also travel, tears and laughter. In the process of working on this book, each of us has constantly been thinking of the years spent with each of these strong women, whose contributions become more and more significant in our practice and research.

The book grew out of a conference organized by World Dance Alliance–Asia Pacific and School of Women's Studies, Jadavpur University, Kolkata. We would like to acknowledge Professor Samita Sen of School of Women's Studies, Jadavpur University, for her support and encouragement in organizing the conference. Her interest in the emergent field of dance and performance studies by bringing it within the academic rubric of Women's Studies has been a source of continuous motivation.

We are thankful to the critical thinking of our colleagues, the brilliant queries of students, the inspiring and supportive team of School of Arts and Aesthetics, Jawaharlal Nehru University, New Delhi, and School of Women's Studies, Jadavpur University, for fuelling our thoughts throughout the conference that finally led to the idea of this book.

For the photographic descriptions we are especially indebted to Avinash Pasricha for giving us the prints and his permission to use his photographs in our book. The editors are thankful to Sadanand Menon; Maya Krishna Rao; Priyadarshini Govind, the Director of Kalakshetra Foundation, Chennai; Pinaki Chaki; Jonaki Sarkar and Parbati Gupta of Dancers' Guild; and Poulami Das of Jawaharlal Nehru University for sharing invaluable material and rare photographs with us. We owe a lot to each one of them.

Priyanka Basu deserves a special mention for the first round of editing she did for us. We acknowledge the contribution of Madhurima Guha for transcribing interviews included in the section on dance activism.

Urmimala acknowledges the critical engagement and encouragement of her parents, Vidya and Sunil Munsi, both of whom were part of many conversations during the conference and the beginning of the book but are not around to see it in print. She would like to thank Manasi, Namrata and Aditya for providing emotional, editorial and intellectual support.

Aishika remembers her mother Shipra Chakraborty for making the *extra*-curricular intrinsically central to the everyday curriculum as she thanks her father Amulya Ratan Chakraborty for his endless love and support. A word of thanks to Bhomra for being a constant source of digression and for undertaking, willy-nilly, long travels with his mother in search of dance.

URMIMALA SARKAR MUNSI
AISHIKA CHAKRABORTY

Plates

Introduction

URMIMALA SARKAR MUNSI
AISHIKA CHAKRABORTY

This book is an attempt at understanding the journeys of women in dance today, their past and the spaces they have created for themselves. It acknowledges the fragility of their social presence and the duality of the reception they receive, which continue to draw the attention of scholars. It also focuses on their contribution to history, one that remains submerged in discourses of aesthetics, culture, and tradition.

Indian dance has come a long way since the beginning of the twentieth century, from the time when dance reforms were initiated to the present. Scholars of dance history and women's/feminist studies have written about the historical trajectories of dancers' journeys, drawing upon individual histories of women dancers—temple dancers, nautch girls, and classical dancers. This study covers a larger area to include Bollywood heroines and item girls, bar dancers, and the popular local/regional women dancers. It often straddles sociology, dance history and women's studies together, and ventures beyond, to look at the multifaceted life/live stories of embodiment, empowerment, exploitation, subjugation, and subversion repeated across social space and time.

Dance genres as well as dancers in India are set apart by the spaces they occupy. The spaces are varied, and are marked by the physical location, the identity they represent, the class and caste affiliations of the audience and the dancers, and the politics of the patronage the space represents. For instance, tribal women, celebrating the birth of a new child or welcoming a new bride home, occupy space in a private domain, culled from within the everyday structure of community life. In contrast, dancers from the classical forms of high art specifically meant for the proscenium also occupy a space which is public and framed within the aesthetic understanding of the norms of presentations linked to such performances. The popular Bollywood form that has become the country's identity, through its screen presence, refers to an altogether different space, one that is structured and controlled by market-led saleability. Public/private, commercial/aesthetics, ritual/secular, national/international, and last but not least, male/female, are a few of the binaries that may be used to contextualize the dance space, if there is any such specifically demarcated space in India.

This volume contextualizes the woman dancer and her performance practice within the changing sociocultural rubric of Indian society. It asks two principle questions simultaneously: (1) How does the woman dancer negotiate and shape the space/s she lives, trains, and performs in? (2) What role does the space play in constituting her gendered identity and consequent sexualization, as the ground where her art is shaped by the spatial norms, directing or controlling her, as both person and performer? To this end, the chapters in this volume bring together scholarships that look at the space as a moving, ever-changing entity, shaped through the range of practices of the woman dancer and which in turn also constructs and shapes her as well as her art.

Traversing the history of Indian women dancers—from the past through to present-day realities around identity and agency, and between tradition and transition—this volume brings together a range of original scholarship. The study of dance and dancers here thus furthers some of the current preoccupations of feminist scholarship, examining relationships among women located in very different and hierarchical social positions, the relationships between the body and the social, and, especially, concerns about gender and performance. Likewise, the principal concern within dance studies reflected here is centred around the aesthetics and counter-aesthetics that have shaped the world of women dancers, their bodies, and their dance.

Thematic Concerns

This volume highlights the ideas of the social, political, material, and metaphorical spaces created/inhabited/negotiated by women in Indian dance, and strives to create an area of conversation between women's studies and dance studies, to strengthen discourses already generated by studies in both areas.

The idea of this volume was crystallized after a conference, 'The Moving Space: Women in Dance', organized jointly by Dance Alliance India and School of Women's Studies, Jadavpur University, Kolkata, in 2013, which brought together scholars, activists, and practitioners from multidisciplinary backgrounds. The common thread among this group was the effort required to generate a conversation between ongoing research on and around dance within the disciplines of dance studies, women's studies, history, and social anthropology. As one can see, the choreographed structure of this volume gains strength from scholarships in diverse disciplines.

While it does not assume the responsibility of becoming a reader for dance studies in India, it contextualizes dance in contemporary India, highlighting the complexities of categorization, visibility and the relationship between tradition and transition in the micro spaces of some regions and contexts and the macro space of the nation state. It views dance as a natural and critical starting point of contemporary discourses on the body and space because it is one of the few art forms in which feminist theory is actually embodied.

Fracturing the conventional reification of body image it however shifts the discourse away from the body to the 'space(s)', historically accorded and culturally framed, to trace the physical experience of the dancer—her somatic and kinaesthetic world, her choreographic agency, and her subjectivity. Constructing new identities, new bodies and new feminist spaces, it maps the public revelation of a woman's subjective/personal/somatic/erotic/political experiences by recording her own life/story in her dance. The reference to training and articulating as a continuous process in dance practices and performances opens up the scope and necessity of using feminist theories in understanding complex relationships between individual experiences, gendered representation, and cultural constructions. Susan Foster writes that the 'initiative within dance studies to approach dance as a historically specific cultural practice rather than an ineffable celebration of a universal human condition has taken place alongside and with the aid of feminist studies'.[1] This argument strengthens the connections between the essays in the four sections of this volume, principally divided on the basis of methodologies of historiography, performance studies, biographical analysis, and practice-led research—focusing on gender and dance together—with one leading the other in different reflections. Foster says:

> Over the past twenty years, dance scholars have used the kinds of interpretive strategies implemented in feminist theory to distance sex from gender as a way to denaturalize the dancing body and historicize dance as a practice and profession. The pertinence of feminism to dance studies has long been apparent. The professions of both dance and dance scholarship are made up almost entirely of women. Dance, the object of study, is feminized within our society. The dancing body is aligned with and central among a whole host of entities similarly defined as feminine: it is most often construed as natural, authentic, spontaneous, fervent, chaotic, and evanescent. Whether primordial or decorous, it is always insubstantial. At the same time, gendered divisions of labor exist within the discipline such that producers and artistic directors are most often male and dancers are most often female.[2]

A feminist historiographical reading of some of the important moments in dance history is essential here, as it widens the scope of a range of readings of the same histories in the existing academic and coffee-table publications. What distinguishes this study from other publications on gender and dance is the inclusion of some established and well-known scholars from theatre studies, media studies, social sciences, history, and women's/feminist studies. This multidisciplinary construct is what extends the scope of this volume beyond dance or into other subject specializations.

'Every social space is the outcome of a process with many aspects and many contributing currents, signifying and non-signifying, perceived and directly experienced, practical and theoretical.'[3] A range of spaces as outcomes of different processes of engagements of dance and their very gendered presence in society—directly or indirectly experienced, perceived through practice or theory—is conceptualized through the framework of the book. This will help the reader navigate through the historical contestations, and contemporary experimentations, surrounding women dancers, allowing, in the process, for gendered identities to emerge as the principal thread tying together the various contributions to this volume.

Judith Butler saw gender identities coming into being through the reiterative and coercive tools embedded within the structures of repetitions that are embedded within systems of teaching and following social norms and value systems.[4] The expectations, thus, being enforced within the everyday embodied practices also bring out certain performative structures, whereby such doings and beings can never be taken as separate or independent of the controlling structural base, which is invisible by itself, but are made visible through the performances themselves. But the world of dance chooses its projection carefully, showcasing aesthetics rather than back-breaking labour, beauty rather than enforced near-violent selective mechanisms, and fulfilment of the dancer rather than the heartbreak of rejection and the precarity of a short career. Constructions of normative structures of gender, that remain at the very base of all projections, remain well hidden by the overt function of dance as the embodied tool for aesthetics representation—of national culture, tradition, and history.

I Become the Space

The French post-structuralist Michel Foucault once claimed that 'the present epoch will perhaps above all be the epoch of space'.[5] Many followed his prediction by heart which is evident from the present preoccupation with space, as emerged from a range of disciplines. In recent post-structuralist and postmodern theory there has been an almost obsessive interest in ideas and theories about space—the ways in which space is experienced and its characteristics as a social construct. Doreen Massey conceptualized space as a dividing line, a differentiating colonial developmental model associated with temporality. She argues that the geography of modernity is the repression of the 'spatial', it is also the repression of the possibility of other temporalities.[6] In a fascinating study of dance, space and subjectivity, Valerie A. Briginshaw, with a focus on space in dance, explores the various ways in which dance can challenge, trouble and question the fixed perceptions of subjectivity.[7] In contrast to a place which is always bound to a location, culturally mythical or experiential, writes Olivia Ainsworth, space is an abstract concept that is continuously expansive, philosophically and geographically describing the area that surrounds and envelops life.[8]

Several dance theorists use the broader concept of space in relation to the body. Carol Brown observes that choreography generates 'a sense of place through tangibly manipulating space as a material of the dance'.[9] Exploring the dynamic engagement between space, corporality and architecture, she states that 'space' is 'no longer conceived as a three-dimensional continuum, space becomes a discontinuous, plurality of spaces containing multiple dimensions'; that is in itself 'performative'.[10] Through dancing, space is experienced as a continuum between inside and outside, outside and inside. A dancer traces the embodied experience of both these spaces 'in rotating the undersides of corporeal surfaces, in (dis)embodying the narratives of place, in measuring space through experiencing bodily articulations, in mapping body parts to points in space; in extruding lines, in shifting scale, in changing orientations; in hollowing volumes, in scribing geometries, in drawing spaces and in spiraling dimensions.[11] To align contemporary dancing bodies with the ordinances of contemporary spaces requires a rethinking of inherited conversations about the practice and making of spaces. In a significant observation Brown comments:

> Choreography is situated in the corporal, social, institutional and conceptual spaces. In its discovery and embodying of spaces, choreography makes places as temporary cartographies of energy and force rather than fixed forms. In its practice it embodies a multiplicity of understandings of space as physical, psychic, metaphoric and virtual. Today dance spaces are continuously expanding and extending to unfamiliar and untried spaces, reversing the parameters of performer-audience exchanges, challenging conventions of spatial practices within dance and opening new sites and situations for choreography. As choreographers increasingly mix dance with other art forms, going vigorously multi-disciplinary, new genres of performance practice emerges such as dance installations, screen dance, site-responsive dance, place-sensitive dance, dance architecture and interactive dance.[12]

The Kusilavas and their Vanishing Space of Performance

Historically, the space of public performance in India remains a tricky one, ostensibly devious, where discourses on politics, morality and aesthetics are densely imbricated. Kautilya's *Arthashastra*, the famous text on ancient Indian politics and statecraft, describes the theatrical stage as a 'magic-space'—a 'space' open to manifold manoeuvring and manipulation. Revisiting the text, otherwise an unconventional source to start a discourse on gender and performance, Sibaji Bandyopadhyay untangles it as a 'treatise on stagecraft' where the Kusilavas, a heterogeneous band of performer-entertainers, play-acted limitless imaginary and fantastic events by recreating a slice of real or imagined life.[13] The Kusilavas (from the word *Kushil*, meaning a person of bad lineage) embraced a cross-section of artist-performers, comprising not merely actors, dancers, singers, and musicians, but also trumpeters, storytellers, acrobats, jugglers, clowns, artisans, and mendicants, who offered a lavish spread of amusement, luxury, and human desire. It was with regard to the latter that the performance of the Kusilavas overlapped with another performer's—the ganika or the prostitute/courtesan, who with all her expertise in dancing, singing and acting also allowed men to have 'free' and 'private' access to her body for a fee or a favour. The state which extracted revenues from the ganikas, many of whom lived independently, bore the expenses of training them in several accomplishments including singing, dancing, acting, playing musical instruments, conversing, writing, mind-reading, and also the art of lovemaking.[14] And since there was not much difference between the craft of a Kusilava and a ganika, the *Arthashastra* enjoins the *Ganikadhyaksha* or the Head of the Department of Courtesans/Prostitutes and 'Leisure Control Officials' to ensure that official regulations regarding prostitutes and courtesans also extend and apply to *nata-nartaka-gayana-vadaka-vagjivana-plavaka-saubhika-charana* (and such other Kusilava).[15]

Though not equating performers ostensibly with prostitutes, another fabled text on Indian performance, Bharata's *Natyashastra*, dubs women performers primarily as sexual objects, setting down explicit rules to control their sexual and performative spheres and entrusting men with the duty of disciplining women through power and even violence. Dealing with drama, performance, and sexual behaviours of men and women, the *Natyashastra* also describes several roles and functions of the *nayika*, the heroine of the play, who primarily portrayed three characters—the *Swakiya* (the wife), the *Parakiya* (the beloved or other's wife), and the *Swadhina* (the prostitute). Epitomizing different imageries of emotions, *astanayikas* play out eight different moods and bodily expressions, each related with contentment and frustration of their romance with the *nayaka* (hero). Recent scholars consider the recommendations of the *Natyashastra* as representative of various patriarchal strategies, on and off stage, for controlling and suppressing women.[16] Even today, the *Natyashastra* is a seminal text not only on performativity and techniques of performance, but also as a rule book of gender and caste to fix social norms and boundaries for different classes, castes, and communities.[17]

Without offering any aesthetic advice to the persons engaged in this occupation/trade, Kautilya, however, had a very different perspective. He crudely described the Kusilavas 'as being artful', the ones who 'regale the audience by putting up shows'. As entertainers the Kusilavas had the necessary skills to impersonate both the real and the imagined, to enchant and captivate their audience with innate expertise in duping people. For their clever act of masquerading, the Kusilavas were also portrayed by the author of the *Arthashastra* as quintessential 'thieves'—'if not in name, then certainly in effect'.[18] As fellow citizens of the 'world of thieves', performers were clubbed together with the *chor* (thief) and the ganika (whore). The space of performance was turned into a space of clandestine politics, connivance, allure and mystery, as the *Arthashastra* metaphorically described the 'stage' in terms of the 'whore's bed' and vice versa. As in every society, the double standard of patriarchal morality sanctioned both a 'sanctified marriage-bed' and a 'whore's bed' to hold the family in place, says Sibaji Bandyopadhyay:

> [B]eing a space which is alternate to the real world, an unavoidable dream-space where much that is regularly repressed in the arena of real-experiences gets to be randomly expressed, the 'theatrical stage' is like a pillar holding the centre in place—in the final instance (although 'noxious'), both the 'whore's bed' and the 'stage' are innocuous; neither of the two can really contribute to any programme, which aims to change the world.[19]

Though not considered a very loyal subject of the state, the policy of policing the Kusilavas' performance is grounded on incitement—motivating instead of silencing and sanctioning instead of prohibiting. The entertainers were incited to poke fun at the state, at religious customs, and caste and sexual practices, by 'ridiculing and rubbishing the Order'.[20] The state's incitement, it was believed, put a damper on the carnivalesque critique as performers were allowed to laugh at their set rules. Taking the actors as 'the only honest hypocrites', the system of governance 'formalized' their subversion which was founded on the principle called 'submission-through-transgression', hence rendering the 'resistive' entertainment harmless by elevating the non-official and the extra-political to the official status. But the state also struck a 'deal', observes Bandyopadhyay. Taking extra care to safeguard the artist 'from the wrath of the mighty' the same Kusilavas were employed for the purpose of spying on behalf of the state, hence turning 'the artist who is officially anti-statist' to be loyal to the state, to be 'unofficially statist'.[21] Kautilya, notorious for advocating the 'immoral' and the 'unethical', also adds reasons and qualification for recommending such policies.[22] He makes it explicit, without hypocrisy, what nation states, ancient and modern, always practised.

The moral and political anxiety around the space of performance continued well into modern times, but with some major disjunctions. Sumanta Banerjee's study of nineteenth-century Calcutta's elite and popular culture can be read as a microcosm of the wider Indian scenario where the progressive elite, backed by the alien state, systematically evicted the indigenous popular cultural manifestations from their status, space and livelihood. Unlike the liberty enjoyed by the Kusilavas in ancient India, popular performers of colonial Bengal faced virtual extinction when the colonial administration, joined by the colonized elite, clamped down their 'explosive' topics for performance. On 20 September 1873, the 'educated natives' gathered at Calcutta Town Hall and established the 'Society for the Suppression of Public Obscenity' to 'salvage' their culture from becoming 'polluted and polluting' and to aid the government in putting in force the sections of the Penal Code and the Printing Act to preserve public purity.[23]

A wedge was drawn between the amorphous cultural world of women, shared equally by the elite women or *bhadramahila* and their low-caste/-class counterparts. Sharing the imperial moral anxiety over woman's body and sexuality, the metropolitan elite not merely distanced their private chamber from the contaminating popular culture but also banished the entire subgenre of popular song and dance from the streets and marts. While winds of change swept through the middle-class homes under the influence of enlightenment, the low-class popular performers had to move to the 'dangerous society', dissociating themselves from 'their sheltered sisters', curled up within the upper-class *andarmahal*s.[24] Ironically, though not unsurprisingly, in this ideological crusade the Indian male elite found 'their biggest allies' in their newly emancipated wives and daughters. The respectable women conformed, in varying degrees, to the models offered, to validate their incorporation into the new social and cultural world. At one level it meant curtailing their freedom in the public productive world, but at another it facilitated their participation in a wide range of activity—from literary to performative—leading to the emergence of a new breed of performance culture absorbed in the male moral-intellectual space isolated from that of the lower-class women. By the late nineteenth century, the *khemtawali*s, *jhumurwali*s or the *bai* dancers, thriving so far in the *majlis* and *mehfils*, in bazaars and village marts, were pushed to the fringe as the centre (stage) was overtaken by an exalted modern elite culture of the *bhadramahila*s.

Women performers who inhabited a liminal social-sexual space outside the pale of marriage fell within the loose uncritiqued category of 'prostitute', a moral threat to the identity and integrity of the society and nation. A series of acts, like the Contagious Diseases Act and the Cantonment Regulation Act included bai and tawaif (courtesan) within the category of prostitute and relocated them outside the city space, stripping them off their status and livelihood. And, ideally, when the nation was refurbishing its 'identity' with sharpening focus on honour, morality and purity, prostitutes could not be performers and vice versa. Fixing women in their respective 'proper' places was on the cards.

Partha Chatterjee's persuasive argument on the nationalist resolution of the women's question redefined the material (public) and the spiritual (private) divide in the construction and demarcation of spaces where men were free to contest and collaborate with the colonial masters in the public realm, and women, representing the quintessential inner core of the nation, were placed firmly within the private domain. The demarcation of the family, as the arena of nationalist resistance to colonial intervention, and the home, as a place of retreat, 'resolved', according to Chatterjee, the 'women's question', by reconstituting her as the authentic representative of tradition and the symbol of India's identity.[25] The creator-organizer of this space was the iconic 'new woman', fashioned by the 'new patriarchy'. She would preserve India's cultural heritage in the domestic realm while carrying an antithesis of sexual provocation or any kind of public sexual display in the 'public' sphere.

Although Chatterjee's argument of the nationalist gendering of separate spheres draws on the Bengal example, it holds true, argues Janet O'Shea, of India as a whole, and especially in the process of the refiguration of Bharatanatyam in south India.[26] Bharatanatyam dancers grappled with the reformist and nationalist discourses that had brought the 'women's question' to centre stage, O'Shea maintains, while the campaigners had pushed dance to the margins of public life.[27] When elite women turned to the same dance (even erotic), once performed by the devadasis, Bharatanatyam was recrafted as the emblem of the nation, and subsequently emerged as a 'national treasure', confirming the feminine and cultural propriety of the women. Intertwining dance with nationalist strategies of gender construction, it was also represented as symbolic of the 'domestic' values of tradition, religiosity and spirituality functioning as a symbol of pan-Indian, and, in some cases, pan-South Asian middle-class feminine propriety.[28]

In this process of coming in and fading out, Bharatanatyam had to shift from a public woman's form, associated with prostitution, courtesanship, temple dance—everything falling under 'extradomestic sexuality', to quote Amrit Srinivasan[29]—into a public representation of symbolic domesticity through its performance of tradition and spirituality. Rukmini Devi's choreography and pedagogy further enabled a move of 'family woman' into public spaces as she purified the form by eradicating the stigma of courtesanship, erasing traditional practitioners from the newly sanitized space.

The culture of exclusion continues unabated from the pre-colonial to the colonial and then to the postcolonial time under the neo-liberal state. A recent study by Anna Morcom notes a line of continuity in the interventionist policies of the state that once launched anti-nautch campaigns to ostracize the devadasis and the tawaif and then under its neo-liberal garb put a legal ban on bar dancers, driving them all underground and denying them their status and livelihood. In a state where culture is embedded firmly within relations of power, domination and hierarchies such exclusions help the upper-caste/-class performers to retain their control over the 'official' national sphere of performance and to erase simultaneously the 'aberrant' and 'transgressive' dancing bodies that failed to fit into the storied space of the modernist nation. Hence performance 'tradition' was separated from performers themselves, forcing courtesans and dancing girls to disappear from 'high profile and in nationalist terms, legitimate, cultural life'.[30] The colonial deduction that an erotic public performer who existed outside the ambit of marriage 'is a prostitute and therefore is not a performer'[31] further undermines the labour and artistic status of performers with changing dynamics of market economics and class stratifications.

Interesting is the parallel trend of appropriation and appreciation of these 'illicit' forms of dance and desire by the regional and national film industries in post-independent India. The growing demand and popular acceptance towards the sizzling cabaret numbers from the 1950s to the 1970s or the pervasive marketability of the more recent item girls demonstrate the popular demand for this 'tabooed' desired dance. The embourgeoisement of performing arts continues, with the emergence of 'respectable' Bollywood dance with a simultaneous exclusion of public/erotic dancers from their space, which now involve increasing sexualization of performance and more transactional sex. Hence, Helen and Bindu, the dancing icons of the Bollywood film industry, rose to stardom winning accolades across the nation while Miss Shefali's sleazy cabaret in Calcutta hotels was viewed as a signifier of a depraved culture as was the case with the bar dancers who were banished from Bombay's nightclubs. The bourgeois capitalism of the new liberal democracy on the one hand appropriates a variety of dancing bodies, from the colonial cabaret to the global hybrid item dancing, as saleable commodities to a wide range of consumer audiences, while on the other hand it disciplines and downgrades sexuality and occupations of low-class women dancers by throwing them out of the public space. The paradox (of inclusion/exclusion) continues.

Our effort, in this anthology, is never to undermine the dancer and her engagement, however critical our understanding may be of the appropriation that may have happened thereafter of her art. Instead we find that the chapters create a discursive space around the women dancers, where some presences are seen as homogenizing and homogenized, while others are seen as the resistive ones, who have attempted collapsing 'the old points of reference'.[32]

Historicizing Spaces: Text and Context

Many writers within historical discussions as well as within the specific area of dance history have discussed the real as well as the discursive space divide to a point when concerns over modernity, classicism, nation and culture merged together to reinvent new models of aesthetics. The revival of classical Indian dance in twentieth-century India as embodied by the classicized Indian women reflected deep patriarchal concerns over female sexuality and her exposure before the public eye. 'Just as performers and promoters inserted dance into nationalist discourse', Janet O'Shea observes, 'as an emblem of cultural pride, they also engaged, through performance, with debates over femininity, respectability, and gender subjugation in Indian cultural practices.'[33] The entire process of historicizing Indian classical dance is born out of these competing and conflicting discourses on the role of dance, women, class, caste, and nationhood at the cusp of an encounter between the colonial civilizing mission and reformist-nationalist responses.

At a highly charged moment of cultural nationalism, issues like caste, sexuality, work, and sex work became part of a new discourse within the emerging and expanding public sphere of the new nation state. Underlining the tension around art, sexuality, and the making of 'classical' Bharatanatyam, Uma Chakravarti (Chapter 1) looks at the disparate yet parallel journeys of the two legends—Balasaraswati and Rukmini Devi Arundale—locating them respectively at two different spaces of the national stage—marginal and central, peripheral and pivotal, depraved and elevated. While Bala, representing the devadasis, was systematically denied her place in the dance system before getting erased from the gloried and acceptable history and heritage of the nation's entertainment industry, Rukmini, embodying the best and new aesthetics associated with Bharatanatyam, created a new 'national' cultural sensibility which in turn virtually killed the traditions that Balasaraswati lived through. Chakravarti chronicles how women dancers negotiate and cope with the private and public spatial divides of life conforming and compromising their artistic and economic flairs with the unyielding patriarchal family forms.

Spawning a plethora of images of the dancers-prostitutes—nati, ganika, baiji, and randi—drawn from a variety of ancient and medieval literary/aesthetic/sensual texts, Ratnabali Chatterjee (Chapter 2) analyses the roles and rankings of these dancers-artists-prostitutes within a well-defined hierarchic order. Her essay narrates the long journey of the nautch girls, the highly sexualized Oriental exotic beauty who suddenly turned diseased and depraved by the end of the nineteenth century.

Placing the 'deviant' woman at the centre of her discourse, Pallabi Chakravorty (Chapter 3) brings in overlapping themes of morality, sexuality, aesthetic labour, and ownership of dance. The essay deliberately reshuffles and disarranges the medieval tawaif or baiji and the present-day bar dancers and item girls, reading them both as icons of illicit dances and excessive sexuality. The essay, charting the history of the tawaif, claims her space in Indian artistic heritage as the creator-bearer of Kathak dance, countering the nationalist hegemonic narratives that either erase or degrade or put her name as a footnote in history.

In Anurima Banerji's essay (Chapter 4), the 'queer' specifically includes an assemblage of gay, lesbian, and bisexual subjects, hijras, prostitutes, nautch girls, and also devadasis. Banerji travels back in time to find out how the colonial state punished 'queered bodies' and 'abnormal' movements as embodied by hijras, dancers, and homosexuals. Banerji not only contemplates the colonized and criminalized bodies as a 'space of renegade actions' but also considers the colonial law as a 'mobile space' which exerted over those unruly 'choreographies of desire and self' the normative principles of colonial command.

Framed in Spaces: Presence and Representation

Dance has been available to theatre and films for a long time in India, besides being an important form of art in its own right. Dance, theatre, and film have given very different spaces to the women trained in these art forms. While there have been crossovers between the three, the mythicized history of women dancers across geographies, age, linguistic affinity, class, caste, and ethnicity has created a specific discourse, emphasizing the aesthetic engagement, extreme dedication and bodily involvement of the dancers, in contrast to the thinking and often more political woman artiste of the theatres and the commodified woman dancer's performance and labour in the consumer culture of the Indian film industry. Keeping this as the historical reference point, this section brings in three chapters on women dancers from varied spaces in contemporary India, striving to balance out equally effort, agency and 'labour', to critically engage with notions such as the display of women dancers as signifiers of the nation and national culture.

Urmimala Sarkar Munsi's essay (Chapter 5) is framed around the different ways the conceptual frame of gendered 'space' is constructed in relation to dance. From the physical space where the performance itself takes place to the metaphorical sense of space that the performance creates in the minds of the audience—such actual or referential presences generate different codes for the gendered body of the dancer to be projected and viewed. Sarkar Munsi problematizes the subsuming of the woman dancer either within architectural sites/sights, which create an aesthetic legitimacy for the female dancer's presence in the celebratory festival structure that initiates a certain form of public gaze. It also critically engages with the idea of the masculinity of spectacular spaces, created specifically for exhibiting the nation's identity such as the Republic Day Parade, trying to embed the ideas of such spaces within the gender discourse.

As a scholar of theatre studies, Bishnupriya Dutt's engagement with dance (Chapter 6) comes out of her readings of the negotiations different 'aesthetic' codifications of the gendered vocabulary that are used as performative tools in dance and theatre. By way of a case study, her essay also looks at the use of gestures in Maya Rao's work, which defies the codification that the canonization of Indian dance has created for classical dance forms. Dutt's essay thus also creates an additional layer of analytic writing that hopes to offer the conceptual groundwork for reading Maya Rao's own interview, in the latter part of the book, where Rao analyses her own creative process in terms of the training as well as creative nurturing that she sees in her current performance work.

Priyanka Basu (Chapter 7) looks beyond the stereotyped and demarcated domain of dance as an essentially 'feminine' space by extending the idea of the feminized space beyond the realm of the classical to that of the popular, encompassing films and other media such as television, by focusing on the participation of the female (and male) bodies in mass consumption through reality TV shows. Her quintessential question starts from the idea of the construction of the 'feminine' spaces in popular realms of dance to debate whether they are pre-constructed or created, trying to understand the processes through which the bodies of women dancers are disciplined to produce an affect upon the audience-consumer.

Choreographing the Space: Identity and Creativity

Foster's uneasiness about having a single dance theory, instead of theories of dance or dance theories, as reflected in her seminal chapter 'Dance Theory?' in the book *Teaching Dance Studies*[34] has strengthened the editorial choices of this volume as it did the curatorial process of the conference bearing the same name. Her understanding of the reciprocity between culture and dance—where she asserts that it is equally important to see dance as shaping cultures as it is to know that the dances are products of specific cultures—also shapes the four sections in this volume. The space, as the hegemonic structure that constricts, restricts, or at least shapes embodied presences such as the dancers, acquires a complex layering of understanding as soon as we think about the 'production' of space as an agency and outcome of the dancers' negotiations with art, skill, creativity, passion, and imagination. As discussed earlier, the specific case of the woman dancer is even more precarious now. As given, cultural policies and the gender-specific positions in the Indian social system, the stereotyping of such psyche (however dated it might seem to the few in the urban circles) and the public (male) versus the private (women) dichotomy, are more complex to understand in the present context. These constructs, or the obvious signs thereof, may be hidden or covered with many other images such as those of the Bollywood female item dancer, who may imagine herself as the 'free' woman to make her choices to do/dance what she wishes, but the text of her bonded-ness finds proof in the media coverage, or the way she is mentioned in the media as the titillating tool responsible for box office success. The fixity and the severity of such social structures become even more evident in the resistance that some contemporary feminist choreographers faced, which in turn drove them to create a different and powerful woman's body and presence on and off stage.

Aishika Chakraborty (Chapter 8) leafs through the dancers' memoirs to see how their lives can be read from their bodily performances and vice versa. Bringing her own personal memory into play, Chakraborty moves from stage to page, as she looks at the double narrative of life and dance inscribed by contemporary dancer-choreographer Manjusri Chaki-Sircar. In revisiting Manjusri's signature choreography, *Tomari Matir Kanya*, as an expansion of her cultural habitus and an accumulation of her cultural memory, the essay reads between the lines/movements of the dancer-author. Delving further, Chakraborty brings out the interpersonal dyad between Manjusri and her daughter Ranjabati, in the way they complimented and contrasted each other not merely as mother-daughter, but also as representatives of two generations of feminist thinkers, writing their bodies/lives in two distinctive signatures.

Space as a concept, as a physical presence, a restrictive political structure, remains at the centre of dance practice and discourses. The process of production and alteration of spaces remains as important to creative practices including dance as does the histories of dance and dancers' experiences of their creativity through their negotiations of those different ideas of space. Nirmala Seshadri's work (Chapter 9) draws on her own performance work to explore the relationship between the prescribed notions of the body emerging through dance training and her own experimentations with ideas of freedom from structure and form. Her contribution in this particular collection emphasizes the importance of the voice of creative processes of practitioners, leveraging embodied practices as the spaces for contestations between binaries of gender.

At a time when hyper-feminization of the woman's body was becoming the trend, set by the nationalistic vision of the normative visuality of the upper-class/caste woman's body in Indian classical dance, Chandralekha stopped performing her traditional repertoire of Bharatanatyam, according to expectations of the national cultural construct. Sadanand Menon (Chapter 10) looks back at her choreographic history and underlines the feminist strength that Chandralekha drew from other forms of art practices as well as from the creative intensities of people like Harindranath Chattopadhyay and Dashrath Patel.

'Is the dancing body/the dancer's body necessarily a body in free space? To what extent is the performance defined and structured by the space in which the body operates/acts?' Samik Bandyopadhyay (Chapter 11) raises concerns about the general indifference to the politics of the space where a dancer, knowingly or unknowingly, negotiates between her 'physical' stage space, the organizational/presentational 'ambient' space, and the 'public' space where she meets the invited or ticketed audience. Bandyopadhyay locates the politics in the 'live theatre' of Kanhailal of Manipur where 'the dancing/acting body' is playing out a history, and making history at the same time. Beyond the rigidly defined and scripturally authorized, authoritarian space, Bandyopadhyay shows how this resistive politics of Manipur theatre draws strength from the indigenous Meitei-Maibi culture where the woman performer takes centre stage as the mother, the rebel, and the warrior.

Transformative Space: Empathy and Activism

Can dance be a space or tool to initiate social/political intervention? There have been debates about whether dance can remain comfortable as an aesthetic form of artistic practice or if it can become more than that while retaining its claim to be an art form. Kolb's Introduction in her edited anthology *Dance and Politics* takes the debate further, discussing whether or not dance should be a political form and tool in order to retain its validity within the world of performing arts. She writes: 'The question here is whether dance which is *politically* motivated can actually have an impact on external reality or manage to inaugurate societal change.'[35]

Can dance then be considered art, a tool for generating and expressing empathy, and also an important form to use for political activism and social work at the same time, without reducing it to a form and tool, and also without acknowledging its creative capacity that in and for itself is available to humans as a communicative tool? The section 'Transformative Space: Empathy and Activism' contains interviews that reflect dance-related experiences ranging from ideas shifting between specifics and generalizations about aesthetic manipulation and cathartic experiences, between political expressions and kinaesthetic corporeality.

In her interview in Chapter 12, Maya Krishna Rao acknowledges her training in Kathakali as the beginning and continued understanding of movements as language. In her discussion with Urmimala Sarkar Munsi she mentions the learning process as a way in which one arrives at an understanding of the nuances of the body and its limits. 'Sitting in My Skin: Kathakali as the Transformative Space' is a transcribed piece, from conversations around Rao's relationship with dance—and her experience of learning, understanding, performing, and embodying, where Rao analyses herself as 'a creature of circumstance' and 'a very political person'.

In a continued engagement with practice, Chapter 13 presents a set of three interviews conducted by the volume editors with Sohini Chakraborty, Alokananda Roy, and Lubna Marium, each having donned many hats during their lifelong engagement with dance. The common passion that brings them together in this chapter is their belief in the power of dance as a tool for social change. All their works are with different communities, where they utilize their training as dancers/choreographers/therapists/activists/entrepreneurs through performative interaction with different sections of marginalized communities.

Chakraborty sees her own work with Dance Movement Therapy (DMT) as 'taking dance beyond the studio and stage' to explore 'the potential of transforming dance into a medium to heal the bodies of survivors of sexual violence and trafficking'.

Roy discusses her work with the inmates of correctional homes of Kolkata as her offering to society, by 'touching and transforming' the lives of people who were in prison for different reasons and for different durations. As a 'reformer of souls', Roy's prison-based intervention brought back rhythms to the lives of the 'convicts', enabling the proscribed bodies to express and transform their emotional experiences through dance in a cathartic relief.

Marium speaks of her work on women's empowerment, using dance as a tool for building consciousness and collaboration, 'as most participants are unfamiliar with the idea of collectively determining the content and form of performance' for self-expression.

Removing dance from its traditional space, dancers move from everyday to proscenium, from temple to the profane, courtyard to screen, street to street theatre, studio to gallery, and further into landscape and digital infrastructure. Quoting Brown, one may say that 'through dance, movement unfolds and actualizes space, opening space to time and making space particular, distinct'.[36] Space, one can agree, cannot be conceptualized as 'a neutral medium, a container or a passive receptacle'. Alternatively, one can view space more 'as a heterotopic way, as an opening to a proliferation of other spaces, or as a labyrinthic passage from one space to another, a space of mutability that changes over time'.[37]

Notes and References

1. Susan Leigh Foster, 'Choreographies of Gender', *Signs: Journal of Women in Culture and Society*, vol. 24, no. 1, 1998, pp. 1–33.
2. Ibid., p. 17.
3. Henri Lefebvre, *The Production of Space*, Oxford: Blackwell, 1991, p. 110.
4. Judith Butler, *Gender Trouble: Feminism and Subversion of Identity*, New York: Routledge, 1990.
5. Michel Foucault, 'Of Other Spaces', *Diacritics*, vol. 16, no. 1, 1986, p. 22.

6. Doreen Massey, *For Space*, London: Sage, 2005.
7. Valerie A. Briginshaw, *Dance, Space, Subjectivity*, New York: Palgrave Macmillan, 2001.
8. Olivia Ainsworth, '"The Echoes of a Place": An Investigation into the Notion of Place in the Work of Dan Canham', research paper, 2014, http://dspace.library.uu.nl/bitstream/handle/1874/298976/PDF%2'The%20Echoes%20of%20a%20Place'%20Thesis%20Olivia%20Ainsworth%203910717.pdf?sequence=2, accessed 12 November 2015.
9. Carol Brown, 'Making Space, Speaking Spaces', in *The Routledge Dance Studies Reader*, ed. Alexandra Carter and Janet O'Shea, London and New York: Routledge, 2010, p. 29.
10. Ibid., p. 59.
11. Ibid.
12. Ibid., p. 71.
13. Sibaji Bandyopadhyay, 'Introduction: The Laughing Performer', in *Sacred to Profane, Writings on Worship and Performance*, ed. Anjum Katyal, Kolkata: Seagull Books, 2005.
14. L.N. Rangarajan, ed., *Kautilya, The Arthashastra*, Kolkata: Penguin Books, 1992, 2.27.25, p. 351.
15. Ibid.
16. Priyanka Sharma, 'Communication of Women's Discrimination and Sexuality', *Natyashastra, Global Media Journal-Indian Edition*, vol. 4, no. 2, 2013.
17. Bishnupriya Dutt and Urmimala Sarkar Munsi, *Engendering Performance: Indian Women Performers in Search of An Identity*, New Delhi: Sage, 2010, p. 168.
18. *Arthashastra* 4.1.65.
19. Bandyopadhyay, 'Introduction: The Laughing Performer', p. 20.
20. Ibid., p. 16.
21. Ibid., p. 20.
22. Rangarajan, *Kautilya*, p. 38.
23. *Friend of India*, 25 September 1873, cited in *Sumanta Banerjee, The Parlour and the Streets: Elite and Popular Culture in Nineteenth Century Calcutta,* Calcutta: Seagull Books, 1989, p. 184.
24. Sumanta Banerjee, 'Marginalization of Women's Popular Culture in Nineteenth Century Bengal', in *Recasting Women, Essays in Colonial History*, ed. Kumkum Sangari and Sudesh Vaid, New Delhi: Kali for Women,1989, p. 129.
25. Partha Chatterjee, 'The Nationalist Resolution of the Woman's Question', in *Recasting Women: Essays in Colonial History*, ed. Kumkum Sangari and Sudesh Vaid, New Delhi: Kali for Women, 1989, p. 239.
26. Janet O' Shea, *Bharata Natyam on the Global Stage: At Home in the World,* Delhi: Motilal Banarsidass, 2009, p. 108.
27. Ibid., p. 23.
28. Ibid., p. 109.

29. Amrit Srinivasan, 'The Hindu Temple Dancer: Prostitute or Nun', *Cambridge Anthropology*, vol. 8, no 1, 1983, pp. 73–99; idem, 'Reform and Revival: The Devadasi and Her Dance', *Economic and Political Weekly*, vol. 22, no. 51, 1985, pp. 2225–8.
30. Anna Morcom, *Courtesans, Bar Girls & Dancing Boys: The Illicit Worlds of Indian Dance*, Gurgaon: Hachette, 2014, p. 31.
31. Ibid., p. 41.
32. Lefebvre, *The Production of Space*, p. 308.
33. O'Shea, *Bharata Natyam on the Global Stage*, p. 104.
34. Susan Leigh Foster, 'Dance Studies?', in *Teaching Dance Studies*, ed. Judith Chazin-Bennahum, New York: Routledge, 2005, p. 19.
35. Alexandra Klob, 'Introduction', in *Dance and Politics*, ed. Alexandra Klob, Bern: Peter Lang, 2011, p. 20.
36. Brown, 'Making Space, Speaking Spaces', p. 72.
37. Ibid.

PART I

Historicizing Spaces: Text and Context

1 The Devadasi as an Archaic Historical Artefact

Culture and Nation in a Transitional Moment

UMA CHAKRAVARTI

By Way of a Beginning

If I look back on my growing years, with the understanding I now have, I am not surprised that dance and artistic activities formed an integral part of my childhood because the new nation, the nation-in-the-making, was strongly marked by creative forms that could express the '*spirit* of the nation' in the understanding of its intellectual elites regardless of its material condition. So, for example, in the school that I first studied in, which in its earlier incarnation was evocatively named Naveen Bharat High School we had a couple who for a while taught us dance; they created ballets for us children which were almost always variations on the theme of the 'spirit' of India. Later, as someone growing up in central Delhi near Connaught Place, close to where the cultural hub of the capital actually has come up with the various academies, theatres schools, and auditoriums, we literally watched the transformations happen. Therefore, when the Triveni Kala Sangam was set up by the Shridharanis with classes in Manipuri dance my mother sent my elder sister and me to these classes, perhaps only for the summer to maybe get us out of her hair. But thinking back I wonder—why Manipuri? It was not something my mother would have been familiar with coming from the South as she did. Therein lies a tale about the emergence of particular dance forms in the public sphere, capturing most effectively the diversity and essential unity of the nation—Bharatanatyam, Kathak, Kathakali, and Manipuri. These dance forms spanned the length and breadth of new India, and delving back into time might produce answers to why these dance forms in particular were promoted before say the regional dance forms.[1] But, in any case, for a few months I swirled around imagining myself a *gopi*, and did my *dhin tin taki ta takita takita-takita dhin tin takita taa* even as my younger brother, who did not go to the classes as we the girls did, tried to do the same whenever I practised but also got laughed at. By the end of that summer, the brief affair with Manipuri dance was over and I never did wear the beautiful costumes again (till a fake performance with an improvised costume many years later in a boarding school I taught at, which required its teachers to perform quite regularly). Manipuri dance was popularized by the talented Jhaveri sisters and Tagore's dance dramas in Bengal. Manipuri was also one of the three dance forms taught rigorously in Uday Shankar's dance school in Almora in the late 1930s and early 1940s.

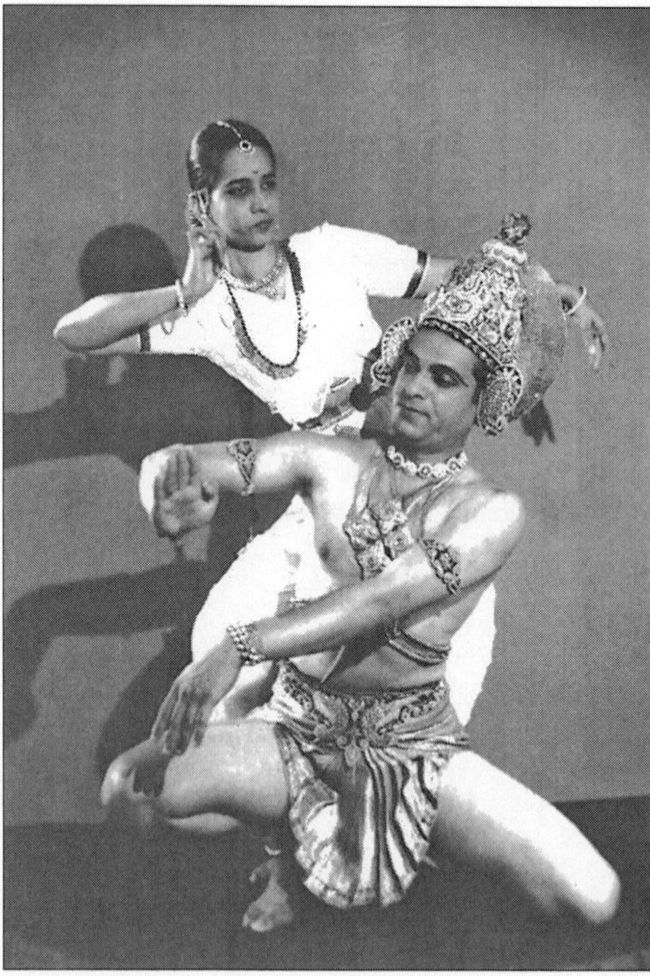

PLATE 1.1: U.S. Krishna Rao and Chandrabhaga Devi in a Duet
Source: Personal collection of Uma Chakravarti.

My real engagement with dance, however, came with an unexpected encounter with Bharatanatyam in the late 1950s and early 1960s in Bangalore where we had moved to after my father's retirement. A college Chemistry professor, U.S. Krishna Rao, at my sister's college was a Bharatanatyam dancer as was his wife Chandrabhaga Devi (Plate 1.1).[2] They were for their time among the rare couples who danced together as well as individually and taught Bharatanatyam to a host of middle-class, mostly brahmin, girls in the city. They had also, at different times, taught Indrani Rehman and Sonal Mansingh. First recruited as a chorus girl for a choreographed dance sequence in the film *Shola aur Shabnam*—a mad episode in which the 'sir' and 'aunty' (that is how they were referred to by their students) tried to maintain the pure traditions of classical Bharatanatyam which was sought to be combined with the *jhatkas* and *matkas* directed by a Madras film choreographer, who had brought four 'extras' with him, and which played out the tensions in combining forms that were antithetical to each other—I ended up becoming a sort of hanger on at the Sunday morning dance classes conducted by the Krishna Raos. Though quite enchanted by the dance form, at the time I could not formally be a student because my family could not afford to pay even the modest fee charged by the Krishna Raos. And so I just sat and watched various girls, including Sonal Mansingh and C.S. Lakshmi (the Tamil writer Ambai), learn various items over many years. What I did pick up this way was not only an understanding of the dance form and its various teachers, each with their own traditions, but also a great deal of everyday information that I heard from the Krishna Raos—about the history of various dance forms in India, creative innovations and experiments from the 1930s onwards in these traditions, anecdotes about dancers as well as their lives, their loves, their successes, and their failures. I soaked in all of what I heard as the ideal 'listener': my sense of history, my sense of someone growing up in a new cultural world, made me an engaged listener, even though I was on the margins of this world of dance. For years I went to watch performances of which there were many in Bangalore: possibly every performance of the Krishna Raos or their students, all the rising stars and the older dancers who danced in the city during the period, including the young and marvellous Kamala Laxman (the best performer of her generation who disappeared from public view somewhat suddenly) as well as the older Balasaraswati emoting the amazing rendering of *Krishna ni begana baro*, which has remained unparalleled in the history of Bharatanatyam. All this I soaked in as experience. That Balasaraswati was an impressive persona who would brook no nonsense and was completely immersed in her art made her unforgettable; at the performance I witnessed in the early 1960s she suddenly stopped in the middle of the piece of music that she was dancing to and told the photographer (who was flashing bulbs at her as he took her pictures) that she would stop dancing if he continued clicking as he was ruining the performance.

Years later, I began to read whatever I came across on dance, its varied histories in recent decades, and the massive transformations in its traditions, consciously enacted by many individuals but more importantly its changed social and material context. Anthropologists like Amrit Srinivasan, Saskia Kersenboom, and Kalpana Kannabiran analysed the changing social contexts of dance and its performers; Priyadarshini Vijaisri outlined the caste-specific nature of the transformations; and dancers like Avanti Meduri have tried to plot the history of the transformations from temple art to secular art.[3] Feminist scholars have collected narratives, translated them and brought the voices of the devadasis into the public sphere, the term by which temple dancers were known in the Tamil region. Drawing from all these and other writings I will try and analytically summarize the complex processes of constructing dance traditions in India through the story of Bharatanatyam. There may be some insights there that have relevance today as issues around art, women performers, caste, work, and sex work have assumed a new urgency as the 'nation' decides what is acceptable and what is not in the context of the entertainment industry. How much and what kind of erotics do we want in the public sphere: how do we define obscenity and vulgarity, what is classical, and what is tradition? And when did our classical traditions come into existence? Was tradition pure at some stage and when exactly did it degenerate if it did so at all? Who makes the canon, and who decides what good art is and what is bad art? Who is a good bearer of tradition and who is not?[4] A close analysis of how Bharatanatyam came to occupy and achieved its iconic status in contemporary India allows us to explore some of these questions.

The crucible of change in the construction of dance traditions can be traced back to south India in the late 1920s and through the 1930s. The emergence of a literati that was simultaneously regional, national, and international in its orientation—comprised almost entirely of the upper castes, especially brahmins—played a critical role in the debates on Bharatanatyam and the need for its reconstruction, to salvage it from its social location in temples, where its earlier 'high' traditions were regarded as having degenerated. The Theosophical Society led by Annie Besant and Colonel Olcott had been invested in the regeneration of a spiritual India since the first quarter of the nineteenth century and this was the context for Rukmini Arundale's creation of an institutional space called Kalakshetra from where this regeneration was to take place.

But at the same time there was a strong lobby led by Muthulakshmi Reddy, herself from a devadasi family, who demanded a reform of the pernicious system of dedicating girls to the temples and an end to temple dancing. The community of devadasis were non-brahmins, and came to be known as the Isai Vellalar. Caste was, therefore, central to the debates on temple dancing and the reform movement whether from the reformist end or the regenerationist end. In a sense the spiritual/classical traditions project was the answer to the demand for reform: one wanted the traditions ended, the other wished to purge tradition of its 'excesses' and return it to its pristine glory which was critical to the creation of the national identity. Caught in the middle of these processes was the community of devadasis, its dancers in particular, and this part of the story has not been told as it should have been. The story is most aptly represented by bringing in the best dancer of her times, Balasaraswati. Her life and times are fortunately now available to us in the form of a well-researched biography which was started by her daughter Lakshmi but completed after Lakshmi's death by Balasaraswati's son-in-law Douglas Knight.[5] This allows one to look at the history of Bharatanatyam over a transformatory moment—*c.* 1920s to the 1970s—sympathetically from the inside, that is from within the community of dancers, as well as from the outside, from the attack on the structures that had sustained Bharatanatyam over many centuries and, therefore, changed the ground on which it had rested.

History, Anthropology, and the Structural Location of the Devadasi

As a feminist historian looking at early Indian texts at the beginning of the decade of the 1980s I was struck by the way tropes of women classified female protagonists of the narratives in three distinctive categories: the wife, the courtesan, and the *bhikkhuni*. The largest number of women fell into the category of the wife as reproducer of children and mistress of the household; almost as her structural counterpart was the courtesan who did not marry, cultivated the arts, enhanced the value of the city where she practised the arts, and was accessible to all the wealthy men who could patronize her.[6] The courtesan provided pleasure, and also reproduced the household of the courtesan, called the ganika in early texts.[7] As a contrast to both these figures was the *bhikkhuni*, the one who renounced both marriage and her sexuality and sought individual salvation, living off alms and teaching the dharma in return to those who maintained her.[8] These three figures were the protagonists, or the subject matter of the narratives. There was also a fourth figure, that of the dasi, the woman who provided labour and worked in the fields and the household. However, she was almost never the proper subject of drama or prose although she did figure in the margins of the narratives in various ways.[9]

In the twin Tamil classics *Silappadikaram* and its sequel, *Manimekalai*, the three tropes of wife, the courtesan/dancer, and the *bhikkhuni* make up the main female protagonists of Kannagi, Madhavi, and Manimekalai. Kannagi, the wife of Kovalan, a prosperous trader, is devoted to him. She is the epitome of virtue and possesses *karpu*, a sacred power that she uses at the end of the narrative in the *Silappadikaram* when her husband Kovalan is wrongly accused of theft and executed for his alleged misdemeanour by the king of Madurai; in turn, when Kannagi discovers the wrong done to her husband and herself by the king, she curses him and the city of Madurai to burn down for the injustice. But before the denouement, and before Kovalan regrets his errant ways and returns to Kannagi, Kovalan has whiled away his time and his fortune with the beautiful dancer Madhavi, who bears a child by him named Manimekalai. Denuded of wealth, Kovalan and Kannagi then set off for Madurai hoping to build another life on the basis of capital raised against Kannagi's beautiful and rich jewels before tragedy overtakes them. Kannagi therefore never reproduces the normal household: when Manimekalai grows up she is caught between the two poles of the erotic/sensuous life, available to her through her mother's profession of dancing and providing pleasure—a choice that Madhavi's mother tells her to pursue as part of their traditional vocation of providing many types of pleasure—and the celibate life of a Buddhist *bhikkhuni*—renouncing the erotic as well as her own sexual pleasure because the pursuit of the erotic is temporary whereas salvation represents a goal that is permanent. It also allows a person to strive for the well-being of others; Madhavi had already shown her the way as she chose the life of a *bhikkhuni* at the end of the *Silappadikaram*. Finally, Manimekalai renounces her sexuality, the arts, and the household through which the elite patrons enjoy the urbane life, and opts for the life of a *bhikkhuni*.[10]

From the point of view of this essay what is interesting is the account of the *arangetram*.[11] It is at this first public performance of the dancing girl Madhavi, who is the most beautiful girl of the Chola kingdom, that Kovalan sees her for the first time; smitten by her beauty he woos her and wins her as his mistress.[12] In later tradition, the devadasi was often the object of love of those interested in music. For example, Kshetrayya, who is regarded as taking the *padam* (a devotional song mostly in the *sringara rasa*) to great heights of sophistication, fell in love with the devadasi Mohanangi who was attached to a temple; she did not reciprocate his love and asked him to turn his attention to Lord Gopala instead, which he did. Mohanangi then became his disciple and translated his *padams* into dance.[13]

The spectacular rise of Vijayanagara provided the backdrop for a display of wealth and patronage to the arts. Krishnadevaraya, the king of Vijayanagara, was the son of a dancing girl and married his favourite courtesan. There are other examples of such marriages. Even the great Shaiva saint Sundarar married Paravai, a dancing girl.[14] The prototype of the dancing girl has very ancient roots in both 'north' and 'south' India. The early medieval complex in Tamil Nadu in the great centres like Thanjavur, Madurai, and Chidambaram provides evidence of dance and music as integral to everyday temple rituals and its annual calendar. There is inscriptional evidence of *devardiyals*—the nomenclature by which devadasis were known in pre-twentieth-century writings, also meaning slaves/servants of the gods—making gifts to the temples.[15] After the fall of the Vijayanagara kingdom, the centre of cultural patronage shifted to Thanjavur, which was ruled by the Marathas from the eighteenth century until the early nineteenth century and it is here that the devadasi system in the temple structure as a ritual and cultural space began to be documented by both cultural anthropologists and social historians, thus allowing us to understand the recent cultural history of the Tamil region as well as its dramatic transformation.

The Devadasi Household

Since the devadasi was integral to the ritual structure of the temple she also had a place in the economic structure of the temple which, in turn, was based on land grants made by the kings and landholders in a given region. The devadasi household was a matrilineal one in which the lands and resources owned by the devadasis transmitted from one generation to the other through the devadasi. The importance of this transmission in the female line was fully acknowledged in that if a devadasi did not have a daughter she could adopt one and thus continue the functions of the devadasi—the music and the dance that was vested in her—as well as its material basis through the inheritance. The men of the devadasi household were musicians and *nattuvanars*—the teachers of the Sadir (one of its meanings is beauty), the name by which the dance form was known before it came to be called 'Bharatanatyam' (it was also sometimes called *dasiattam*).[16] They also managed the landholdings. Not all the women became devadasis; some married the men of the community and were like the other wives, reproducing the households of the community which came to be known as the Isai Vellalars, a non-brahmin caste in the system of castes. When a devadasi had learnt the art, she had her *arangetram* and was married to the presiding deity of the temple. She therefore remained a *nityasumangali*, one who was always auspicious because she could never be widowed unlike other women who were married to ordinary mortals.[17] Once she reached maturity she could take a sexual partner from amongst the upper castes including brahmins[18] and through him she reproduced the devadasi household which was maintained by the lands that she inherited.[19] Artists were also patronized by the royal families and were expected to bring honour and distinction to the court through the practice of their art.[20] The structure outlined here was an 'ideal type': by the time the histories of the devadasi households began to be documented the entire material basis of the system had begun to be dislocated, as kingdoms such as that of the Marathas at Thanjavur were taken over by the British. Devadasi families like Balasaraswati's were forced to leave Thanjavur in search of patronage with many of them moving to Madras (now known as Chennai) or to places like Trivandrum (now called Thiruvananthapuram) where royal establishments still survived. Balasaraswati's family history shows us that her great-great grandmother Kamakshi may have been part of the temple complex at Trivandrum[21] and then moved to Madras where the family 'settled' and where Balasaraswati was born as decline of patronage had already set in by the 1860s. The connection with Thanjavur was, however, not broken as it survived as the place of origin in the names of all the children of the devadasis.

Social Changes in the Early Twentieth Century

When Balasaraswati was born in 1918, dance Sadir was still very much located in the families of the traditional artistic community; in fact, there were no performers who were not from the community. There was a tradition of both singers and dancers within her family: her great-grandmother was a dancer and her grandmother was the well-known and renowned veena player Veena Dhanammal. Balasaraswati thus had access to both art forms—indeed she could sing very well and was awarded the Sangita Kalanidhi from the Madras Music Academy for her artistry. In fact, she was known to break into song while dancing. According to family folklore, as a child Balasaraswati was witness to a beggar who would come and dance at the gate of her house and she would dance along with him. Years later she thought of him as a yogi of sorts who came to initiate her into the love for dancing.[22] The matriarch of the family, Dhanammal, was not so keen on dance—she may have sensed the winds of change—but came to be persuaded to give Balasaraswati permission to be trained in dance.[23] However, soon after she had her *arangetram* at the age of 7 at the Kamakshi Temple in Kanchipuram, in the presence of elders, public debate began to rage on the art form, in particular over the temple dancer and the devadasi system. Many currents fed into this debate: the anti-nautch movement of the late nineteenth and early twentieth centuries, the non-brahmin movement in the Tamil region, reformist strands within the devadasi community, but, more importantly, the emergence of a strong cultural nationalism that located its notion of a purist culture in the 'ancient' past of India—in a reconstruction/construction of that past as a culture imbued with a spiritual quality which was in essence the hallmark of Indian-ness.[24] The Tamil elites, particularly those influenced by the Theosophical Society, provided intellectual leadership to what might otherwise appear to be a narrow puritanical missionary attack on the debaucheries associated with Hindu temples which were hardly sacred spaces anymore: instead they were dens of prostitution. All these strands, distinctive though they were, played themselves out in the introduction of a Bill to end temple dancing in 1927, spearheaded by Muthulakshmi Reddy who was a public figure by then. Trained as a doctor she was very much a part of the Tamil political scene; she was also the first woman legislator in the Madras Presidency and she worked tirelessly for social reform, even opening a school for the children of the devadasis so that they could leave their traditional occupations and move into professions that were not stigmatized. And stigmatized the devadasis were: for example, one critic and journalist who was attending a dance concert in 1913 as part of wedding celebrations described the reaction of the audience to the dancers: 'During the dance program I saw two things that made a deep impression on me; the first was the heckling by toothless old men in the front row and the second was the gossip of youngsters . . . about who had at various times [had the dancer]. The revulsion towards dance which I felt as a result stayed with me until just recently.'[25]

The revulsion was broken only when the critic saw Balasaraswati perform for the first time. Clearly, the art of the devadasi tradition had undergone many changes under declining patronage and the break-up of the system in which the art was originally located and newer forms of patronage that did not have the ethos of the older structures of patronage.[26]

The non-brahmin movement led by Periyar also reflected the new ideological moment with its critique of the traditional religious and cultural structure of the temple, but his opposition came from another end. An atheist, a breaker of icons, and far ahead of his times on many issues including marriage and the valorization of reproduction by just about everyone, it was the caste-specific nature of the devadasi tradition that led him to make his famous response to those brahmin men who wanted to keep the tradition of temple dancing going as it would mean an end to the culture that kept it alive. 'Let the Brahmin girls take to dancing then!', he retorted. And in the end that is what happened under the transformation of Sadir into Bharatanatyam led by E. Krishna Iyer and Rukmini Arundale, unfortunately with disastrous consequences for the traditional community associated with music, but more specifically dance as it lost the material base upon which the practice of the arts was founded; tragically, the community's relationship with the art itself was effectively broken. It was the conscious project of the cultural nationalists to turn Sadir into Bharatanatyam that led to the demise of the devadasi's relationship to art within the precincts of the temple and, thereby, open the doors to large-scale distress for the community. In the words of a devadasi from Andhra Pradesh:

> Our art lost its sanctity and some women from our community turned to unsavoury methods to sell their art. . . . Society took full advantage of this but the more determined amongst us obtained special permission from the district administration to perform outside the temples. This was mandatory otherwise we faced the threat of imprisonment. As it is some of us had to face the wrath of our kin and some of our family members began to pressure us to stop practising our art as we had lost the protection of the temple, and this is how our numbers dwindled.[27]

E. Krishna Iyer and Rukmini Arundale apparently took a middle position in the reformist debate, working however within the framework set by the reformers that the tradition of the dance as practised by the devadasis *had* become degenerate: for Krishna Iyer the mission simply was: 'Let temple dancing end but let the art form, the Bharata Natyam be saved.' As part of this position he publicly performed the dance dressed as a woman to show its highly evolved aesthetics. Rukmini Arundale completed Krishna Iyer's mission by patronizing some of the *nattuvanars* who began to teach Bharatanatyam at Kalakshetra. She herself learnt the art from Meenakshi Sundaram Pillai and for a while he taught Bharatanatyam at Kalakshetra.

Divergent Journeys: Balasaraswati and Rukmini Devi

The tensions in this charged moment of transition in the practice of dance and its teachings is encapsulated most effectively in the parallel journeys of Balasaraswati (also see Plate 1.2) and Rukmini Devi: the former representing the best tradition of Sadir/Bharatanatyam and Rukmini representing the new aesthetics associated with the dance form and its *institutionalization*, which ultimately played its own role in ending the traditional structure by creating a new 'national' cultural sensibility and which virtually killed the traditions that Balasaraswati lived through her life and dance till the very end of her days.

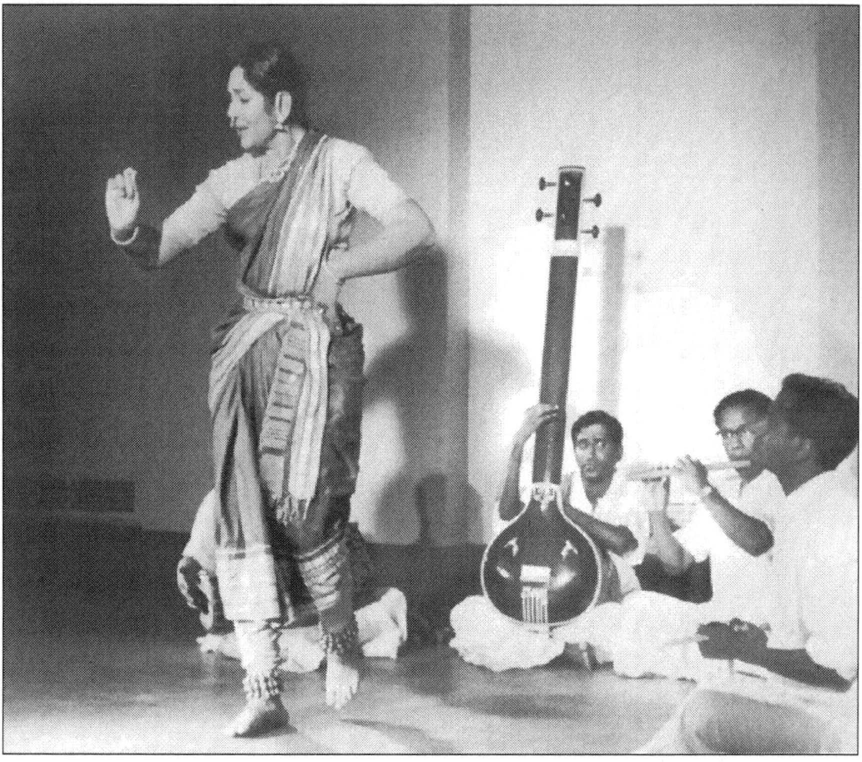

Plate 1.2: Balasaraswati Performing Abhinaya.
Source: Jacob Pillow's Dance Festival Archive.

Rukmini Devi was born Rukmini Shastri in a brahmin household of Thanjavur in 1904. Her father was closely associated with the Theosophical Society which was quite influential in a segment of the newly constituted educated brahmin community[28] in the late nineteenth and early twentieth centuries. As a young girl Rukmini was introduced by Annie Besant to George Arundale, a colleague of Besant's in the Society. Much older though he was, Rukmini married him in 1920 when she was just 16 years old. Arundale eventually succeeded Besant as leader of the Theosophical Society in 1934. Rukmini was therefore well-poised to lead the society to play an important role in the 'rescue' of Bharatanatyam from its 'fallen' position as the earlier Sadir and in reconstructing it as 'Bharata Natyam',[29] the epitome of the dance tradition of India, able to capture the *essence* of Indian culture in the art of dance. Theosophy itself was a reconstruction of the best in ancient Indian philosophy without having to bear the burden of all that was degenerate in the larger Indian cultural-intellectual tradition, but it was also capable of being eclectic, absorbing other philosophical and intellectual traditions wherever they may have originated from. The Theosophical Society's philosophical position had until the 1930s been interpreted by its four great former presidents;[30] to this the 'artistic traditions' were now to be added as a fifth position. A piece written by George Arundale published soon after Rukmini gave her first public performance, captures the almost messianic location of Rukmini Devi at this great transitional moment in the artistic traditions of India:

> We are at the beginning of a new era . . . [when] the beauty aspect of life, will be much more definitely stressed . . . We are hoping that Theosophy as beauty will incarnate in actual forms . . . so that we [may] perceive Theosophy through dance, through music, through painting and culture, through architecture and through ceremonial, the essential beauty of life amidst myriad divergences of colours, sounds, gestures, postures . . . [And] I have reason to believe that Mrs Rukmini Arundale will largely dedicate herself to this work, attempting to exemplify the great truths of life, especially through the medium of dance.[31]

Widely travelled, and with friends like Madame Pavlova, Rukmini could bring various currents sweeping the world in the arts into her work of 'regenerating' the ancient gold behind the degenerate dross that had accumulated over Indian dance. E. Krishna Iyer had committed himself to the cause of ensuring that the form of the arts practised by the devadasis survived even as they themselves died out as practitioners of the art; Rukmini completed the agenda for the nation's middle classes by making dance in the form of Bharatanatyam *respectable*. How could it be otherwise when a beautiful and cultured Tamil Brahmin woman was publicly dancing, thereby transforming its performance and its acceptability to new audiences imbued with a new zeal to make the arts a part of the emerging nationalism-based culture of India?[32] In an excess of sentiment one writer described Rukmini's performance thus:

> Rukmini Devi has great beauty of face and form, great grace of movement, but . . . it was not these qualities of which one was most conscious. The performance was so utterly impersonal and so spiritual in its feeling that the bursts of applause at some unusually beautiful or skilful movement seemed incongruous and out of place; as soon might one applaud a priest at the altar.[33]

Similarly, S. Sarada, the granddaughter of a Sanskrit scholar, wrote:

> Rukmini appeared on the stage like a damsel come alive from the ancient Indian sculptures . . . The dancer was not only beautiful . . . but her complete identification with the spiritual message which she was endeavouring to convey through her dance made for complete rapport between her and her spectators. She had proved that this physical art when presented with purity, devoid of vulgarity could convey the soul uplifting message of ancient India.[34]

Rukmini Devi herself termed her regeneration of dance at Kalakshetra 'as transforming art into what it was intended to be by the divine being himself . . . [and] to impart to the young the true spirit of that art, devoid of vulgarity and commercialism'.[35]

All the while, in the 1930s, the attack on the institutions that had supported the Sadir before were collapsing with the introduction of the Devadasi Abolition Bill in the Madras Legislative Assembly in 1927 which meant that the devadasi performers of the dance were in effect written out of the moment of transition, except for Balasaraswati—but for the moment we will leave her story and return to it later. It also had terrible consequences for the *nattuvanars*, who lost their institutional space for teaching, choreographing, and helping to reproduce the tradition over time. Without that space they tried to fit into the emerging structure of performers and audiences. For example, Kandappa Pillai, Balasaraswati's teacher and *nattuvanar*, was invited to teach in the dance school established by Uday Shankar at Almora,[36] an invitation that he accepted, breaking Balasaraswati's heart as she could not match the terms offered by Uday Shankar since she herself was looking for ways of keeping her dance performances alive. Pillai left Almora after two years but died soon after his return to Madras (now Chennai) and so Balasaraswati lost her *nattuvanar* forever. Meenakshi Sundaram Pillai, the famed teacher of his time whose own family situation had been deeply affected by the changes put into place without fully understanding the implications, is a good example of what was happening to traditional devadasi and *nattuvanar* families. The end to temple dancing meant a loss of lands and, therefore, the secure base upon which the arts were founded. Working on the model of the normative Hindu patrilineal family, the inheritance in the female line ended: it was achieved in one stroke of the pen, with no mechanism or thought given to ways in which the economic autonomy of devadasis, through female inheritance, to pursue art could be retained. Under the new dispensation women in the devadasi households then had perforce to conform to the model of the dependent Hindu/bourgeois wife who was 'maintained' by her husband. They were turned into good chaste wives deprived of their art (as Sadir was regarded as degenerate because the devadasis practised it), were not sexually contained within a monogamous marriage, but instead took partners from many of the upper castes. This was in total contrast to the upper-caste woman who married within her community and reproduced legitimate children within the caste system, who in turn upheld the normative property systems. No one thought that there were other ways in which the art and the economic structure might be salvaged so that women's economic autonomy could be assured—all that Muthulakshmi, struggling against her stigmatized condition, could think of was a home for the children of the devadasis which she opened in Madras.

And so Meenakshi Sundaram Pillai's beautiful and talented daughter simply disappeared from public view as she married the raja of Ramnad and never danced before an audience again, whether in its traditional or newly constituted form. Amrit Srinivasan captures these issues very well when she points out that the devadasis, whether dedicated or not, could not get married during the days of change. She writes:

> At the time of the reform campaign some eminent men did take dasis as wives in symbolic assertion of their emancipation and public spirit. But these exceptions . . . only served to prove the rule [since] it was the very beautiful or gifted dasis alone who managed to make good matches . . . Jayalakshmi the famous dancing girl of Pandanallur became the Rani of Ramnad. For the majority, however, marriage became an expensive and difficult proposition.[37]

The fate of Mylapore Gowri Ammal, a devadasi in the Mylapore Kapaleeswarar Temple, and famous as the queen of *abhinaya*, is even more heart-rending. Writing in the 1950s, a dance critic described her condition thus:

> The queen of bharata natyam who held undisputed sway over the hearts of dance lovers . . . is now living in obscurity. Her family had been attached to the Mylapore temple . . . with the abolition of the devadasi system in the temple her family property and house were confiscated and she was turned out on the streets. Now she resides in a hut in an obscure place, old and partially blind, under the shadow of starvation. She is out early in the morning, almost groping her way for miles to give tuition for a paltry sum of money. Yet such as the dignity of this great lady that she would never stretch her arms in front of disciples.[38]

Gowri Ammal taught *abhinaya* to Balasaraswati and to scores of other dancers even after her fortunes declined. Years later, the Krishna Raos recounted to me the way she trained her students after she could no longer see: her fingers would 'feel' the face of the student to let them see the expressions that they were evoking. Yamini Krishnamurthy captured the contradictions of the moment very aptly: 'While frail old Gowri (of Mylapore) . . . beset with family troubles, was dying in penury, her art was becoming vibrantly live again.'[39]

The vulnerable situation for the men is also captured well in the example of Jayalaksmi, Meenakshi Sundaram Pillai's daughter, who may have acquired a new respectable status because of her talent and beauty but was lost to the world of art and aesthetics, or of continuing the Pandanallur traditions after him.[40] Eventually, her father was invited to teach at Kalakshetra and he trained Rukmini Devi in Bharatanatyam (as mentioned earlier). The association ended very soon as Rukmini insisted on giving her first public performance in just over a year, a decision that Meenakshi Sundaram did not agree with because Rukmini wasn't really trained enough in his view, and so they parted ways after her performance.[41] Their views on the passing on of tradition were perhaps irreconcilable, especially at this transformative moment in the way the arts and its distinctive aesthetics were perceived by the teacher and his student.[42]

It was thus not easy for either the women or the men to make a transition into the new system, keeping their dignity and their art intact. It is possible to understand the enormous challenges that confronted Balasaraswati, the only devadasi who managed to keep her own understanding of the devadasi tradition alive, at this moment of forced capitulation of a whole way of life. In contrast to Rukmini Devi, Balasaraswati had been listening, absorbing music, and practising both dance and music ever since she was four. Trained by a *nattuvanar* chosen for her by her mother (who routinely used physical punishments to achieve his goals of training her to be a dancer), she simultaneously lived the traditional ethos of the devotee who danced to please the lord in the temple. When she was little she used to dress and go before a Thanjavur glass painting of Krishna in the hall downstairs and dance before it, believing that she was awakening him.[43] When she was a little older the family decided to perform her dedication ceremony, conducted with some secrecy, because although dedication was not yet illegal in the 1920s it was already controversial. As the years unfolded Balasaraswati and her family chose to resist the changes in the social world that they had inherited, conforming instead to the values of the traditional system, remaining in the public view, even in global public view, on those very terms, thus showing both courage and tenacity.[44] Gradually the women in the family, along with Mylapore Gowri Ammal (a friend of her mother), and her teacher/*nattuvanar*, carefully crafted a repertoire of dance items including *padams* and *javalis* (musical compositions of the late nineteenth century, mainly in the *sringara rasa*) that Veena Dhanammal had learnt.[45] Her musical training contributed enormously to Balasaraswati's unique skills at *abhinaya*. Ultimately, Balasaraswati was acknowledged as the greatest dancer of her day. Yet the power relations in the new cultural scene in Madras in the 1920s were such that the new elites had positioned themselves as patrons of the traditional dancers, deciding who could or should be promoted. A passage from an interview with Rukmini Devi clearly illustrates this shift in the patronage system:

> I invited her to my place at the Theosophical Society to give one of the finest performances because I recognized that she was talented . . . I saw a large number of dancers [who] were just beginning to come out, because before that, hardly anyone knew of their existence, and I went to them. Some of my friends who knew I was keen took me...to see this little girl learning; she was just learning *tei ya tei*. She looked very bright and intelligent. Of course they were [all] very pleased because very few people went to their house and took an interest in their dance . . . When she was able to dance she came to the Theosophical Society and gave a demonstration there for my birthday . . .
>
> There was some charm about her . . . she had a great tradition behind her, she was very friendly to me. I was very sympathetic to all these professional dancers who were not popular at that time. I felt it was my mission was to not just be a performer but to help others too to do some things in a better taste . . . like costumes [which were all a mixture in those days].[46]

Later, E. Krishna Iyer positioned himself as the discriminating patron who mediated between Balasaraswati's performance and north Indian audiences: '[I invited] Balasaraswati, a talented professional artiste in traditional bharata natyam to [Benares] where [my] discourses on the art and the dance by the Lady artiste helped to bring home to the minds of North Indian connoisseurs also, the greatness, beauty and refinement of India's richest dance treasures.'[47]

The patronizing middle-class/upper-caste elite voice is unmistakeable in both statements. It was, therefore, inevitable that in later years there was a certain tension between Rukmini Devi (whose position was quite similar to E. Krishna Iyer in terms of presenting Bharatanatyam as the epitome of refinement) and Balasaraswati: the latter representing the older tradition and the former representing the new recast tradition. However, this is an issue discussed ahead.

In their personal lives too Rukmini and Balasaraswati represented contrasts: as stated earlier Rukmini married a much older man from among the cosmopolitan elite of Madras and assumed the mantle that thereby fell upon her of turning the Theosophical Society into a space for the emergence of newly refurbished cultural 'traditions' of India in the form of Kalakshetra, the institutional space through which these traditions were recast. Balasaraswati, on the other hand, like her mother and other women in the family, became the partner of R.K. Shanmugham (26 years older than her) at the age of 18, who in turn unhesitatingly supported her dance and music, and was protective of the rights of the devadasi community. He went on to become well known in education, industry, and finance, even becoming the first finance minister of India in 1947. Yet Balasaraswati was not his dependent and her own fortunes went through many ups and downs. While she ultimately became well-known she was often in dire financial straits, supported a large entourage, suffered severe ill health, had many pregnancies but bore only one child Lakshmi, whom she took along as a baby on her travels, and yet through all this hung tenaciously on to dance.[48] In her own life Balasaraswati continued the distinctive conjugality practised by the devadasis in which the women reproduced the devadasi household, keeping alive the traditions of dance and music that were the hallmark of these households.

Rukmini Devi and Balasaraswati must have had many occasions when they met each other, such as the Madras Music Academy's annual performances and other cultural events. One particular stand-off between them has been alluded to in Balasaraswati's biography which captures the tension between the traditional basis of performance in the erstwhile Sadir and the new institutional basis of its recast version called 'Bharata Natyam' (with its claim to represent 'Bharata'—the ancient nation, to be the future Indian nation). The distinctive positions came to be articulated around the place and meaning of *sringara* in the dance form. The controversy erupted in the public sphere in 1945 at the All India Dance festival held in Bombay. The power imbalance in the world of dance was evident from the opening of the festival with a performance by Rukmini Devi who dominated the entire festival, evident even in the festival souvenir. Her profile was summarized thus: 'Rukmini Devi has regenerated this art, rescued it from its degradation and virtual extinction and restored it to its pristine beauty, *by permeating it with religious and devotional spirit*. She has succeeded in dramatizing it with appropriate music and costumes, and rescued it from all monopolies, especially as regards teaching and conducting [emphasis mine].'[49]

No such introduction preceded Balasaraswati's performance. Further, the statement was an insult to the traditional communities in which the dance form was nurtured over centuries but who were being dismissed as 'monopolists' thereby implying that the dance form was now being 'democratized', ignoring the marginalization of the communities whose livelihood was now being taken away in one fell swoop.

But more significant was the controversy over the performance of dance items that portrayed the *sringara rasa*. Rukmini Devi did not completely avoid *sringara* pieces in her performance, but she emphasized non-*sringara* pieces, which was considered more 'dignified'.[50] She saw the need to differentiate between what was *sabhyam* and *asabhyam* and regarded many *padams* then in vogue as too earthy and realistic for her (delicate and refined) sensibilities.[51] Notably, the de-eroticizing project was accompanied by a rhetoric of truth and beauty derived from theosophical principles. For Balasaraswati, on the other hand, *sringara* was at the core of her art, especially of her *abhinaya*. Bala continued to perform *sringara*, fully believing that human love and divine love are both expressive of devotion and surrender—*sringara* itself meant that which creates ecstasy, and when the *abhinaya* was subtle it was divine.[52] She forcefully held on to her point of view and her own repertoire, thus making sure that the so-called classicization did not go without contestation. The problem according to Bala was with the performers, not with the tradition of which *sringara* was an essential part. As the art critic Sadanand Menon argues, the import of the onslaught on the traditional communities had been ruthless: Balasaraswati's biography amply demonstrates the anger experienced by Bala and her family for the systematic denial of their place in the dance system and their erasure from the newly emerging nation state.[53] By the end of 1947, when the Act to end temple dancing was finally passed, 'the defamation of the devadasi had been legislated, and both the art and the artist [of Sadir] had been banished and replaced'.[54] The controversy around *sringara* has been rendered irrelevant by the new generation of dancers who aren't willing to engage with the import of the differences between Balasaraswati and Rukmini and so we have Leela Samson, the official biographer of Rukmini Devi and former director of the Kalakshetra, regard the whole controversy as needless, kept alive by dance critics. Yet even as she sums up the period of Balasaraswati and Rukmini she seems to reconcile the tensions by separating Balasaraswati from the rest of the devadasis and condemning the latter, rationalizing the demise of the devadasi as attributable to society which had decisively rejected her.[55]

But could a whole way of life, a deeply internalized system of thinking and performing, just disappear simply because some people thought it was a degraded and corrupted way of being? And what of the devadasi herself, her devotion to the Lord and the art form through which she worshipped her God? What the onslaught on the traditional system meant in the life of the devadasi is poignantly brought out by an incident in Balamma's (as Balasaraswati was affectionately called) life. In 1954, racked by ill health and declining fortunes, she was driven by a desire to fulfil an earlier vow to dance before Murugan at the temple in Tirutani but temple dancing was now forbidden by law. Balasaraswati carried her ankle bells and was accompanied by her mother, who always sang for her when she danced, and her 11-year-old daughter to whom she hoped to pass on the traditional art that she herself had been trained in. She arrived at the temple when the formal rituals were over. Manipulating the priest, she bribed her way through to have the doors of the sanctum closed, thus leaving her and her entourage in the intimate sphere of the sanctum. Then, putting on her ankle bells, she danced before Murugan as her mother sang for her. Following 'years of quiet yearning', Bala had fulfilled her vow, and fully experienced the joy of that moment.[56] After this incident, she believed that she was always dancing for Murugan.[57] It is chastening to think of what the traditional artist was suddenly being denied after 1947: her own mode of expressing devotion. No more a deity in a temple for her—only an image of Nataraja on stage—almost as a stage prop—and an audience that was quite removed from the world of the 'performer'.

Epilogue

In conclusion it might be instructive to bring in, the way others from devadasi families as well as the new troupe of performers of Bharatanatyam handled the tension between their performing lives and their personal lives. The life and career of M.S. Subbulakshmi, the most famous daughter of a devadasi of her times, is a stunning contrast to that of Balasaraswati, with whom she shared a deep life-long friendship (beginning with an adolescent sharing of adventures captured in an amazing studio photograph with Bala and 'M.S.' in striped pyjama suits sporting cigarettes hanging from the mouth). While Bala went on to shape the repertoire of Bharatanatyam performances with her strong emphasis on *abhinaya* including the *sringara* items with its focus on *padams* and *javalis* that the singers in Bala's family kept alive, refusing to be cowed down by Rukmini Devi's sanitized re-invention of Bharatanatyam, 'M.S.', as she was popularly known, reinvented herself to become not only the most famous singer of her times, but the most famous singer of Meera's bhajans. M.S. was married to T. Sadasivam, a brahmin widower with two children, who carefully crafted her move from an actress who played Shakuntala to G.N. Balasubramaniam's Dushyanta, and with whom she is said to have fallen in love, to a Meera devoted to the god Krishna, a move in which he fully succeeded. Her reinvention achieved the erasure of her otherwise tainted birth in a devadasi family. Sadasivam managed her professional career, even sitting in front of her at her performances and gesturing his suggestions to her as he decided what she should sing and for how long. He also managed her finances and her world of friends and admirers, consciously cutting her off completely from her natal family. In sum, M.S. was a full participant in the reconstruction of an Indian culture that was permeated with religious devotion that became the hallmark of the new Indian national culture.[58] It was only late in her life, while receiving the award of the Bharat Ratna, that M.S. publicly acknowledged her debt to her mother, and that too only after the death of her husband, with the words: 'At this hour of honour I cannot but think of the loving care and guidance I received from my late husband all through my life and the blessings of my beloved mother.'[59]

The new post-devadasi generation of dancers has struggled to reconcile the tension between traditional Sadir and Bharatanatyam: Chandralekha, known for her rejection of the conventions of Bharatanatyam and her experiments with new dance forms and themes, nevertheless choreographed a dance titled 'Devadasi' and dedicated it to both Bala and Rukmini Devi who were invited to its first performance.[60] The Krishna Raos were taught dance by the famous Meenakshi Sundaram Pillai who is said to have been particularly generous to them as they were a 'Brahmin dancing couple' which was very unconventional in the 1940s.[61] Kalanidhi Narayanan, who is now famous for her *abhinaya* training of young students, recounted how her mother, who was very talented at music and dance, could not learn these arts formally because she was a young married woman—she was from a brahmin household—and so she taught her daughter dance instead. Kalanidhi performed publicly but only at benefit performances (so that the stigma of dancing for money would not be attached to her). Though she got rave reviews she stopped dancing when she married; her husband was addicted to films but did not care for either music or dance and so she stopped attending all performances. Her husband remained critical of Bharatanatyam because of its association with the devadasi and therefore considering it not quite respectable.[62] Sudharani Raghupathi, a well-known Bharatanatyam dancer from a brahmin family, lives in two separate worlds: her husband and son have never seen her dance on stage.[63] The respectability question that Balasaraswati and the devadasi dancers had confronted in the 1930s has never really been settled by Rukmini Arundale's recasting of Bharatanatyam; it had left a bitter legacy for Balasaraswati too who was scathing about the false dichotomy between respectability and vulgarity in dance.[64] Consequently, she also had a conflicted relationship with the state where the new arbiters of the destinies of dancers might commission you, or offer a trip which could be withdrawn because somebody younger or smarter would out-manipulate you in the name of middle-class respectability.[65] Indrani Rehman records the internalized sense of stigma in the traditional *mahaaris*,[66] the devadasis who danced Odissi because they were regarded as polluting. The famous Gangubai Hangal was invited to sing at the

Congress National Conference; though happy to do so, her greatest fear was that after the performance she would be made to sit and eat separately from the delegates. She is also famous for her sardonic remark—when a man sings well he becomes known as a pandit or an ustad; when a woman sings well she gets the epithet of a *bai*.[67]

Tensions in the artistic traditions of India remain: family forms, art and aesthetics, economic basis of artists, caste, and social background still impact cultural forms in India. Yet the way Bharatanatyam has come to stand for a pristine ancient Indian cultural tradition that all of India can claim for itself is evident in an advertisement of the Bihar Tourism Department. Titled 'Blissful Bihar' it has vignettes of Nalanda, Buddhist monks, wrestlers, a tribal village scene, a *jatra*, and modern crooners. But the dominating image is that of a pretty little Bharatanatyam dancer, dressed in the costume devised by Rukmini Devi and striking a post-Kalakshetra *adavu*, providing evidence of history in Bihar as reviving culture and tradition under the new political dispensation there.[68] Could they have used an image of an aging Balasaraswati performing her incredibly powerful *sringara abhinaya* against the music of a *padam* or *javali* to claim the same revival of cultural tradition?

Notes and References

1. For example, Odissi and Kuchipudi which have upstaged, to a certain extent, from among the four dance forms listed, Manipuri.
2. Chandrabhaga's life and career as a dancer have been documented in C.S. Lakshmi, *Mirrors and Gestures: Conversations with Women Dancers*, Delhi: Kali for Women, 2003, pp. 64–92.
3. Kalpana Kannabiran, 'Temple Women in South India: A Study in Social History and Political Economy', unpublished Ph.D thesis, Jawaharlal Nehru University, Delhi, 1992; Saskia Kersenboom, *Nityasumangali: Devadasi Traditions in South Asia*, Delhi: Motilal Banarsidass, 1987; Avanti Meduri, 'Nation, Woman, Representation: Sutured History of the Devadasi and her Dance', unpublished Ph.D thesis, New York University, New York, n.d.; Amrit Srinivasan, 'Reform and Revival: The Devadasi and Her Dance', *Economic and Political Weekly*, vol. 20, no. 44, 2 November 1985, pp. 1869–76; Priyadarshini Vijayashree, *Recasting the Devadasi: Patterns of Sacred Prostitution in Colonial South India*, Delhi: Kanishka, 2006.
4. Some of these issues have been debated with some heat and a lot of passion in the banning of bar dancing in contemporary times and has divided the women's movement which is just learning to factor caste and class into issues of sexuality and also to listen to different positions without using blanket condemnation for those who seem to stand in opposition to each other in how we may think about work, sex work, caste, and

performative traditions.

5. Douglas M. Knight, *Balasaraswati: Her Art & Life*, Chennai: Tranquebar, 2010.
6. The Buddhist texts have a marvellous account of how Ambapali, patronized by kings and princes, became a famous courtesan of her times. She was found in a mango grove and when she grew up into a beautiful young woman all the Licchavi princes wished to marry her to possess her. And so they fought among themselves. Finally, to settle the conflict, it was decided to install Ambapali as a courtesan, a *nagaravadhu*, so that she was accessible to all the men equally rather than be in the sole possession of one. Ambapali was drawn to the Buddha and joined the sangha where she composed some verses about her reflections on her own life which form part of the *Therigatha*. See Uma Chakravarti, 'The Rise of Buddhism as Experienced by Women', *Manushi*, no. 8, 1981, pp. 4–8.
7. The structural opposition between the wife and the courtesan/devadasi is stunningly captured in Sharada Ramanathan's film *Sringaram* (2007). A sequence shows the preparations for a 'normative' marriage with a girl being inspected by her prospective in-laws. She is modestly turned out, singing a devotional song, married and sent off to her marital home while parallel cuts capture the devadasi dancing uninhibitedly to a charged erotic song at a temple, exulting in her own sexuality.
8. Chakravarti, 'The Rise of Buddhism as Experienced by Women', pp. 4–8.
9. I have drawn from various texts, primarily the early Buddhist texts which have a rich tradition of storytelling and are peopled by scores of characters—kings and queens, merchants, travellers, brahmins, philosophers, monks and nuns, ordinary householders, workers, ploughmen, and artisans. Each person is located in a village, a city, or a region. This is in contrast to the Brahminical prescriptive texts which are less concerned with people and more with codes of responsibilities, rituals to be performed, and penances to be observed.
10. Summarized from the twin Tamil classics *Silappadikaram* by Prince Ilango Adigal and *Manimekalai* attributed to the late Sangam period.
11. Indira Menon, *The Madras Quartet: Women in Karnatak Music*, Delhi: Roli Books, 1999, p. 13.
12. Ibid., p. 43.
13. Ibid., p. 18.
14. Ibid., p. 43.
15. Leslie C. Orr, *Donors Devotees and the Daughters of God: Temple Women in Medieval South Asia*, Delhi: Oxford University Press, 2000.
16. Knight, *Balasaraswati*, p. 5.
17. Menon, *The Madras Quartet*, p. 41.
18. For example, M.S. Subbulakshmi's father was an Iyer; what is significant is that she was always known by her mother's name—Madurai Shanmukhavadivu Subbulakshmi—and even if the mother ultimately contributed little to her transformation into the nightingale of India, she is acknowledged as the person through whom she derived her

genius. Gopalkrishna Gandhi, *Of a Certain Age: Twenty Life Sketches*, Delhi: Viking, 2011, p. 107. Menon also writes about the specific features of the devadasi lineage system, pointing out that unlike other patriarchal communities the devadasi women took their mother's name which was prefixed by the name of her ancestral village. Menon, *The Madras Quartet*, p. 44.

19. The structure, though in a sense non-normative, was very much within the compulsory heterosexual relationship framework because it was as invested in reproduction and the passing on of property as normative marriage was. We have no evidence of a devadasi choosing to remain single and being allowed to do so (I owe this point to a question raised by Shad Naved, to whom I am thankful for bringing this issue to my notice).
20. Knight, *Balasaraswati*, p. 10.
21. Ibid., p. 13.
22. She said later, 'if I am dance mad now how it could be otherwise, my first guru was a mad man'. Knight, *Balasaraswati*, p. 18.
23. Veena Dhanammal was part of a group of devadasi women who formed an association to counter the reformists bent upon ending the devadasi system: the group included her daughters and the famous Bangalore Nagaratnammal (who left all her money to be spent in the work of restoring the site of Tyagaraja's *samadhi* at Tiravarur) and Mylapore Gowri Ammal. Later, when the festival was being held at Tiruvarur, Nagaratnammal is said to have proudly proclaimed, 'I am a devaradiyal', and the crowd assembled there applauded her. She also put in a clause in her will that everyone irrespective of caste, creed or sex should be allowed to participate in the festival. Menon, *The Madras Quartet*, pp. 46, 69–70.
24. Uma Chakravarti, 'Whatever Happened to the Vedic Dasi', in *Recasting Women*, ed. Kumkum Sangari and Sudesh Vaid, Delhi: Kali For Women, 1990, pp. 27–87.
25. Knight, *Balasaraswati*, p. 24.
26. Given the changing contexts and the consequent changes in audiences for the dance, it is difficult to criticize Muthulakshmi Reddy's movement to end temple dancing; one can understand from where her reformist drive was emanating. It was from personal anguish and anger at the stigma associated with the children of the tradition—those were her own roots. She wrote her own stigma into history in a speech in the Madras Legislative Assembly: 'The appellation (of the devadasi) as every one of us knows, whatever the original meaning might have been, now stands for a prostitute. None of us familiar with the custom can dispute the fact.' Menon, *The Madras Quartet*, p. 46.
27. *The Hindu*, 25 June 1995, cited in Menon, *The Madras Quartet*, p. 49.
28. The leaning towards the brahmin intelligentsia in Madras Presidency of the Theosophical Society and in particular of Annie Besant may be discerned in a variety of ways; Besant had a very brahmin-centric notion of caste, even claiming that Manu's system had preserved the

race in India, was conservative with regard to reform of women's status, opposed widow remarriage. It is no surprise that the boy chosen to be the new messiah of the theosophical movement was from a brahmin household.

29. It was E. Krishna Iyer's suggestion to the annual conference of the Madras Music Academy that led to the renaming of the art. Menon, *The Madras Quartet*, p. 54.
30. They were Madame Blavatsky, Col. Olcott, Annie Besant, and Jiddu Krishnamurthi. Knight, *Balasaraswati*, p. 104.
31. Ibid.
32. Ibid., pp. 104–6, 124.
33. Leela Samson, *Rukmini Devi: A Life*, Delhi: Viking, 2010, p. 90.
34. Ibid., p. 87. We see here the rehearsing of the theme of ancient glory, medieval degeneration, and twentieth-century regeneration by the respectable upper-caste reformers which dominated discourses from the nineteenth century and which is the subject of my essay, 'Whatever Happened to the Vedic Dasi', cited in n. 24 (in this chapter).
35. Samson, *Rukmini Devi*, p. 96.
36. Institutional learning at the new centres for the performing arts may not have been intended to produce dissatisfaction with the traditional forms of teaching but they did and added to the collapse of the family- and community-based teaching and practice of the arts, especially of Bharatanatyam. Knight, *Balasaraswati*, p. 103.
37. Srinivasan, 'Reforms and Revival', pp. 1873–4.
38. Govind Vidyarthi, pp. 52, 54, cited in Menon, *The Madras Quartet*, p. 50.
39. Menon, *The Madras Quartet*, p. 55.
40. A passing conversation that I had in the late 1950s brings out the meaning of the changes in the tradition of Sadir/Bharatanatyam. When I was hanging about the Krishna Rao's in Bangalore I remember being told of their days as students of Meenakshi Sundaram Pillai, who was very forthcoming with his skills in choreography as he composed a special *tillana* for this unusual couple who danced together. They could see the changes wrought by the times upon this great teacher whose losses were immense; according to them he had two beautiful and talented daughters, one died young and the other married the raja of Ramnad. He was broken by both 'losses'.
41. Knight, *Balasaraswati*, p. 106.
42. Ibid.
43. Ibid., p. 25.
44. Ibid., p. 30.
45. Ibid., p. 31.
46. Ibid., p. 105.
47. Cited in Knight, *Balasaraswati*, p. 99. Knight also adds that Krishna Iyer's claims of facilitating Bala's performance in Benares annoyed her to no end but neither she nor others in her family were in a position to refute him because they had no access to the middle-class forums that were

creating public opinion.

48. Summarized from Knight, *Balasaraswati*, pp. 112–26.
49. Ibid., p. 130.
50. Ibid., p. 119.
51. Sankara Menon in Samson, *Rukmini Devi*, p. 120.
52. Ibid., pp. 101–2.
53. Sadanand Menon, 'Beatification of the Erotic', *Outlook*, 29 December 2011.
54. Ibid.
55. Samson, *Rukmini Devi*, p. 125.
56. Balasaraswati's secret venture is made more poignant by Rukmini Devi's open performance at the Chidambaram temple with the consent of the priest as a fitting tribute to the Lord, dissolving centuries of prejudice because 'she was a Brahmin woman'. Samson, *Rukmini Devi*, p. 102.
57. Knight, *Balasaraswati*, p. 151.
58. C.R. Rajagopalachari wrote some of her songs; Gandhiji inspired her Meera renderings especially *Hari tum haro* and *Vaishnav janato*; and Nehru referred to her as the Nightingale of India. She was also awarded the Bharat Ratna.
59. Menon, *The Madras Quartet*, p. 130.
60. Lakshmi, *Mirrors and Gestures*, p. 114.
61. Ibid., p. 81.
62. Ibid., pp. 1142–4.
63. Ibid., pp. 314–15.
64. Ibid., pp. xxvi–vii.
65. Knight records an incident where Bala was supposed to take her troupe to Russia for a festival of sorts. She prepared her troupe to weather the cold, spending considerable money to equip the troupe with warm clothes, and then suddenly found that she had been replaced with another artist compounding her humiliation with a financial loss. Knight, *Balasaraswati*, p. 178.
66. Lakshmi, *Mirrors and Gestures*, pp. 174–5.
67. Personal communication from Vijaya Mulay.
68. From an advertisement in *Indian Express*, 26 December 2011, Delhi edn., p. 5.

2 The Nayika and the Nautch Girl
The Courtesans in the Colonial Gaze

RATNABALI CHATTERJEE

> Native Public opinion would not go with us in an attempt to put a stop to prostitution. . . . Prostitutes danced before Yudisthir and Ram and in the guise of dancing girls and singers they are a necessary part of most domestic ceremonies today.
>
> —From Major C.A. Mc Mohans to C.M. Riwaz, 7 June 1892, Home Judicial File no. 48, p. 1143

The mid-nineteenth century, characterized as the Victorian age, brought overlapping themes of morality, imperialism, and philanthropy within its historical rubric. It was also said to have provided a paradigm of sexual and moral hypocrisy. Yet, as Michel Foucault pointed out, it was from this period that there was a proliferation of discourses on sexuality rather than a repression. The centres of debate, which he maps out, are as varied and wide-ranging as medicine philanthropy, criminal justice, and political strategies.[1] Acceptable and deviant forms of sexuality radiating from these centres created a further incentive to discussion. All this represented a moment when the deviant woman was at the centre at the discourses. She was named 'the prostitute' and defined through a special language linking imperial political ethics to a universal moral code, so that a fall from virtue was seen to symbolize the end of an empire.[2] In this the Indian dancing girl acted as a special example.

Though the nineteenth century marked the climax of imperial glory, it was in the eighteenth century that social boundaries including race came to be reshaped in Europe within the existing distinctions between classes and gender. It involved the growth of a world system based on European economic, political, and cultural dominance which brought in increased contacts between Europeans and non-Europeans. This also threw up the need to define European officials as superior and civilized in comparison to the superstition and barbarous practices of the subject races.[3]

Further, it was through a demarcation of space and physical stereotypes that the Western nation states began to systematically codify their history. As a land of the 'natives' began to assume specific geographical locale (India, China, Egypt, etc.), the spaces inhabited by men and women also came to be marked as 'public' and 'private'. Women, like natives, were not allowed to step out of their ordained territory. Great Britain's emergence as a nation state coincided with the process of colonization which had been well set in motion from the eighteenth century. Through their officials (mainly British) they began a process of codifying and legitimizing which were often based on theories built in England and worked out in India. British prejudices and attitudes acted as guiding factors for the colonial officials, as in the case of statistical surveys conducted in India. Though this was supposed to bring into effect European scientific knowledge regarding demographic assessment, it was clear from the beginning that all the European travellers' tales of merchants turned rich and missionary accounts of mysterious pagan rites had been assembled to create an 'Orient' which no amount of statistical knowledge could dislodge.[4]

Among the many themes that developed in the European imagination about the Orient, two appear to be most persistent. The first claimed the East to be a place of 'lascivious sexuality' and the second that it was a realm characterized by inherent violence. Both themes had their origin in the medieval period, but gave the Western imperialists (particularly in the eighteenth century) their greatest justification for invasion and establishment of control over an alien people.

From the beginning of their rule, the discomfort of British officials when they directly came in contact with their 'native' subjects was quite apparent. This, according to Bernard Cohn, was most evident in their categorization of groups who threatened the prescribed sociological order. These were people who by the very conditions of their existence tended to wander beyond the British concepts of civil society. In India, sadhus (mendicants), fakirs (Muslim divines mainly Sufis), nats (acrobats), musicians, and women dancers (generally known as 'nautch girls') were recorded by the British officials as belonging to special categories.[5] No notice was taken of the existing hierarchies and the women were all herded together in the official records as 'prostitutes'. Yet this term did not give an objective description of an already determined group, but rather overlaid some of the indigenous categories like 'Devadasis' (temple dancers) or baijis (courtesans). It also denied these women their histories as performers and artists.[6]

This chapter traces that trajectory through which one set of women artists were ousted from their social moorings to be appropriated as colonial subjects.

I

The earliest term discovered in the East India Company's official records demarcating the professional prostitutes in Bengal is *Nootee* or dancing girl (Plate 2.1). They were grouped with the indigenous merchants and shopkeepers in the markets of Dacca and Murshidabad.[7] Textually nati (from which 'Nootee' is obviously derived) can be traced to the classical manual on erotics and dramaturgy. Vatsyayana's *Kamasutra*, composed around the second or first century BC, mentions 'Nati' as an actress.

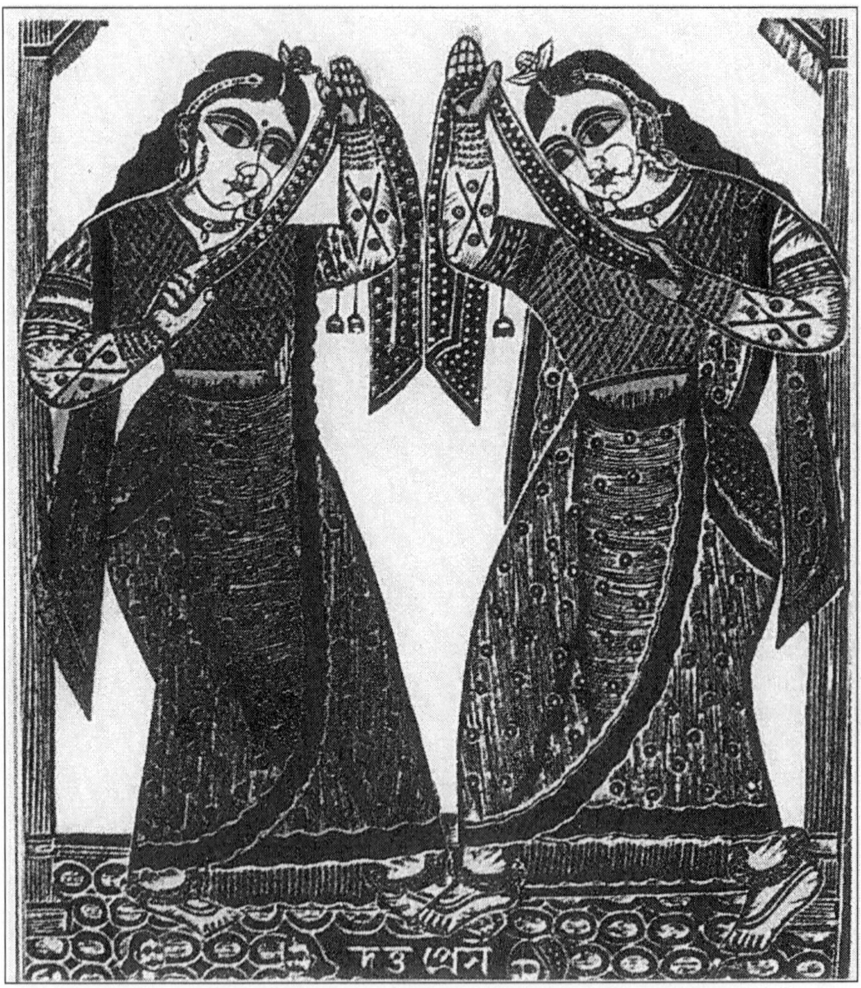

PLATE 2.1 Visual Representations of Public Dancers in Nineteenth-century Woodcut Painting
Source: Courtesy of Ratnabali Chatterjee.

The text in its table of daily sexual rituals and its classification of all men and women into physical types provided a formula for Sanskrit court poetry. This classification was elaborated in Bharata's *Natyashastra* (third century AD), one of the earliest Sanskrit works on dramaturgy and poetics where women's erotic presence was accentuated by attributing to each a particularly amorous mood. Categorized as nayikas (heroines) and nayakas (heroes), men and women were situated in a world of 'amour' for which the courtesans' salon provided the actual setting.[8]

A number of other synonyms characterized women who could loosely be classified as selling their sexual labour for money. Among these, ganika merits attention as an accomplished courtesan—who was taught music, dance, and the arts at the expense of the state. In Kautilya's *Arthashastra* mention is made of the uses to which not only the women but their kin were put: 'They, the teachers shall train the sons of prostitutes to be chief actors (rangopajarin) on the stage. The wives of actors and others of secular professions who have been taught various languages and the use of signals (Samjna) shall along with their relatives be made use of in detecting the wicked and murdering and deluding foreign spies.'[9]

The *Arthashastra*, considered to be complementary to Vatsyayana's *Kamasutra* and written around the same time, concentrated on the Hindu *tribarga*—*dharma*, *artha* and *kama*. In the hierarchized social order dreamt by Kautilya, prostitutes were categorized in strict accordance with their relations to the ruling class. He considered prostitution to be an art. Dancers, actresses, musicians, and acrobats were all listed according to their merits. They all paid taxes to the state. A supervisor called *ganikadhyaksha* controlled these performers, both men and women. Within this structured social order where patriarchy and class provided the norms of conduct, courtesans, and randi (common prostitutes) occupied separate zones. The 'ganika', because of her youth, beauty and expensive training in the arts, occupied that public space where men gathered, leaving their wives in the confinement of the *anthapura*. The power of the courtesan, who charged high fees, and even salaries by the state, was held as valid, and both in Buddhist and Jain texts they serve as the central icons through which an entire historical era is formulated.

Temple prostitutes or devadasis belonged to another group of female dancers whose training was provided by the religious institution to which they had been dedicated. Though Dhoyee in *Pabandutam* and Kalhana's *Rajatarangini* extol the charms of the temple dancers—they were dependent to perform before the deity—they actually acted as concubines to the priests and kings.[10] The *Kuttinimata*, an early medieval text, mentions them as being maintained by the temple but it probably never exceeded beyond clothes and ornaments. Interestingly, a number of these women who gained a certain amount of wealth donated it to the temples. Rich prostitutes, mainly courtesans, also set up works of public utility such as wells, tanks, and gardens. Though living as the 'other' to the 'wife', courtesans carved out a niche for themselves in ancient Indian society through acts of charity.

In Sanskrit literature carried into the medieval period, erotic significance of idealized feminine stereotypes was recognized by contemporary readers by their association with court or temple dancers. The representations of the heroines, nayikas, depended centrally on the male presence (the nayakas). Yet, in spite of the desires for sexual gratification implicit in the literary (or visual) constructs the nayika in medieval court poetry and art remained mainly an aesthetic concept, her representation strictly guided by artistic and literary canons.[11]

In Bengal, the post-Chaitanya Bhakti movement (sixteenth century), with its anti-ritualistic attitudes, offered a powerful religious alternative, within which the woman-image assumed a special symbolism. The Gaudiya Vaishnava theology (as it came to be known), structured into a philosophical system by the six Goswamis, had as its central theme the concept of Bhakti. Bhakti was conceived of not simply as devotion but as a state of bliss in which the devotee is aware of his complete surrender and merger with deity. In its conscious departure from notions of 'reason' and 'knowledge', Bhakti became synonymous with spiritual realization, with the establishment of a mystic personal relationship with god. Given the abstractions and intangibility of this mystic experience, the Vaishnava devotee required the outward manifestations of certain rituals: rituals which required, in turn, a personal definable god. The Bengali Vaishnavas following Chaitanya adopted Sri Krishna as their deity. The text of *Bhagavata Purana*, particularly the tenth *skanda* describing Sri Krishna's childhood plays and amorous adventures with the *gopinis*, was prescribed as the mystic narrative of god's divine manifestation of power. The Gaudiya Vaishnavas, while deifying Chaitanya as an avatar of Vishnu, used his various moods to construct their own image of the devotee. Among the various modes in which the devotee offered himself to God—*dasya* (servant), *sakhya* (friend), *vatsalya* (mother), and *madhurya* (lover)—the last was considered to be the most important.[12]

In the mythic structure that was erected, Vrindavan appeared as a geographical expression of a blissful infinite, and the Vaishnava in turn regarded his own body as the mystic Vrindavan where Krishna resided. And as the supreme embodiment of the 'lover devotee', in his longing for divine union, Sri Chaitanya was deified as the physical manifestation of Radha. Bhakti now expressed itself through a crop of highly erotic poetry. The *rasa* or the moods evoked rested on the theory of merger—where the physical is subsumed within the spiritual and the divine.

One of the early texts which served as a grammar of aesthetics for Bengali Vaishnava poetry was *Ujjala Nilmani* by Rupa Goswami. Here, aesthetics, including all literary exercises, stood as description of the divine love play between Radha and Krishna. In *Ujjala Nilmani* the devotee as Radha and the supreme being as Krishna were worked into an aesthetic formula in which the concept of *Parakiya*—the 'other'—of the *patibrata* (good wife) and *kumari* (chaste virgin) was fully developed. In the devotional poetry of Vidyapati and Chandidas, Radha as the *abhisarika nayika* journeyed to meet her lover, escaping from social restrictions of a married life. Through this single image the poets projected the intensity of a woman in love. She was valorized as the *bhakta* who crosses all difficulties in her/his spiritual passage to reach the supreme bliss of her reunion with God. Radha as the 'main *gopi*' steadily assumed the importance of being the central icon in Vaishnava poetry: at the same time the concept of *Parakiya* gained ground, helping to create an alternative to the role model imposed by the family on women in general. By the seventeenth century, Vaishnava women preceptors emerged as a significant force and women like Jahnavi and Sitadevi (the wives of Nityananda) headed their own sects as 'gurus'.[13]

It was around this time that two divergent trends were seen in the post-Chaitanya Vaishnava movement: appropriation of the movement by orthodox Brahminical orders, and, at the same time, the launching of a number of popular religious sects—the Bauls, Sais, and Fakirs. While the former, known as Gaudiya Vaishnava dharma, came to be recognized by the ruling Muslim sultans as one of the major Hindu sects, the Radha-Krishna legend woven into lyrics and sung as kirtans pervaded Hindu popular culture. Vasudeva Krishna divested of Puranic mythologies and losing his heroic and kingly visage was transformed into the hero of a pastoral romance. The mystic resonance of these lyrics cast its spell on Bengali society right till the nineteenth century.

At the same time, the erotic implications of the mythic narrative were played out in Bharat Chandra's courtly poetry—the *Vidya Sundar* inspired by Bhanudutta's *Rasamanjari* (dated around the fifteenth century). Bharat Chandra also attempted an exposition of the 'Rasa-Shastra' in the context of the romantic imageries of Radha and Krishna. In these texts an elaborate set of literary classifications of romantic erotic moods for the nayika were prescribed—like the *abhisarika* (one who goes to meet her lover), *birohini* (one whose lover is away), and *khandita* (the jealous woman). These were grounded in elaborate cycles of time and space, season and ritual that produced series like the *Baramasyas* (series of twelve months) of the *Ragamala* (musical melodies). In all this, in art and literature, the heroine or the nayika emerged as a central aesthetic category.[14]

It is this ideal of the nayaka and nayika, literary, aesthetic and sensual, which found its way into the court, art, and literature of the provincial Mughal courts of the eighteenth century. A syncretic culture composed of the residual Vaishnava mysticism and the Muslim Sufi ethos came to prevail in the courts of the Bengal nawabs right till the end of the eighteenth century. With the dispersal of Mughal imperial power Murshidabad became the capital of Bengal and an alternate centre of the aristocratic patronage where painters, poets, and musicians, fleeing from a disintegrating Mughal empire, sought refuge.

Recreating the pomp and splendour of the imperial style, the Murshidabad court culture thrived on a Mughal elan, even as it fed on the local syncretic traditions. The demands for secular imagery coinciding with the prevailing repertoire of literary mythic images of Radha and Krishna, nayakas and nayikas resulted in the creation of a genre of ideal portraiture. The images of the nayikas, derived from court paintings of Mughal and Rajput princes, were subsumed into the courtly perception of the 'noble beauty', while the courtesans and the dancing girls provided the actual visual model, the idealized feminine form symbolizing divine grace, which was clearly idealized and removed from the flesh-and-blood women of real lives. The nayaka was usually modelled on the male patron (Nawab Sirajuddaulah was depicted as a nayaka in a series of nayaka-nayika *bhed* paintings of the Murshidabad School). The male viewer was thus able to identify with the protagonist by his recognition of the actual physical setting—the architectural space of the palace, or the inner garden of the zenana mahal. This iconography of Murshidabad court paintings, more than any other genre, in aligning the real and the mystic, the secular and religious, helped to create a physical stereotype of the ideal feminine beauty. The courtesans, by providing the actual model, came to be situated at the core of the courtly vision.[15] She was constructed through the aesthetic and erotic discourses of the court. As a product of the feudal society which the courtesan also aesthetically represented, she appeared even in real life to be the centre of the sensuous world of 'amour'.

II

The hierarchy that was built into the core of feudal relations regulated the lives of the courtesans and their aristocratic clients. Strict differences existed between the baijis (courtesan), dasi (slaves concubines), and the randi. The court dancers and musicians not only participated in public rituals, they also moved into the zenana mahal to entertain the inmates. This practice continued well into the eighteenth century. Often some of the courtesans were granted patronage by rulers and through contract marriages entered the royal harem. Nawab Wazid Ali Shah of Oudh, known as an accomplished poet and musician, had turned his entire harem into a dancing school which he called the *Pari-Khana* (the place of fairies). Every dancer was connected to the nawab through the contractual form of *muta* marriage.[16]

In Bengal, the cases of Mir Jafar's two wives, Munni and Babbu Begum, provide interesting instances of how courtesans could aspire to important social positions in the harem. The career of Munni Begum is well charted in British records. Munni was born in a village called Balkunda near Sekausha. Her poverty-stricken widowed mother, unable to bring her up, sold her to a dancer called Bishu. Bishu brought up Munni with her own daughter, Babbu, to become an accomplished dancer. The troupe, though based mainly in Delhi, used to move around the country performing, and often stayed for months in a place if they were treated well. Bishu and her two daughters arrived in Bengal in 1746. They were invited to perform on the occasion of the wedding feast of Nawab Alivardi Khan's grandson Ekram-ud-daulah. Here Munni attracted the attention of Mir Jafar who was a grandee in Nawab Alivardi's court. He offered both Munni and Babbu his patronage including asking them to stay on in Murshidabad. After a short while both the dancers became a part of Mir Jafar's harem through the *muta* marriage. Soon, Munni became the favourite of Mir Jafar and when in 1757 Mir Jafar, with the help of the British, became the nawab of Bengal, Munni's fortunes increased.[17]

By this time Munni had given birth to two sons, Nizam-ud-daulah and Saif-ud-daulah. After acquiring the throne of Bengal, Mir Jafar placed Munni's son in the post of the governor of Chattogram. Whispers were rife in the court circles as Mir Jafar's other wives—women of aristocratic birth who had greater dynastic claims—were set aside in favour of Munni.[18]

Around 1760, Mir Jafar, who had failed to live up to the Company's expectations of how much he could deliver, was deposed and his own son-in-law Mir Kasim placed on the throne of Bengal by the British. Mir Jafar was forced to leave Murshidabad and take up residence in Calcutta. According to the rumours in the court and the Company's official circles, it was at this time that Mir Jafar was able to lay his hands on the traditional jewels of the Bengal nawabs from the Hirajheel palace, which he passed on to his favourite consort Munni Begum. It was believed by some historians that this was the main source of Munni's rise to power.[19] After 1763, when Mir Jafar became the nawab of Bengal for the second time, his dependence on Munni grew to the extent that he declared her son Nizam-ud-daulah to be his heir. For Munni the passage was set from being a mere courtesan to becoming the head of the *zenana* mahal which she soon proved to be.

After the death of Mir Jafar in 1765, problems cropped up over the question of Nizam-ud-daulah's succession. Questions were raised by Mir Jafar's relatives over the propriety of placing a courtesan's son on the throne. Names of Miran's son and Mir Jafar's sister's grandsons were put forward as legitimate successors to the dynastic claims. Munni Begum with her usual foresight stepped in, bribing the Company's officials with huge sums of money and Nizam-ud-daulah was granted the position of the Nawab Nizam of Bengal. On Colonel Robert Clive's return in the same year Munni Begum presented him with Rs.500,000 to further secure the position of her son. Unfortunately for her, Nizam-ud-daulah died within a few days of the *punia* ceremony (coronation festival). Though a number of people suspected Reza Khan of being instrumental in murdering Nizam-ud-daulah, Reza Khan could extend very little influence over Munni's strong presence. In 1766, the Company officials placed Munni's second son Saif-ud-daulah on the throne of Bengal. Being a minor the latter's allowances were decreased, and Munni Begum, in spite of inner resistance from the 'harem' and outer resistance from men like Nanda Kumar, reigned supreme as the 'Gaddinasin Begum'.[20]

After 1775, when the trouble between the Privy Council and Warren Hastings reached its peak, the members of the Council began to attack Munni Begum as his main support. Her past as a courtesan was raked up. It was declared that her rise to power was through careful means and she was not a fit person to be in charge of the nawab's household. Munni Begum's allowances were reduced in spite of Hasting's objections. In Company circles, Munni Begum's fortunes were considered to be linked with Hastings and so her defeat, in a way, signalled Hastings's failure. That they were wrong was proved by Munni Begum, who stood firm even after Hastings left. Her position as the head of the nawab's household was recognized even by the Muslim society at large. When a number of Muslim students were arrested for being involved in the skirmishes of 1789, and the consequent Hindu-Muslim riots, the leaders of the Muslim community approached Munni Begum to mediate on their behalf. She readily forwarded their petition to the Governor General.[21]

On 10 January 1813, Munni Begum died.[22] The Company officials showed their respect with ninety gun salutes and keeping the flag at half-mast on Fort William—a respect which they reserved for royalty. It is paradoxical that the woman who virtually ruled Bengal for all these years with the help of the Company could not make it evident to the Company's officials that different social norms existed in India, which allowed a courtesan a certain mobility which was incomprehensible to the protestant ethics of the Anglo-Saxon middle class.

Munni Begum was considered the exception, she (and her dance) focused on those thousands of other unfortunate women in India who were caught between two worlds of the dying Mughal and the emergent colonial culture. Veena Talwar Oldenburg in her book on Lucknow and in a later article on the lives of courtesans of this city gives a vivid account of the courtesans and their patrons, once British rule was established in the area.

> Under the generous patronage of the Nawabs of Oudh and the town notables during the eighty odd years that Lucknow served as the Nawabi capital the apartments in the Chowk bazaar where these women lived and entertained in decadent opulence were centres for musical and cultural sources.
>
> A courtesan was usually part of a household establishment under the chief courtesan or chaudhrayan. The latter owned and maintained extra apartments having acquired wealth and fame through her beauty and musical and dancing abilities. Typically a wealthy patron, often the king himself, would set her up in agreeable quarters and support her household in the style in which he wished to be entertained and she would recruit budding young singers and dancers to compete with other reputable establishments. Every reputable house maintained a team of skilled male musicians or gharanas of musicians thereby enhancing the prestige of the establishment. Doormen, touts and other male auxiliaries screened the clients at the doors.[23]

Thus the courtesan's house did not open its doors to every common customer. For the petty shopkeepers and poor workers, the women who offered their sexual service in the bazaars 'thakais', women without the accomplishments of the courtesan, the randi sufficed. The latter was divided from the former through their class position into two completely separate spheres, yet the British refused to recognize these hierarchical divisions among women they generally lumped together as 'prostitutes'. This completely alienated women who saw themselves as the pivot of aristocratic cultural practice. 'The soldiers', they said, 'had no tamiz (manners) or tahzib (culture). We could not speak their language, nor they ours. For them we were no different to randis and they seldom wanted to stay for the nautch.'[24]

By the middle of the nineteenth century, Calcutta had become an important centre of cultural activities as more and more deposed rulers of Indian states were forced to take up their exiled residence in the city.

With the migration of a number of musicians, dancers, and poets once patronized by these nawabs, parts of Calcutta were landmarked as the Mughal city. Here the dancers of Wazed Ali Shah and the poets of the Delhi Durbar mingled with the aristocratic members of Tipu Sultan's deposed family to create the cultural ambience for those who came in a nostalgic search of the grand old days.

It added to the already existing Indian fashion of arranging nautches for family occasions (of a son or a daughter's wedding) or even religious festivals like Durga puja. The dancers were invited from Agra, Benaras, and Lucknow to Calcutta. The rich families in Calcutta vied with one another to get the highest paid baiji. Local newspapers in Bengali as well as the British journals reported these social gatherings (Plate 2.2). Thus, in 1815, a Bengali journal reported that the famous baijis Niki and Ashroom went to the houses of Nilmani Malik and Raja Ram Chandra. On the occasion of the Dol Jatra (the festival of colours) in the same year the *Asiatic Journal* of 15 March reported, for instance: 'At the Nautch parties held in the garden house of Babu Motilal Malik, the two major attractions of the evening were Begum Jan and Hungul.'[25]

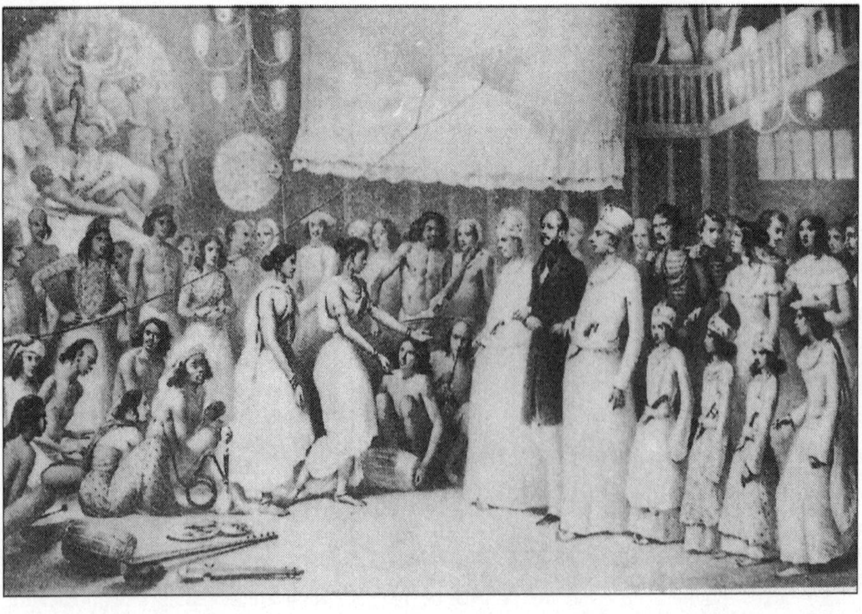

PLATE 2.2: Indigenous Women Performers Dancing on the Occasion of Durga Puja, organized in honour of the Prince of Wales at the Belgachia Villa of Calcutta. *Source*: Woodcut painting by J. Nash, 1 May 1876. Courtesy of Ratnabali Chatterjee.

III

In the early days of the East India Company the 'native' way of entertaining the sahibs was through a feast following a nautch. This was recognized by the British as a social event which was integrated as a 'custom' in the new rituals of ruling.

From 1757, when the East India Company gained military control of Bengal, their positions changed from merchants seeking trade concessions to a national power within the state system of the eighteenth century. By 1803, Lord Lake had captured Delhi, the Mughal capital. This was seen by Wellesley and others as legitimizing British presence in India. By proclaiming the East India Company the protector of the Mughal Emperor, the British thought of coming into the possession of the nominal authority of the Mughals. In 1858 India became a part of the British empire. This ended the paradoxical situation when the vast number of people subjugated by the British still owed allegiance to another ruler, the Mughal emperor in Delhi. Between this period, i.e. 1757–1858, India, for the Company officials, was a vast theatre of power which needed to be managed. The ritual preceptors who were chosen to lay down the norms varied in their decisions. It is through these fractured perceptions of Orientalists and officials that the colonial narrative was constructed. Indian dancers, the nautch girls, were only some among many of the characters that crowded the colonial stage.[26]

For European artists like Solvyns the 'nautch' offered a colourful opportunity to look at the native household and its luxuries of which the dancing girls formed a part. To visitors like Fanny Parkes it was part of an oriental adventure. She went into raptures over one of the dancers, Niki, calling her the Cataline of the East.[27] Solvyns recorded the different groups of dancers whom he distinguished by their dresses, fascinated by their embroidery and design. Among many categories, he mentioned two groups in particular—the Bayadari and the Domni. The last comprised lower-caste women who came in groups to perform at marriages and were mainly folk singers. Solvyns further recorded (after a conversation with Colonel Gardener) that while Domnis' songs were always full of ribaldry, the baijis were strictly against obscenity.

According to Solvyns, both Colonel Gardner and his son had their own groups of nautch girls. By 1810, the East India Company officials were coming under certain censorship from their peer groups in England. The East India Vade Mecum or Complete Guide to Gentlemen Intended for the East India Company by Captain Thomas Williamson (1810) laid down the norms of behaviour that members of the ruling race should follow. One of the strictures was to beware of 'native' dancers.

> If we add the allurements held out by the stable beauties some fellow who can speak English begins by describing the elegance of the native women and their great perfection as singers and dancers and rarely fails especially with youths under such circumstance to excite something more than curiosity. The dancing girls are introduced and consequence follow over which I shall draw the veil, simply observing that nothing can be more dangerous than the irregular indulgence; it never failing to drain the purse and in a few days or weeks the constitution also.[28]

Thus, the dancing girl became a symbol of that exotic Orient which wanted to lure the occidental youth into every kind of moral and physical disorder.

This theme is elaborated by Richard Burton, the translator of the *Arabian Nights*, and in Vatsyayana's *Kamasutra*. Burton, like other military officers of his time, had been served by an Indian who looked after his house and met his sexual needs. Burton noticed that she never expressed any love for him. This led him to come to the moral conclusion that Indian women were driven by sexual needs which could never be satisfied by a European. He further concluded that in recognition of this, native men got their daughters married before puberty. Burton was a typical upholder of Victorian polarized ideas on women and looked upon Indian women as comparable to the working-class women at home who were doomed through their sexual desires to be prostitutes. In direct opposition, the asexual women of the British middle class were seen as fit companions and loving wives who sacrificed everything for their husbands.

Yet, in spite of these views, British patronage of dancing girls continued till 1857. In their desire to adopt the indigenous forms of authority, the British adopted many traits of the nawabi culture. In *Nashtar*, a novel written by Hasan Shah in 1790, the author relates the tragic story of an impoverished writer and his lover Kharem Jan, a dancing girl who has to entertain unwillingly English officers of the East India Company. Hasan Shah traces the breakdown of the old patron client structure that existed in the nawabi court and the new relationship that emerged once the East India Company took over. The narrator is a *munshi* (clerk) in the household of the young English officer who patronizes the dancing girls. The narrative marks out the individual and human aspect of the relationship that binds Kharem Jan to the young Englishman, eager to learn about his country from where he has come to make his fortune. His friendship with the author highlights his sensitive nature and brings to mind those positive features of individual Englishmen for whom Indians were not only subjects to be controlled but men and women in an alien society who should be understood.

In comparison, in *Umrao Jan Ada* (1899), a novel by Mirza Mohammed Hadi Ruswa, the setting is both pre- and post-Mutiny. His heroic Umrao

Jan is a product of her time. Her friend Khurshid Jan is picked up by a Raja Sahib and moves up the social ladder only to be rudely dashed down once the Raja loses his estates in the mutiny. Umrao becomes an associate of a rebel leader and has to hide once the rebellion is over. This marks the major shift that occurred in the relationship between the dancing girls and their British patrons—the colonial state, haunted by the fear of an uncontained rebel population, could no longer trust any 'native', and the eighteenth-century sexual myths of the women were now eclipsed by this of the rebel who was out to destroy all white men.

IV

In the trajectory of the Indian courtesan from one who belonged to the 'highest' tax bracket to the position of a common prostitute, Veena Talwar Oldenberg sees 'a non-confrontational resistance' which continues even today. She traces this resistance from the day the courtesans were ousted from their rightful place in elite culture: 'At all Hindu and Muslim courts in the many kingdoms that made up the subcontinent before the British began to displace the rulers, the courtesans were an influential female elite. The courtesans of Lucknow established themselves as a notable group of women in the eighty-odd years that the Awadh dynasty had Lucknow as its capital city.'[29]

They were recognized as preservers and performers at the high culture of the court who actively shaped the developments in Hindustani music and Kathak dance styles even in the nineteenth century. Their style of entertainment was widely imitated in other Indian court cities. Association with them bestowed prestige on those who were invited to their salons for cultural soirees. It was not uncommon for the young sons of the nobility to be sent to the best known salons for instruction in etiquette, in the art of conversation and polite manners, and the appreciation of Urdu literature.

During the period of the nawabs, these women could manipulate powerful courtiers and the nawabs themselves; even the most powerful patron did not have control over their lives. The executive authority and managerial functions were the exclusive preserve of the Chaudharayan and her appointees. 'An angered patron had options because he had made material investment in Kotha and there were no refunds or exchanges; his *izzat* too would be on the line since gossip about him would quickly and freely circulate in the bazaar.'[30]

These tactics were improved upon during the changed situation initiated by the Contagious Diseases Act. The Acts were passed in 1864 and amended with a view towards greater effectiveness between

1866 and 1869. In an immediate sense the legislation developed in response to the growing pressures on doctors and officers after the Crimean War when the alarming numbers of British soldiers suffering from venereal disease were published. Since venereal diseases were considered controllable, the colonial authorities were now engaged in the formulation of a policy to ensure the safety of the soldiers. Their models for providing institutional checks, such as the setting up of Lock Hospitals were derived from England. Once transported to the colonies, the Act became more binding upon the prostitutes than their clients. A key element of this measure was the compulsory examination of prostitutes; the colonial authorities first turned their attention to those women who were visited by the British soldiers. They were picked up and examined within hospitals. Later, as British soldiers could not be confined within the cantonments, the Act was enlarged to cover all the big cities and all prostitutes, brothel keepers and pimps had to be registered. In the British records of this period all women who could in any way be associated with commercial sex were to be brought under the registration system and this included the courtesans. Since this was the only way in which the colonial state was sure of providing the British soldiers with sexual commodity, they desired an elaborate apparatus of coercion which hunted down native women, thus liberating them of all other identities by pushing them into the sexual category of the common prostitute.

At the same time, the colonial state did not speak in one voice. It mediated between different interest groups—the government at home, the white planters and merchants, the missionaries, and also the native elites, the latter being their strongest ally in any reform measure.

After 1858, the instruction of distancing themselves from the natives led many British officials to withdraw from the native feasts and nautch parties. Others, however, saw nothing wrong in a nautch. It was seen as a distinguished aristocratic gathering of natives and definitely to be viewed as a revelry which was not vulgar. Reverend Dr Millar, the principal of Madras Christian College, for instance, saw nothing wrong in attending a nautch party arranged in honour of Prince Albert's visit to the city.

In 1890, however, things were changing and both missionary appeals and indigenous public opinion were to call out against official participation in these activities. Sir Charles Elliot was accused by a Bengali annual, *Sanjibani*, for attending a nautch—'His honour has been in this country for a long time, and does he not know to what class these dancing-girls belong?'[31] Interestingly, the charge as it was framed was not directed at the organizers of the orgy, but was based on the character of the women who merely served as entertainers. While the British officials even at this stage did not wish to intervene in what they considered to be an age-old native custom, even though a group of natives was crying out for its removal, they also did nothing to stop the process of registration of courtesans as prostitutes even when the Contagious Diseases Acts were repealed. On one hand, they continued to tax the women to keep the Lock Hospitals functioning. On the other, they were fined for non-attendance.

These new challenges provoked the courtesans to intensify their struggle to keep out an intrusive civic authority that taxed their incomes and inspected their bodies. Characteristically, they responded by keeping spurious account books bribing the *dais* (female nurses) who carried out medical inspection and kept the police happy with money and sex.[32] Though the tactics were new, their survival strategies stood the test of time. The courtesans had managed to survive by absconding from repressive policing authorities and putting up a spirited defence of their rights and privileges.'[33]

Notes and References

1. Michel Foucault, *History of Sexuality: An Introduction*, New York: Penguin Books, 1984, pp. 18–19.
2. Lynda Nead, *Myths of Sexuality*, Cambridge, MA: Basil Blackwell, 1990, p. 91.
3. Rana Kabani, *Europe's Myths of Orient*, London: The Macmillan Press, 1986, p. 51.
4. Bernard S. Cohn, 'Introduction', in *Colonialism and its Forms of Knowledge: The British in India*, Delhi: Oxford University Press, 1997, p. 10.
5. Lakshmi Subramanian, 'Disenfranchising the Devdasis', Occasional Paper No. 2, Women's Studies Research Centre, University of Calcutta, January 2000, p. 5.
6. Cohn, 'Introduction'.
7. Board of Revenue Police, Circular of the Governor General in Council, 15 December 1792.
8. H.C. Chakladar, *Social Life in Ancient India*, Calcutta: Susil Gupta, 1954, pp. 11–35.
9. R. Shamastry, ed., *Kautilya's Arthasastra*, Mysore: Mysore Printing and Publishing House, 1960, quoted in Sukumari Bhattacharji, 'Prostitution in Ancient India', in *Women and Society in Ancient India*, Calcutta: Basumati Corp., 1994.
10. Ibid., pp. 84–5.
11. N.N. Bhattacharya, *History of Indian Erotic Literature*, New Delhi: Munshiram Manoharlal, 1975, p. 98.

12. Ramakanta Chakravarty, *Vaisnavism in Bengal, 1486–1900*, Calcutta: Sanskrit Pustak Bhandar, 1985, pp. 348–9.
13. Ibid.
14. Ananda K. Coomaraswamy, *The Eight Nayikas*, 1914; repr., New Delhi: Munshiram Manoharlal, 2000, pp. 8–33.
15. Ratnabali Chatterjee, *From the Karkhana to the Studio: Changing Social Roles of Patrons and Artists in Bengal*, New Delhi: Books & Books, 1990.
16. Veena Talwar Oldenburg, *The Making of Colonial Lucknow*, Princeton: Princeton University Press, 1984, pp. 134–8.
17. Brajendra Nath Bandyopadhyay, *Banglar Begum*, Calcutta, 1912 CE (1319 [Bangabda]), Mani Begum, Bangiya Sahitya Parishad, pp. 35–7.
18. Home Public Consultations, 20 January 1776.
19. *Calendar of Persian Correspondence*, vol. III, letter no. 123.
20. National Archives of India (NAI), Proceedings of the Controlling Council of Revenue, Murshidabad, 20 December 1770.
21. Bandyopadhyay, *Banglar Begum*.
22. *Calendar of Persian Correspondence*, vol. V, Calcutta, 1930, p. 146, no. 902.
23. Oldenburg, *The Making of Colonial Lucknow*, pp. 134–8.
24. Ibid., p. 137n105.
25. Brajendra Nath Bandyopadhyay, *Sambad Patrey Sekaler Katha*, vol. II, Calcutta: Bangiya Sahitya Parishad, 1977 (1384 [Bangabda]), pp. 772–4.
26. Cohn, 'Introduction', pp. 16–57.
27. Sumanta Banerjee, *Dangerous Outcast: The Prostitute in Nineteenth Century Bengal*, Calcutta: Seagull Books, 1998, p. 14.
28. Kenneth Ballhatchet, *Race, Sex and Class under the British: Imperial Attitudes and Policies and their Critics, 1793–1905*, New Delhi: Vikas Publishing House, 1979, pp. 2–3.
29. Veena Talwar Oldenburg, 'Lifestyle as Resistance: The Case of the Courtesans of Lucknow', in *Contesting Power: Resistance and Everyday Social Relations in South Asia*, ed. Douglas Haynes and Gyan Prakash, Berkeley: University of California Press, 1992, p. 30.
30. Ibid., p. 49.
31. Ballhatchet, *Race, Sex and Class under the British.*
32. Banerjee, *The Dangerous Outcast*, pp. 115–17.
33. Oldenburg, *The Making of Colonial Lucknow*.

3 The Tawaif and the Item Girl
A Struggle for Identity

PALLABI CHAKRAVORTY

Introduction

I went to see Madhuri Devi in Bowbazar, north Calcutta, in 1998. I remember climbing up dark and dusty stairs with peeling walls smeared with *paan peek* (betel leaf spittle). I was greeted on a sunny rooftop by a smiling Madhuri Devi. She disappeared into her room and brought out an album for me. There were many photographs of her dancing *mujra* (soiree). In her earlier life she had been a baiji, and although she still lived in the quarters she had left her profession far behind. She was sending her children to respectable schools. I saw Madhuri Devi perform again in 2006, at the International Kathak Festival—Kathak at the Crossroads—organized by the late maestro Chitresh Das in San Francisco. Madhuri Devi got a standing ovation among one of the biggest gathering of gurus, practitioners, and scholars of the tradition.

We are living in astonishing times as scholars and performers of South Asian dance and music. We see these forms and their histories liberated from their mystical, esoteric, orientalist past, as world art performances of the twenty-first century. Scholars and performers of South Asian performing arts are spread across the globe, and music and dance from the region feature in many prestigious international and national conferences and festivals. Today, creativity and innovation in the performing arts due to technology, media, and the speed of communication are transforming lives, practices, and relationships at an unprecedented rate. So much so that now any dance movement can be copied from YouTube to create a new hybrid vocabulary, any image can arrive from a multitude of visual universes, stripped of history,

*A version of this chapter was delivered as a keynote for a conference titled 'Affective Labor in Dance: South Asia and Beyond' at the University of Chicago, and a section of the chapter appeared in my essay 'Global Dancing in Kolkata', in *A Companion to the Anthropology of India*, ed. Isabelle Clark-Deces, Malden: Blackwell, 2010.

meaning, or context. In this world of blurred boundaries and rapidly changing contexts, I pause to ask how we can think about aesthetic labour, heritage, authority, and ownership today, in relation to the Indian performing arts. I ask this despite the various historiographies of 'invention of tradition' and all the remarkable recent scholarship on Indian music and dance that addresses these questions in different ways and shows the constructed nature of such discourses. I reiterate some of these questions on creativity, innovation, heritage, and history as they have their own ways of staying relevant and leveraging the burning issues of contemporaneity.

I bring up the questions of 'authority' and 'history' specifically in the context of Kathak dance because the relevance of the tawaif or baiji and her fluid identity have resurfaced in contemporary culture as she has converged with the bar dancers and item girls of the twenty-first century, as icons of illicit dances and excessive sexuality. Consider this comment by Devdutt Pattanaik in a recent article:

> Later the dance of the *devdasis*, once as sadar kacheri, became the much sanitized Bharatnatyam (a word that did not exist a century ago, I am told by dance historians) following the outcry of social reformers influenced by both Hindu monastic orders and Christian missionaries in the Madras Presidency. Therefore, the audience sought its entertainment elsewhere, where sexuality and sensuality openly acknowledged—on the screens of cinema as the cabaret performer in the night club, the mujra of the tawaif in her kotha, then around trees in dream sequences, and finally atop tables in bars by the uber confident item-girl.[1]

It is interesting to see how the devadasi was sanctified and restored as the repository of modern day Bharatanatyam in scholarly contexts and the popular imaginary (these include many recent academic monographs as well as programme notes of reputed practitioners), whereas the tawaif, especially as the source of Kathak dance, remains mired in obfuscation (see Plate 3.1). She remains an ahistorical figure whose identity has merged with the modern-day bar girls, cabaret dancers, and sex workers.[2] While Kathak dance is defined by the *gharanedar*, patriarchal Brahminical lineages, the history of the tawaif and her *mujra* continue as symbols of corruption. Consider this comment by Kathak maestro Birju Maharaj recently:

> Hindi cinema has committed a grave mistake by showing kathak as a dance form performed in brothels. It has made some people sitting in jackets and cap, while dancers wear crude and lewd dresses. They dance on songs with unwholesome words with the sole purpose of enticing the audience. Kathak *tawaifs ka naach nahi hai* [Kathak is not the dance of brothels]. This depiction has adversely affected the dignity of the art form.[3]

The sanctification of Kathak dance during cultural nationalism in the early twentieth century and in postcolonial India had purged the tawaif,

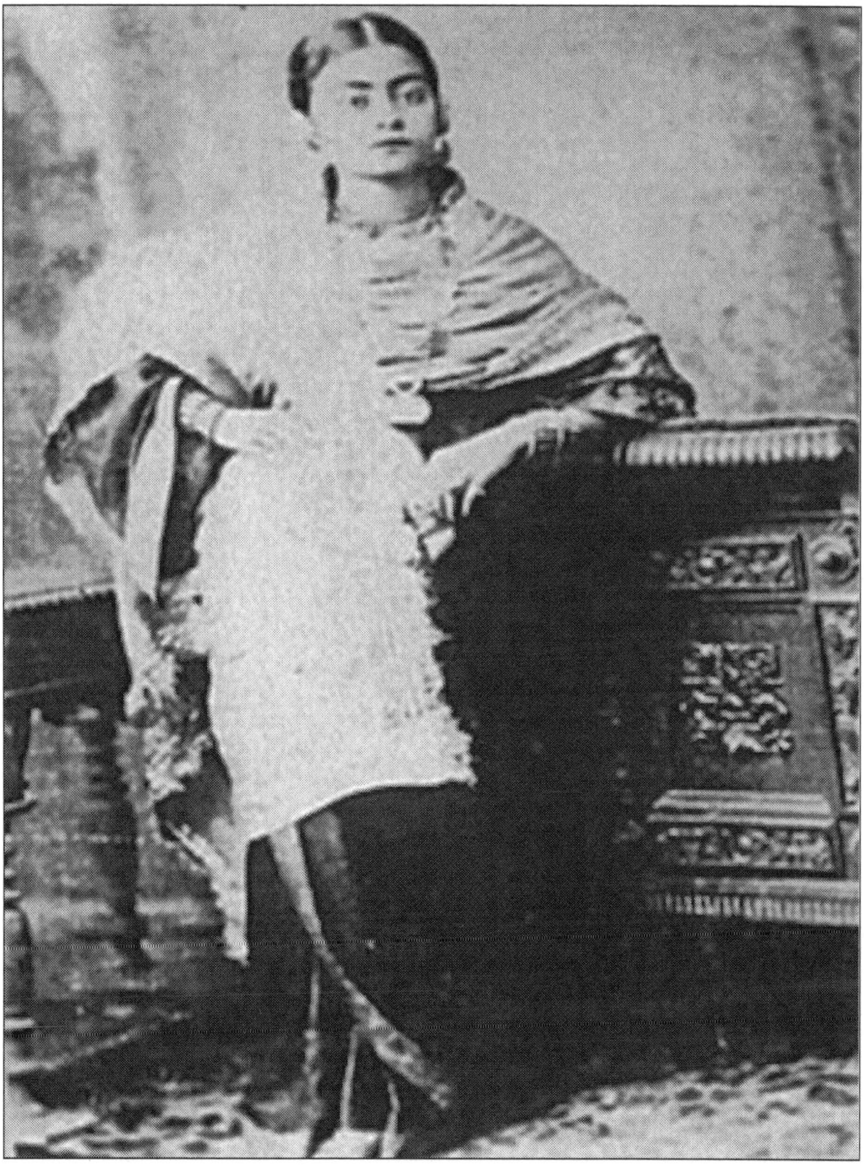

PLATE 3.1: A Postcard Image of a Tawaif (Courtesan), which was circulated at the End of the Nineteenth Century. *Courtesy* of Saba Dewan. *Source*: Kashi Sangeet Samaj, Banaras. *Photo courtesy* of Anurima Banerjee.

not unlike the devadasis, from the historical narratives of classicism. However, unlike the devadasi, the tawaif's female Muslim identity created a double impediment to the male Brahminical Hinduization of the performing arts, so they could not be given any sacred status like the Hindu devadasis to purify their polluted image.

In this chapter I first explore the contribution of the tawaifs as the forebears of Kathak and I argue that their 'affective labour' was crucial to the continuity of the embodied knowledge of Kathak in contemporary times. I trace the tawaif's artistic contribution, from Urdu dance dramas such as *Indra Sabha* in Wajid Ali's court to the creation of the popular music and dance genre *thumri*, giving special attention to the contribution of the renowned tawaif/baiji Gauhar Jan in popularizing *thumri* in the early part of the twentieth century. Second, I show how the discourse of the tawaif and her so-called wanton sexuality resurface through the discourses around the popular dance reality shows in contemporary India as the alluring figure of the 'item girl'. The men and women from underprivileged or non-elite backgrounds in India who participate in reality shows and dance like the 'item girls' of Bollywood films are also targets of derision by the gatekeepers of culture. The overt sexuality of women in these dances and their assertion of a new brand of femininity in public spaces open up yet another new script on the debates on women's sexuality, aesthetic labour and ownership of dance. Throughout these narratives we also see the overlapping worlds of Indian performing arts and Indian cinema.

The Tawaif in History

Despite the high status of the tawaif within the culture of the Urdu- and Bengali-speaking gentry in the past, the tawaif or the nautch girl continues to be associated with the decadence and opulence of the courtly or the zamindari milieu. One could argue that this is a vestige of past colonial efforts to delegitimize Islamic courts in India as places of sexual excess. The tawaif's association with the courts automatically attached her to decadence in colonial and postcolonial India. This association was enhanced by the Hinduization of the arts in India by the cultural revivalists and nationalists in the 1920s who wanted to trace Indian arts and aesthetics back to Sanskrit roots.[4] Kathak's Islamic roots and the identity of the tawaif as a Muslim woman surely created a double handicap for these women in terms of gender and community.

Yet the tawaif was central to an aesthetic Indic identity (the Indo-Islamic traditions of music, dance, painting) that is not only traced back to the splendour of the Mughal court, such as Akbar's in medieval India, but also to the court of Wajid Ali Shah whose courtly traditions of music, dance, and dance dramas gave birth to many modern performing arts traditions, including Parsi theatre, which in turn greatly influenced Bombay films during the early twentieth century.[5] The abrupt end to the rule of the nawabs of Awadh in the nineteenth century, the most prominent of the successor states to follow the Mughal dynasty, was also a watershed event in Kathak's history. I briefly look at the importance of Wajid Ali Shah, the last nawab of Awadh, who was a great patron of Kathak dance, by focusing on the Urdu dance drama *Indra Sabha*, written by Amanat Ali (1816–59), before embarking on the subject of the tawaif lineage in Kathak dance. Both *Indra Sabha* and the tawaif establish a common trajectory of the Kathak lineage and provide historical links to the modern-day performing arts and cinema in India. *Indra Sabha*'s transition from an Urdu play at Wajid Ali Shah's court to Parsi theatre has been analysed in detail by Kathryn Hansen.[6] *Indra Sabha* was made into a Bombay talkie in the year 1932.

Indra Sabha to Kathak

Indra Sabha is significant because it is an original work that assimilates various literary and performing arts traditions, from Urdu ghazal to Braj Bhasha *thumri* to Awadhi folk. All of these are woven into a narrative base to tell the story of Indra's court. The author Amanat Ali creates a court that replicates that of Wajid Ali Shah, where Wajid Ali as Indra is entertained by courtesans or *paris* (fairies) through songs and dances. The royal court or gathering of people in the play is referred to as *sabha*, *majis*, *mehfil*, and *jalsa*, all of which mean public recitals and performances and were associated with Kathak soirees in the colonial period. Wajid Ali's patronage of Kathak dance is wellknown and he himself danced as Krishna. The genres of *thumri*, *battana*, *khyal*, *ghazal*, Kathak, and *tappa* all flourished in his court. Wajid Ali himself wrote *thumris* and *dadras* under the pen name 'Aktar Piya'. Also, two musical treatises from the nineteenth century, *Saut al-Mubarak* and *Bani*, are attributed to him; the latter was written in his court in Metiabruj.[7]

Wajid Ali especially recruited courtesans and trained them to participate in his dance dramas so he could play the role of Krishna. All the theatrical performances in his court were called *rahas*, and he maintained a *rahas khana* or drama hall named after the *raslila* tradition of Vaishnava devotional drama.[8] The language of the songs in *Indra Sabha* embodied the voices of a *pari* (fairy), the *gopi* (cowherd girl) in *Hori* (festival of colours) in Braj Bhasha, and the lament of the *ashiq* or lover in an Urdu ghazal. Hansen writes: 'The voice complains of her beloved's haughty neglect and threatens suicide. The language of the songs moves easily between *Urdu*, *Braj*, *Awadh*, and *Khariboli*. The Hindu and Muslim cultural referents mingle as the king's identity morph from Indra and Krishna to Nawab.'[9]

Kathryn Hansen asks whether the play is a self-consciously constructed syncretic work or a spontaneous reflection of the hybrid culture of the Lucknow court. But she is certain that this courtly secular milieu held a wide appeal for a large cross-section of the public.

After the fall of Awadh, the exodus of dancers and musicians from the court to the cities of Calcutta and Banaras is well-known. Performers who were formerly employed at the royal court turned to theatre, cinema, and recording industries (which were growing rapidly) for economic reasons. The song and dance genres, such as Kathak, *thumri*, and ghazal, had entered the popular arena and were readily accepted by audiences because of the status and prestige associated with these performing arts. In *Bells of Change*, I analyse in detail how the courtly dance was transformed into bai-nautches in the salons of the Calcutta zamindars, and how *bhadralok* (the new middle-class elite) competed with each other to throw the most lavish nautch parties.[10]

The public debate on prostitution leading to the anti-nautch movement in the 1890s crippled the institution of the tawaif and reduced the entire community that had varying social status and artistic skills to a single category of prostitutes. Without going into the details of the various forces that led to the demise of the institution of the tawaif,[11] I explore the complex identity of the tawaif by focusing on a few individuals. My aim is to connect their legacy to the dance now called Kathak.[12] But, first, a few words on the social status of the tawaif community and their artistry in dance and music.

The Tawaif in History

The word 'tawaif', used as a singular in Urdu, is the plural of the Arabic word *taifa*. The word 'tawaif' in common parlance now denotes a prostitute but the complex identity of the tawaif is emblematic of the mosaic culture of India with its bewildering social hierarchies and communal and religious and regional identities. Interestingly, in the colonial census report of 1881, all prostitutes were recorded as Muslims.[13] Siddiqui later writes that the British Government alleged that all Hindu women of 'loose-character' accepted Islam.[14] This curious statement, also from the census report, shows the tumultuous cultural and social transformations taking place in the nineteenth century when the highly cultured salons were being homogenized as brothels and an entire community stigmatized. Somnath Chakrabarty identified the different regional communities of nautch girls (all the different communities of dancing girls were simplified as 'nautch girls' by the British) to shed some light on the diversity of the artistic communities in pre-colonial India. In the Beria community in Uttar Pradesh, the dancing girls were called Berin. They were called Deogarni among the Gand community in central India, and in Telengana they were called Bogam. The term 'tawaif' was ascribed to the Muslim nautch performers, whereas the communities mentioned here were all Hindus by religion.[15] I should add here that in Bengal they were known as baiji. However, in the book *Ye Kothe Valiyan*, Nagar reports that many tawaifs claimed they were from the Gaur Thakur caste although they worshipped Islam.[16] Their primary identity was according to their matriarchal *biradari* (extended family) whereas their religious identity was syncretic rather than communal. The tawaif community, not unlike other Indian communities, was hierarchical with many regional differences. For instance, the tawaifs of the Deredar caste were the most respectable among the Muslim community and they distinguished themselves from the quasbi or randi (common prostitutes) and held them in contempt.[17] The kaneez and khanaki occupied lower ranks in Bengal like the quasabi and randi, whereas jan was the highest tier reserved for the high-status poets and performers. The other caste identities that were associated with the hereditary flesh trade were the Nat, Bhand, and Mirasi communities.[18]

The highest category of tawaifs learnt the arts of singing, dancing, and classical language from renowned ustads (male teachers) of the time. They marked their distinction by identifying themselves as shagirds (students) of these ustads and the cities from which they hailed. For instance, Janab Atar Badauni is referred to in some verses of Abbasi Jan Ada Tawaif's *quasida* (poetry).[19] Unfortunately, the learning that happened in the zenana (women's quarters) of the tawaif is not recoverable through material traces such as in the verses they wrote or in colonial travel records or photographs. As a result, it became easy to deny women the status of ustad or teacher later and their banishment from artistic history became certain under the reformed Brahminical patriarchy of the arts. The famous recording artist Gaisberg, who was visiting India at the beginning of twentieth century, had written in his dairy about this other kind of knowledge transmission:

> Songs and dances were passed by word of mouth from mother to daughter. They began public appearances at the age of 10 to 12 years. The clever ones went up to the top and sometimes travelled all over the country in great demand at the wedding feasts of the wealthy. As they began to make names for themselves, many of them insisted that the word 'amateur' should be printed on record label.[20]

A rare example of women's acknowledged status as teacher is Zeba-un-Nisa of the Benaras *gharana*, whose son, also a musical artist, said he learnt everything he knew from his mother.[21] Anindya Banerjee writes, during a discussion with the late Kumar Mukhopadhyay, that the ustads never shared their most cherished *bandishes* (musical compositions) with the tawaifs; rather these were reserved for their own family members or their students from respectable families. The tawaifs often got their most intimate musical knowledge from their sarangi players who usually occupied the lowest status in the musical hierarchy.[22] The sarangi players were very close to the tawaifs as their accompanists and this kind of transmission of knowledge was perhaps inevitable.

The mother-daughter transmission of knowledge (or female-to-female knowledge transmission) is evident if one considers the lives of the famous tawaifs Mah Laqa Bai Chanda (1768–1820) and Gauhar Jan (1873–1930). The former, known to have been trained by her mother, also trained her adopted daughter Husn Laqa Bai or 'Madame Beauty Cheek' in dance. Her first biographer in Urdu, Gawhar, wrote in 1896 that as long as Husn Laqa Bai was alive, the courtesan's way of life continued in good order. After her, the courtesans split into separate groups under the leadership of Pyaran Ji and Banu Ji whose female lineages have been traced by historians and one of them can be found near Charminar. These courtesan groups are supported with stipends and land grants out of the fond memory of Mah Laqa Bai. Scott Kugle further writes that 'this legacy may complicate the history of Indian classical dance, for it provides information about women teaching other women to dance. Modern histories of Kathak and other forms emphasize that male dance masters passed on the classical traditions.'[23]

Gauhar Jan is one of the most important examples of the tawaif legacy, showing it to be the forebear of modern-day Kathak. Among her teachers were Bindadin Maharaj, considered to be the founder of Lucknow *gharana* of Kathak. Consider this passage from Amiyanath Sanyal: 'In the *mehfil*, Gauhar threw her first arrow—she stood up and danced to a *darbari tarana* and sang along. It was followed by the fireworks of her *tan*. Then she sang a *thumri* and performed *bhao* from Bhaia sahib's *gharana*.'[24] Here she sings and dances both to *tarana* and *thumri*, two very different components of the Kathak dance repertoire.

Gauhar Jan and her mother Malka Jan (whose real name was Victoria Yeoward) came to Calcutta from Benaras in the latter part of the nineteenth century. They were both famous for *bolbanao thumri* and other north Indian musical forms such as *hori*, *chaiti*, *kajari*, and *dadra*. These forms were practised and preserved almost exclusively by the tawaifs who excelled not in just performance but also in penning their verses. The verses were about ecstatic passion, pangs of separation, jealousy, longing, anger, and playful love. The tawaifs' contribution to Urdu poetry is evident from the life history of Maha Laqa Bai Chanda who belonged to the court of the Nizam of Hyderabad and was the first female poet to author a *diwan*, a collection of Urdu ghazals titled *Gulzar-e-Mahlaqa*.[25] The literary journal *Payam-e-Yar* (1898) also regularly published *ghazals* and *quasidas* by courtesans from many parts of north India.[26] Gauhar Jan wrote *thumris* and *ghazals* under her pen name 'Humdum' and 'Gauhar Piya', and her mother Malka Jan wrote more than 600 poems (in a book which was published in 1886 titled *Makhzan-e-Ulfat-e-Mallika* or 'Treasures of Mallika's Love').

The artistry of *bolbanao thumri* is unique as it involved both singing and dancing and rested on the ability of the performer to tease out multiple interpretations of a given phrase. The ultimate artistry was about evoking a sensuous mental space of intimacy and emotion through *abhinaya/bhao* (facial expressions), hand gestures, and the slow lilting movements of *gatnikas* (a particular style of moving and expressing emotion). Vikram Sampath writes in detail about how Gauhar Jan, already a famous artist in Calcutta, begged to learn *bolbanao thumri* from Mauzuddin and Bhaia Sahib after hearing the former in a rendition of a *Banarasi-ang* (Banaras-style) *thumri*.[27] Sampath highlights Gauhar Jan's ability and open-mindedness to absorb and assimilate the various musical renditions of the ustads and teachers she heard and learnt from. The women musicians and dancers of the time were not bound by the stylistic and geographical boundaries of the *gharanas* and believed in the healthy interaction and intermixing of styles to create their own individual styles.[28] I would like to add that the creation of 'purity' of styles in the form of *gharanas*/lineages was an aspect of the social reforms and cultural revivalism of the early part of the twentieth century. These movements Hinduized both music and dance and gendered the art forms into patriarchal *gharanas* of Muslim and Hindu lineages.

Gauhar Jan acquired star status early in her career and was the most sought-after artist of the time (see Plate 3.2). Abdul Halim Sharar, who wrote on Lucknow, witnessed Gauhar Jan's performance in 1896 in Calcutta and observed:

> It is unlikely that anywhere else there were more perfect demonstrations of dance than the courtesans of Lucknow. At one performance, I witnessed her (Gauhar Jan's) skill in *batana* on the same theme for three full hours. All those present at the gathering including the most expert dancers and distinguished people of Matiyaburj were spellbound.[29]

Gauhar Jan's fame was not restricted to Calcutta or north India but spread to the south. She also trained women like Indubala who became

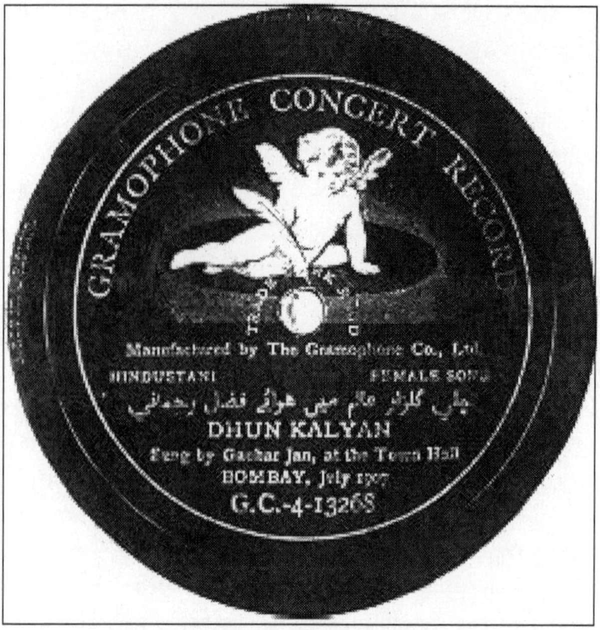

PLATE 3.2: Writing on Gramophone Record of Dhun Kalyan by Gauhar Jan in 1907. *Source*: Women on Record, Centre for Media and Alternative Communication, http://www.womenonrecord.com/wp-content/uploads/2011/05/gauhar-jan-5.bmp, accessed 26 July 2016.

a famous baiji in Calcutta. Although I focus on Gauhar Jan here, and she was by far the most famous courtesan whose voice has been captured for posterity by the Gramophone Company, there were many others like her. Sasimukhi—the first artist to be recorded by the Gramophone Company with her colleague Phanibala in Calcutta by Gaisberg—and Phanibala were also famed courtesans of the time.[30] We get information about their soirees from invitations (called tickets) that were sent out to zamindars, in newspaper accounts of lavish parties, and in some travelogues and photographs of the times. Some other tawaifs of the time include Wazir Jaan, Sugan Bai, Niccki Usharan, and Jaddan Bai (mother of the famous Bombay film actress Nargis). These women, too, were carving their niche during the late nineteenth and early twentieth centuries. Their repertoire was varied and eclectic, and they performed solo, in teams, and in duets.[31]

However, the anti-nautch social reform movement of the 1890s forced them to seek work in the new industries of theatre, music, and cinema, but many had to give up their artistic profession and turn purely to the flesh trade. It is a travesty that the tawaifs of Lucknow, who in a fledgling nationalist fervour banded to foment sedition against the colonial government during the uprising of 1857, were later denounced as a corrupting influence by nationalists and cultural revivalists, including Gandhi. The tawaifs were specifically targeted by the British because of their active role in the rebellion of 1857. The British were determined to control them and tax them heavily. This resulted in the latter's avoidance in registering for government records to evade heavy taxation.[32]

In 1921, when the tawaif community organized a meeting and offered to be part of Mahatma Gandhi's non-cooperation movement, Gandhi is reported to have unequivocally rejected this 'obscene' proposal.[33] The discrimination continued even after independence. The then home minister, Sardar Patel, issued orders to All India Radio (AIR) not to permit 'those women whose public lives were a public scandal' to enter its studios.

India's ancient civilization, heritage, and culture were to pave the way for a purified present, rescued from the debased tawaif, so that tradition could be recast in the garb of modernity. It was considered important to unite India under a national identity of a spiritual Hindu past derived from Sanskrit roots. The art practices of Indian dance and music created the much needed civilizational lineage. A 1959 issue of *Marg*, on Indian classical dances, begins by qualifying Kathak as etymologically related to *katha* (which is how it is usually introduced now as part of a continuous tradition of male singing minstrels associated with the art of storytelling), going on to connect the dance to several Sanskrit sources including the epic *Mahabharata*. It lays down the textual sources from ancient Sanskrit texts, traces the *gharana* through male lineages, and through the essays codifies and textualizes the technique for an English language audience. In the same volume, Baijnath Mishra separates the nautch dance as a different category from the classical dances.[34]

In the search for a modern self-identity for India by the nationalists, encapsulated in the word 'swaraj', the Muslim heritage is neither claimed nor refuted. Although the Muslim League (established in 1906) gained popularity in the 1930s by using Urdu language and Islam as unifying themes, the founding members of both the Indian National Congress and the All India Muslim League, products of English Victorian education, rejected the tawaif on the grounds of sexual promiscuity.[35] The women had to be refashioned, educated, and reinvented in the spiritual image of the Hindu goddesses Durga, Radha, Sita, and Saraswati.

The Item Girl on Reality TV

Devdutt Pattanaik writes:

> Every time I watch a Bollywood item number, that is increasingly becoming a sought after art form by both aspiring and waning stars, and I watch 'empowered' women displaying their sexuality, objectifying themselves, tantalizing men with their bodies and their flirtatious gaze, challenging them to accept their invitation, I see beyond them the faces of hundreds of smiling devadasis and nautch girls, women well versed in song and dance who were mocked and rejected by puritanical society as 'prostitutes'.[36]

My current research is on television reality shows and the dancers and choreographers of these shows. I focus, among other issues, on this new kind of femininity through dance that is opening up new debates about women's sexuality, authority, and ownership of culture. Based on ethnographic research in Mumbai and Kolkata, among reality show and Bollywood dancers, I explore how a new generation of dancers and choreographers from underprivileged and non-elite backgrounds are claiming new dance identities, that turn the goddess image upside down. Dance reality shows open up new anxieties and debates about desire, consumerism, morality, and sexuality that affect middle-class sensibilities. Much like in an earlier period of nationalist discourse, women's bodies have emerged as central to these contestations, and dance reality shows have become public battlegrounds for young women and their mothers. (Although males are also well represented in the reality-show genre, my focus is only on women here.) Many young women use these shows to claim a new modern identity no longer bounded by the nationalist construction of *bhadramahila* (respectable women) in Bengal. In fact, the nationalist construction of Indian women as repositories of tradition and spiritual identity is being turned on its head by a new generation of women and men in India, who are engaged in redefining femininity (and masculinity) through the dancing of different narratives of the new Indian market democracy. This became particularly evident to me during interactions with the contestants of dance reality shows in dance classes, dancers' homes, coffee shops, and shopping malls.

Once I talked with one of the contestants in her modest living room in a not-so-fashionable part of south Kolkata. She was one of the youngest contestants (who were generally between 18 and 30). In her miniskirt and highlighted hair, she looked at once ambitious, well-groomed, and vulnerable. Her mother came in during our conversation with tea and snacks for me, and because there was an immediate rapport between us, she invited me to lunch. The stories tumbled out from mother and daughter, and I felt both their conflict and angst and their sense of pride and accomplishment. The mother told me in detail that her daughter was a regular participant in dance contests, and that she had won many gold medals. The dance competition on ETV Bangla called 'Dhoom Machale' (which I was researching) was a great opportunity for her daughter to display her talent. But there were conflicts with the choreographer, she said, and both mother and daughter were unhappy about the choice of costumes for the show. Both narrated their embarrassment over a particularly revealing costume that the daughter had once been asked to wear—a problem that had been compounded by the string of the dress snapping during the performance. Another contestant expressed similar sentiments regarding costumes and a general disapproval of her by her university professors for choosing to be part of a commercial television show. During many of my interviews with the contestants and their mothers, I learnt how schools and colleges have been openly hostile towards these students, even going so far as to encourage other classmates to avoid their company. The sexual morality of the contestants of reality shows has been repeatedly scrutinized and questioned by academic authorities in public schools and colleges, and, generally speaking, the contestants and their families have been treated as corrupting influences on the academic environment. In the context of this ongoing social transformation in India, Ruchira Ganguly-Scrase and Timothy Scrase observe:

> The struggle to preserve middle-class culture and identity in the face of great social change highlights the way in which cultural politics is at the core of middle class opposition to neoliberal reforms and, moreover, these cultural struggles take place as much within the relative privacy of the home, as in the public sphere of the street, the workplace or the tea shop. In other words, while neoliberal reforms have inexorably changed social and economic life, their indirect impact through globalised-induced cultural change has also been an affront to middle-class morals, culture, and identity.[37]

Although this is partially true for a section of the middle classes, the personal narratives of these mothers and dancers actively contest these sentiments and clearly recognize the possibility of class mobility in the new economy—attitudes that were repeatedly apparent to me during conversations not just with mothers and contestants, but also with producers, recruiters, and choreographers. All of them routinely expressed the importance of platforms such as 'Dhoom Machale' (or 'Dance Bangla Dance') in providing opportunities to talented young adults who were not from well-connected or rich families. Many contestants and their choreographers even pointed out that the platform had allowed them to launch their dance or acting careers. Many from the small towns and raggedy suburbs saw these shows as an opportunity to realize their dream of buying an apartment in Kolkata or a car. One contestant's mother and grandmother both asserted that the daughter/

granddaughters's life would not follow their own; according to them, the time had arrived for women to pursue their own desires. Others articulated their ambivalence to past codes of morality by explaining that those codes had denied them opportunities.

Conclusion

The unmooring of Indian dance from the past authoritative narrative of classicism has created new debates surrounding cultural authenticity, authority, and middle-class respectability. The popularity of Bollywood in the global circulation of Indian dance has given rise to new genres such as reality shows and new identities of womanhood. The broadening of the dance platform has allowed young women and men to explore new career opportunities by participating in various dance contexts from reality to corporate shows. However, these opportunities have also been seen as exploitative engines of the neo-liberal economy leading to excessive desire and erosion of morality. Thus, dance reality shows and the image of the 'item girl' have opened up new public spaces where heated narratives of gender, class, sexuality, and democracy are brought into debate. Within this chaotic search for an aesthetic modernity, the spectre of the tawaif and her dance has re-emerged as a shadowy figure devoid of history or agency to be appropriated as debauch and full of excessive sexuality. Her contributions to the making of modern Kathak dance and Indian artistic heritage remains largely a footnote.

Notes and References

1. Devdutt Pattanaik, 'The Nautch Girl Strikes Back', *Mid-Day*, 3 November 2013, http://www.mid-day.com/articles/the-nautch-girl-strikes-back/238752, accessed 3 May 2016.
2. On delegitimizing the hereditary female and transgender practitioners of Indian dance, see Anna Morcom, *The Illicit World of Indian Dance: Cultures of Exclusion*, New York: Oxford University Press, 2014.
3. Quoted in Rana S. Zaman, 'Films Need to Take Kathak Out of Brothels', *The Hindu*, 2 May 2015, http://www.thehindu.com/news/cities/Delhi/films-need-to-take-kathak-out-of-brothels/article7163455.ece#comments, accessed 3 May 2016.
4. Anand K. Coomaraswamy, *Dance of Shiva: Fourteen Indian Essays*, revd edn., New York: The Noonday Press, 1957; Kapila Vatsyayan, *Classical Indian Dance in Literature and the Arts*, New Delhi: Sangeet Natak Academy, 1968.
5. Kathryn Hansen, 'The Indar Sabha Phenomenon: Public Theater and Consumption in Greater India (1853–1956)', in *Pleasure and the Nation:*

The History, Politics and Consumption of Public Culture in India, ed. Rachel Dwyer and Christopher Pinney, Oxford: Oxford University Press, 2001, pp. 76–114.

6. Ibid.
7. Margaret E. Walker, *India's Kathak Dance in Historical Perspective*, Surrey: Ashgate Publishing, 2014.
8. Hansen, 'The Indar Sabha Phenomenon', p. 80.
9. Ibid., p. 85.
10. Pallabi Chakravorty, *Bells of Change: Kathak Dance, Women and Modernity in India*, Calcutta: Seagull Press, 2008.
11. There is plenty of academic work on this but seldom does it connect the tawaif to the artistry of Kathak; one exception is Walker, *India's Kathak Dance*, other than my own work, especially see Chakravorty, *Bells of Change*.
12. This is also demonstrated in Chakravorty, *Bells of Change*.
13. Firdous A. Siddiqui, *A Struggle for Identity: Muslim Women in the United Provinces*, New Delhi: Foundation Books (Cambridge University Press), 2014.
14. Ibid., p. 168.
15. Somnath Chakrabarty, *Kolkatar Baiji-Bilash*, Calcutta: Bookland Private Limited, 1991, pp. 140–4; Shramana Das Purkayastha, 'Performance as Protest: Thumri and Tawaif's Quest for Artistic Autonomy', *Rupkatha Journal on Interdisciplinary Studies in Humanities*, vol. 5, no. 2, 2013, pp. 98–106.
16. Siddiqui, *A Struggle for Identity*.
17. Ibid., p. 160.
18. Ibid., p. 163.
19. Ibid., p. 162.
20. Premankur Biswas, 'A Voice from Long Ago: Sashimukhi, not Gauhar Jaan, was the First Indian Voice to be Recorded', *The Indian Express*, 4 August 2015, http://indianexpress.com/article/lifestyle/a-voice-from-long-ago-sashimukhi-not-gauhar-jaan-was-the-first-indian-voice-to-be-recorded/, accessed 4 May 2016.
21. Siddiqui, *A Struggle for Identity*, p. 172.
22. Anindya Banerjee, 'Kolkatar Sangeet e Baijider Abadan' (The Contributions of Baijis in the Music of Kolkata), paper presented at a seminar for a memorial on Kolyan Mitra, Kolkata, 17 June 2015.
23. Scott Kugle, 'Maha Laqa Bai: The Remains of a Courtesan's Dance', in *Dance Matters II*, ed. Pallabi Chakravorty and Nilanjana Gupta, New Delhi: Routledge, forthcoming. Also see Scott Kugle, *When Sun Meets Moon: Gender, Eros, and Ecstasy in Urdu Poetry*, Chapel Hill: University of North Carolina Press, 2016.
24. Quoted by Banerjee, 'Kolkatar Sangeet e Baijider Abadan'.
25. Scott Kugle, 'Mah Laqa Bai and Gender: The Language, Poetry, and Performance of a Courtesan in Hyderabad', *Comparative Studies of South Asia, Africa, and the Middle East*, vol. 30, no. 3, 2010, pp. 365–85.
26. Siddiqui, *A Struggle for Identity*.

27. *Piya bina nahin avat chayn* ('There's no comfort to my heart without my beloved').
28. Vikram Sampath, *My Name is Gauhar Jaan!: The Life and Times of a Musician*, New Delhi: Rupa, p. 62.
29. Quoted in Sampath, *My Name is Gauhar Jaan!*, p. 63.
30. Biswas, 'A Voice from Long Ago'; Amlan Dasgupta, 'Women Recording Artists', paper presented at a seminar on gender and history, University of Calcutta.
31. See Chakravorty, *Bells of Change.*
32. Veena Talwar Oldenburg, 'Lifestyle as Resistance: The Case of the Courtesans of Lucknow', in *Contesting Power: Resistance and Everyday Social Relations in South Asia*, ed. Douglas Haynes and Gyan Prakash, New Delhi: Oxford University Press, 1991; Idem., *The Making of Colonial Lucknow, 1856–1877*, Princeton: Princeton University Press, 1994.
33. Sampath, *My Name is Gauhar Jaan!*, p. 190.
34. Baijnath Mishra, *Marg*, vol. 12, no. 4, 1959.
35. Ibid.
36. Pattanaik, 'The Nautch Girl Strikes Back'.
37. Ruchira Ganguly-Sacrase and Timothy Sacrase, *Globalisation and the Middle Classes in India*, London: Routledge, 2009, p. 152.

4 The Queer Politics of the Raj

ANURIMA BANERJI

We have an Empire, which extends right round the world, and our service may be, and often is, in many queer and uncivilised countries.

—Health Memorandum for British Soldiers in the Tropics

[T]he nineteenth century witnessed a generalization of the deployment of sexuality, starting from a hegemonic center.

—MICHEL FOUCAULT, *The History of Sexuality*

Queer

Strange, odd, peculiar, eccentric. Of questionable character. Suspicious Dubious. A homosexual. Especially, a male homosexual. Perturb. Unsettle. To put out of order.

To queer the pitch: (originally) to interfere with or spoil the business of a street vendor or performer. To question. To spoil (the reputation or chances); to put (a person) out of favour (with another). Bad. Contemptible. Worthless. Untrustworthy. Disreputable. Counterfeit. Forged. Out of sorts. Giddy. To ridicule. Swindle, cheat, puzzle, flummox. Noun, adjective, verb, intensifier. Origins uncertain. Origins unknown.

—*Oxford English Dictionary*[1]

By now, the question of the queer as a theoretical and political category in the South Asian context has been thoroughly unpacked and interrogated by a range of scholars and activists. The queer, as episteme and as palimpsest, has come to be understood as polysemic rather than embodying a singular connotation. Most commonly, it is a unifying identitarian label considered synonymous with lesbian, gay, bisexual, and transgender (LGBT) subjects and collectives.[2] At another level, the queer is enlarged to index identities and practices that are variously 'non-heterosexual', 'non-normative' in terms of gender and sexuality, embraced by those who wish to evade specific labels, remain ambiguous in their public identifications, or cast themselves as dissidents working against the standard sex/gender system.[3] Finally, in its broadest conception, the queer is deployed as a fluid and capacious container for the marginal, the renegade, the imminent, the precarious, the insurgent—signifying all that is anti-normative.[4] In all of its incarnations, the queer has been reclaimed by its subjects from its unceremonious (Western) history as a derogative, shorn of its pejorative status, and transformed into a symbol of defiance and difference.

A related body of scholarship has opened up nuanced and complex meditations on sexuality and postcoloniality, laying bare the political complications and predicaments which arise when queer and South Asian imaginaries collide or intersect.[5] Their scholarship considers queer acts and representations in South Asia while linking them to present-day politics, proffering novel understandings of how queer subjects and communities are produced in the matrix of aesthetic, social, and institutional performances.[6]

Critically, much of the current discourse considers, in dense and intricate ways, the validity of the queer idea for its presumed subjects, and complicates the category itself as a contested terrain. My essay complements these modes of enquiry but through an alternative historical angle: one that seeks to make intelligible the British colonial perspective on 'queerness' in nineteenth-century India—a direction that has yet to be visited in existing studies. I ask: how was the notion of queerness imagined, constructed, and deployed by imperial forces? What were the discursive strategies delineating queerness for the colonial apparatus and its Indian subjects?

This is a project born out of the familiar idea, chronicled by a host of scholars that queerness in India surfaced as an object of social pathology, moral concern, and state regulation (obsession?) during the British Raj.[7] I am especially interested in the ways that the notion of the queer has changed over time, and how its evocations appeared so exuberantly in laws of the nineteenth century—for the law is a space where discourses of queerness are especially evident and salient. Actors who appear to be fragmented into different social and legal classes today might have been once discursively united under the colonial legal frame as bodies marked by abnormal movement. Thus my analysis privileges the meanings of the queer from the standpoint of hegemonic colonial agents and institutions, as expressed in the epigraph opening this chapter, where the queer is in symmetry with the 'uncivilized', and indicates a zone of ungoverned cultural and sexual incongruity, to be reined in by imperial discipline.

In the context of this study, the queer specifically includes an assemblage of gay, lesbian, and bisexual subjects; prostitutes, nautch girls (professional dancers), and devadasis (female Hindu ritual specialists trained in music and dance); and hijras (a 'third gender' community encompassing self-identified eunuchs, intersex, and transgender individuals) once allied to tribal groups in India. What brings these subjects together, from the colonial vantage point, is their communal refusal to conform to the ideal comportments prescribed by imperial logics and laws, and their emblematic engagements with 'aberrant' actions, with 'abnormal' movements. I argue that the colonial officials saw the hijra, the homosexual, and the devadasi as a continuum of bodies composing a single moving space, synthesizing subjects whose forms of mobility were perceived as political menace. Although many of these minoritarian enactments may have been variously considered normal or exemplary in the social milieus in which they took place, they were uniformly positioned as anti-normative performances under the panoramic colonial gaze (see Plate 4.1).

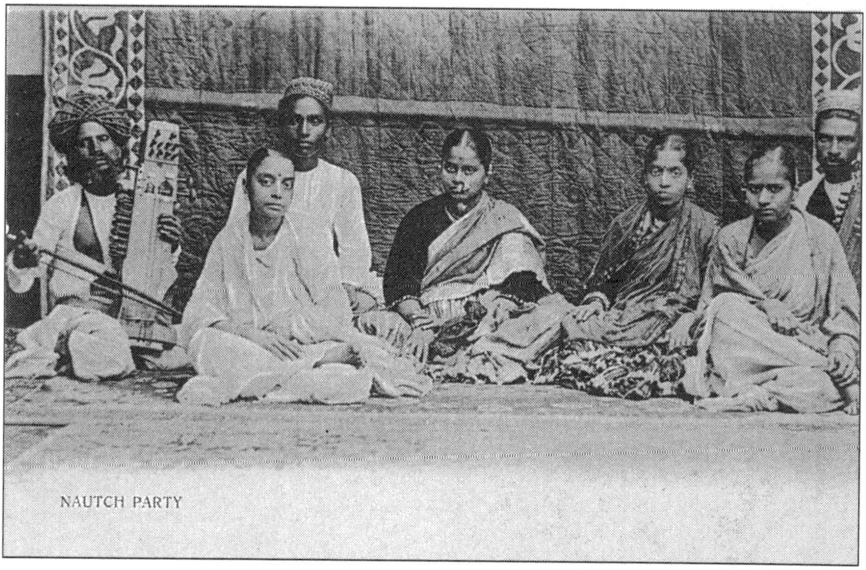

PLATE 4.1 Postcard of a Nautch Party.
Courtesy of Kenneth X. Robbins Collection, Freer Gallery of Art and Arthur M. Sackler Gallery Archives, Smithsonian Institution, Washington, DC: Gift of Kenneth X. Robbins.
Source: Photo courtesy of the Smithsonian Institution, Washington, DC.

I argue that the idea of the queer in India represented a colonial category, intentionally used to stigmatize subjects who were, in the dominant view, sexual deviants and gender outlaws, but also inscribed by such extreme cultural difference that they could not be assimilated into the sphere and machinery of normative colonial thought. So the queer simultaneously signalled sexual perversion and the exotic, the savage, the anomalous.

My analysis focuses on three key laws generated in the post-Mutiny period, after the Crown formally took over the reins of governance from the East India Company in 1858;[8] this was a critical moment, as the salient laws regulating the conduct of hijras, dancers/prostitutes, and 'sodomites' appeared on the books in quick succession as strategies of discursive and cultural domination. I examine here the Criminal Tribes and Eunuchs Act (CTA, 1871), the Contagious Diseases Act (CDA, 1868), and Section 377 of the Indian Penal Code (IPC, 1860), which deals with 'Unnatural Offences'.

I begin with a discussion of the CTA 1871 to suggest that it encapsulates, in a sense, the colonial concerns of the time around the supposed pathologies of indigenous movement (concerns reflected in the texts of the related IPC and CDA), and tethers the figure of the hijra to sodomy and public performance, conceptually linking transgender subjects to homosexuals and dancers. The language of the law thus transparently draws together these three classes, constructing an alibi for this triad to be seen as imbricated positions, as they exist within the purview of the queer.

Let me emphasize one caveat here: nowhere in the text of the laws does the word 'queer' itself appear. However, I want to suggest that the notion of queerness nevertheless haunted the legal texts I am examining, and linked them ideologically while binding together their subjects into an implicitly 'queer' collective. Here I draw from the eminent analyst Akhil Reed Amar's technique of interpreting legal language in relation to its habitus, a position he elaborates in *America's Unwritten Constitution.*[9] Amar exhorts us to consider law in terms of its undeclared supplements, contending that the decipherability of the text depends on the reader's ability to credibly grasp its cultural ambience, the social and ideological space in which the text is located and circulates. Rather than relying on strict originalism, and limiting the universe of the legal statement to the literal written words that articulate it, Amar emphasizes that both the unwritten and intertextual principles undergirding it must be mined and illumined. He evocatively names these symbolic supplements 'blurred peripheries and penumbras' following a famous argument made by Justice William O. Douglas about the US Bill of Rights having 'penumbras . . . formed by emanations' that 'help give them life and substance'.[10] To merge the explicit and the insinuated in this way is to elongate the law's borders of meaning. Taking this route then, of tracing the 'unwritten' in conjunction with the 'written', the textual material and its penumbras, it becomes possible to locate the tacit presence of the queer and all it conjured for imperial authorities in the legal texts showcased here.

Templates of Law

Diverse systems of law predated the imposed British model of legal precepts; Indian law had particularized forms, until the colonial apparatus converted it to a centralized, universalist, and transhistorical doctrine. Prior to colonial intrusion, a mix of formal and informal, customary and written laws, varying across regions, had prevailed in the subcontinent.[11] Pertinently, there are no available records indicating that hijra performance, same-sex relations, and public dancing were contrary to central state regulations.[12] These identities and activities were acknowledged and incorporated into Indian life as auspicious or ambivalent elements, and socially accommodated in line with the general Indian pattern—variously as subjects of cultural respect, neutrality, or censure, depending on the regional and temporal circumstance.[13]

With the arrival of British rule, the legal paradigm changed dramatically. Colonial agents instigated a process of consolidating, codifying, and centralizing a national legal system. These newly instated laws disrupted the cogency of customary practices and imposed legal ideas excavated from English and American codes, ancient Hindu and Muslim texts, and a range of personal laws, enshrining the fixed and single interpretation in place of pre-existing pluralities to aid imperial governance over the heterogeneous populace of the subcontinent.[14] Under this centralized institution, the eunuch (the colonial rendering of hijra), the dancer-prostitute, and the homosexual eventually emerged as criminally marked bodies.

The Criminal Tribes and Eunuchs Act

This Act came into effect with the explicit aim of providing for 'the registration, surveillance and control of certain criminal tribes and eunuchs'.[15] Its overarching purpose was to control those groups who were autonomous and mobile, with 'no fixed residence', and thus had escaped state surveillance, the confines of a colonial mechanism determined to sculpt the native body politic into a position of docility. For those labelled as 'criminal tribes', mobility had meant self-determination and escape from colonial state directives, while for the rulers, mobility translated into evidence of the colonized subject's innate physical and moral instability, a predisposition for subterfuge, an affront to imperial discipline. Thus the law was an attempt to 'fix' these peripatetic subjects—fix their character, and fix them in place.

The task of identifying and designating a group as a criminal tribe was left up to local governments.[16] Descriptions of some of the listed tribes show that they were primarily indigenous and caste-based classes made up of nomads, religious and secular wanderers, forest dwellers, and itinerant performers. The tribes' alleged proximity to 'nature', or *zoe* (bare life)—basically, occupying remote areas that were difficult to police, like jungles, mountains, deserts, and neglected rural areas—paradoxically made them 'unnatural' in terms of their ability to reconcile the rules of *bios*, or politically organized community regulated by the colonial apparatus; their refusal to conform to imperial structures and the derivative moral and social codes gave colonial officials ammunition to dehumanize them (see Plate 4.2).[17]

The tribes' interests and proficiency in certain genres of performance actually caused the authorities to indict them for their carefree movements, and this vision of their chaotic bodily expressions and supposed lack of control over their physical faculties tied up with perceptions of sexual immorality. Because they were seen as innately criminal, caught up in the matrix of cultural and biological determinism, the tribes are tellingly never referred to as communities, but as 'gangs',

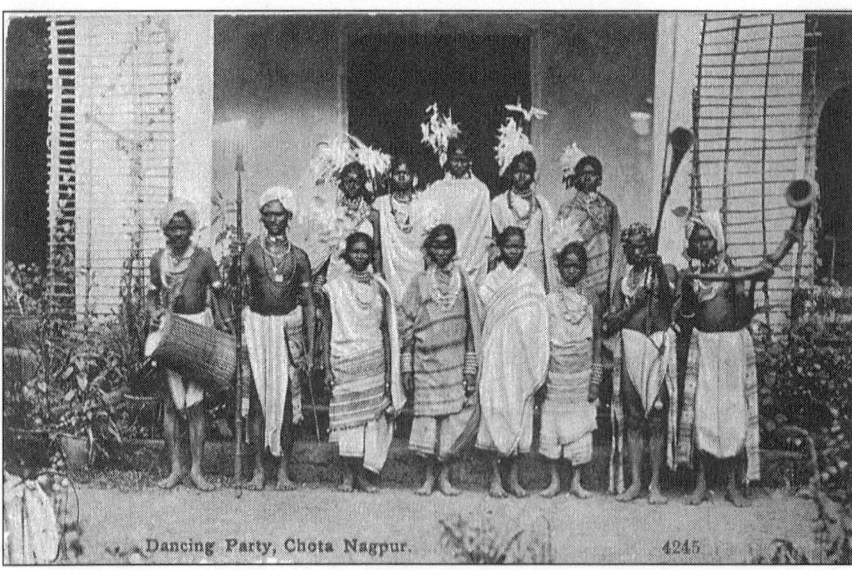

PLATE 4.2: Postcard showing a 'Tribal' Dancing Party from Chota Nagpur. Courtesy of Kenneth X. Robbins Collection, Freer Gallery of Art and Arthur M. Sackler Gallery Archives, Smithsonian Institution, Washington, DC: Gift of Kenneth X. Robbins.
Source: Photo courtesy of the Smithsonian Institution, Washington, DC.

and invariably described as thieves, thuggees (thugs), dacoits (robbers), con artists, beggars, poisoners, killers—a primitive and violent menace, 'savage specimens' outside the realm of the civilization.[18]

Colonial ethnographer E.J. Gunthorpe, for instance, meticulously catalogued what he saw as the deplorable traits of the indigenes in his *Notes on Criminal Tribes* (1882).[19] He speaks of the Hindu Kykarees, for instance, as 'a criminal race well known to the Thuggee and Dacoity Department'.[20] He mentions the Kolhatee tradition where 'a certain proportion of the unmarried females . . . are brought up as dancing-girls and never marry'.[21] And the Kunjurs, 'a well-known wandering, predatory race' of Hindus whose women are 'notorious for their obscene songs accompanied with the most obscene gestures and signs, and also for their grossly abusive language'.[22]

The CTA prescribes that such criminal tribes are to be registered, following which they are to be placed in 'reformatory settlements' and closely supervised in the interest of rehabilitation.[23] The unsettling and unsettled body is thus to be settled through the imposition of corrective colonial manoeuvres. Movement as freedom, movement as chaos: in this condemnation tinted with fascination we find the same tropes and tenor of description as that of the 'noble savage' in the West—with the tribal body prefigured as an object of concurrent romanticization, animalization, and pathologization.

Transgender subjects like hijras, or eunuchs, were similarly treated as adjuncts of criminal tribes in Part II of the same Act, marked by the impression that they shared the same dissembling tendencies and embodied equally irregular, freakish movements. Eunuchs in their very existence were innately destabilizing figures for imperial authorities, for in terms of the dominant gender schema they were 'not this, not that';[24] their physicality and appearance violated colonial propriety (see Plate 4.3). Because of their seeming gender incongruity, their interstitial embodiment, they were regarded as 'criminals, or crime's offspring, since their anatomical disposition, their very being, confounded the law that distinguished the sexes and prescribed their union'.[25]

Notably, the Act qualified eunuchs as 'all persons of the male sex, who admit themselves, or on medical inspection clearly appear, to be impotent'.[26] Thus it is the prospect of the biologically sexed male body in crisis, the loss of phallic reproductive power—'impotence' due to castration, the presence of intersex genitalia, or other medically-ordained abnormalities—that haunted the colonial authors of the text. Further embedded in the Act was the notion that the truth of the body lay in science, extracted through what could only be invasive procedures

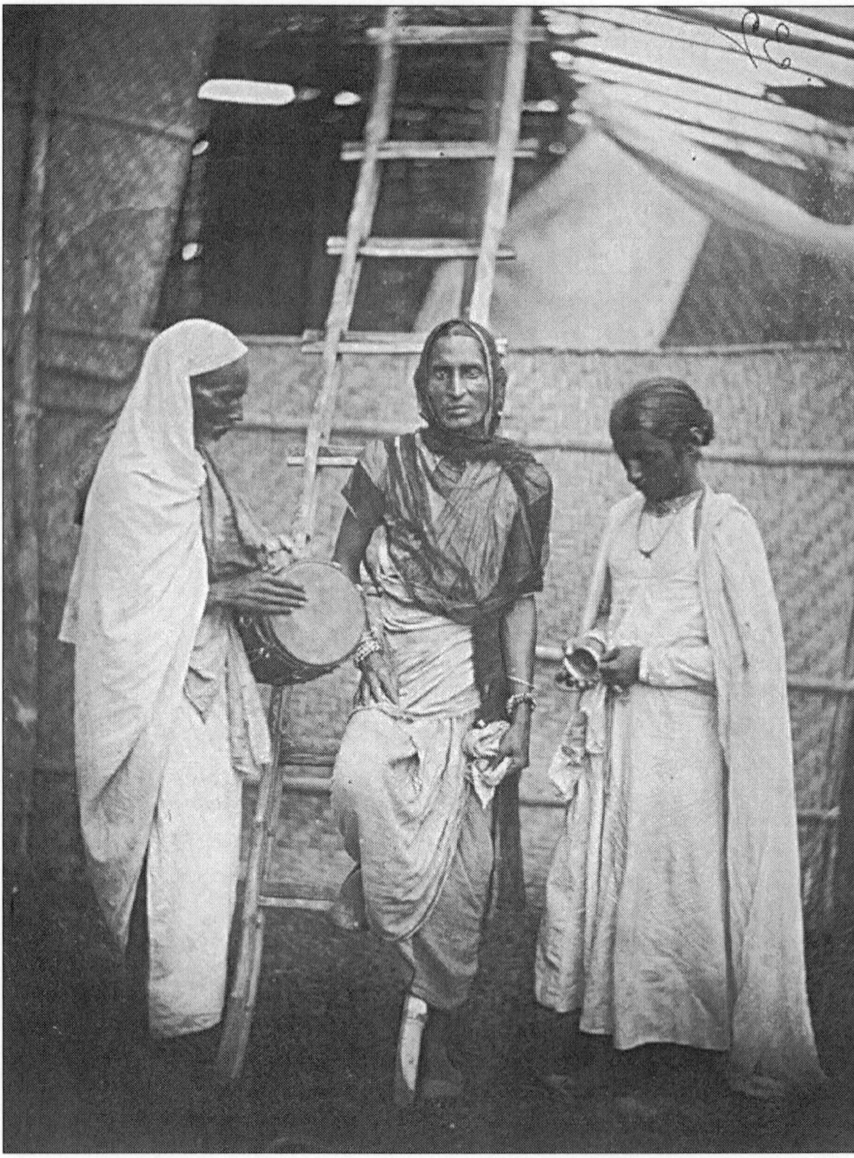

PLATE 4.3: *Portrait of Gurmah, Khunsa, or Hijra*, Reputed Hermaphrodite and Companions, Eastern Bengal. Taken by an unknown photographer in the early 1860s. © The British Library Board, London, Photo 124 (38).
Source: Photo courtesy of the British Library, London.

of verification, exercised by medical authorities to establish the status of the patient's sexual potency or impotence, and thus determine her or his condition as a eunuch.

Under the terms of the Act, the eunuchs' forms of mobility were acknowledged as being different in character from other criminal tribes, though subject to equal restriction. The Act specifically forbade cross-dressing and public performance as punishable violations of the law. It stipulated the following terms:

> 26. Any EUNUCH so registered, who appears, DRESSED or ornamented LIKE A WOMAN, in a public street or place or in any other place, with the intention of being seen from a public street or place,
> or who DANCES or plays music, or takes part in any public exhibition, in a public street or place or for hire in a private house,
> may be arrested without warrant, and shall be punished with imprisonment of two years or with fine, or both.[27]

This legal rhetoric unambiguously highlights three major points: the eunuch is determined to be so by virtue of possessing a male body, rendered impotent—but it is dressing *like* a woman (significantly, not *as* a woman) that crosses the line. The law effectively effaced the self-identification of hijras as transgender agents and as public figures.[28] In other words, if the eunuch had managed to live discreetly and privately, bearing the knowledge of 'his' impotence, s/he would approvingly adhere to colonial codes of sexed modesty. But *appearing* feminine is the truly transgressive act, accompanied by the daring of 'dancing' in particular, 'exhibiting' oneself in general, publicly or privately, whether for personal pleasure or for profit. Assuming a gender position and presentation that refused to correspond to proper 'sex' (in all its senses), at odds with prevailing schemes of thc 'natural' and 'normal', the dancing hijra flamboyantly offended colonial propriety, betraying the rulers' projected sense of Victorian decorum.

Strikingly, dance, rather than representing the summit of grace and cultivation accomplished by a deft and dexterous body, served instead to corroborate native depravity: a lack of reason, an absence of corporeal control, an inherent iniquity. The CTA text intimates that while the bare *presence* of the eunuch body was symptomatic of a generalized illicitness tainting the immediate environs, the *dancing* lifted it into a realm of pure profligacy. (This was as true for the tribal *junglee* as the hijra.) Dance-as-debauchery displaced dance-as-refined-aesthetic in this legal situation. The law thus painted a crooked portrait of tribal and eunuch gestures: Strange. Degraded. Immoral. *Queer.*

Contagious Diseases Act

The ideology of Indian dance as a dishonourable practice, fundamentally bound up with vice, as outlined in the CTA, had a durable prehistory in the form of colonial deliberations on the status of professional performers and ritual specialists like the devadasis (female temple servitors, also called temple dancers), tawaifs (courtesans), entertainers in *kothas* (brothels), and other dance artists (see also Plate 4.4).[29] (And the devadasi nomenclature was itself a collapsing construct that gathered within its folds identities as variegated as the *basavi* and *bhavani* of western India, the *kulavanthalu* and *vilasini* of Andhra Pradesh, the *jogati* of Karnataka, the *mahari* of Odisha, and the *kudikkar* of Kerala, among others.[30]) All of these disparate activities were condensed into the homogenizing 'nautch'[31]—a careless but convenient descriptor for a multitude of choreographic endeavours, synthesized within a solitary frame. The nautch girl, both celebrated and reviled, possessed a talismanic force as the target of imperial allure and antipathy: the spectacle of her seductive but indecent gyrations captivated the colonial gaze. An 1882 *Times of India* article, referring to a series of functions organized in honour of a department colonial official, attests that:

> At one of these, the guests, European and native, sat for hours looking at the lascivious movements of the *nautch*-women and listening to their amatory strains.
> This is the orthodox Hindoo idea of honorific entertainment. Their own ladies are banished to the secrecy of their chambers, while these women of pleasure are brought from the bazaars to occupy the center of the room, while around the walls are seated the grave and reverend signiors who make our laws for us [ironically] and administer them. Hour after hour passes by, dancer succeeds dancer, still the occupants of the couches continue to yield the homage of their presence to these nautch-women. It is a matter of congratulation that the Native Press itself is beginning to give expression to feelings that have been entertained a good while by the educated among them, and is calling for an abandonment of this custom, and the introduction of native ladies into society.[32]

Already tinged with a seductive aura, nautch of all types was readily conflated with prostitution, and the sexual stigma intensified with the introduction of the CDA in 1864. Certainly, in many moments dancing and sex work frequently overlapped, while in others they were strictly separated—though under the aegis of the Act these nuances were principally ignored, and real or imagined prostitutes were subject to its regulations.

The curiously named law came into effect as a consequence of imperial anxieties about the sexual proclivities of British soldiers and the native sepoys. As members of the military lived in close proximity in the barracks over a sustained period of time, they were deemed especially susceptible to the contaminating effects of homosexuality,

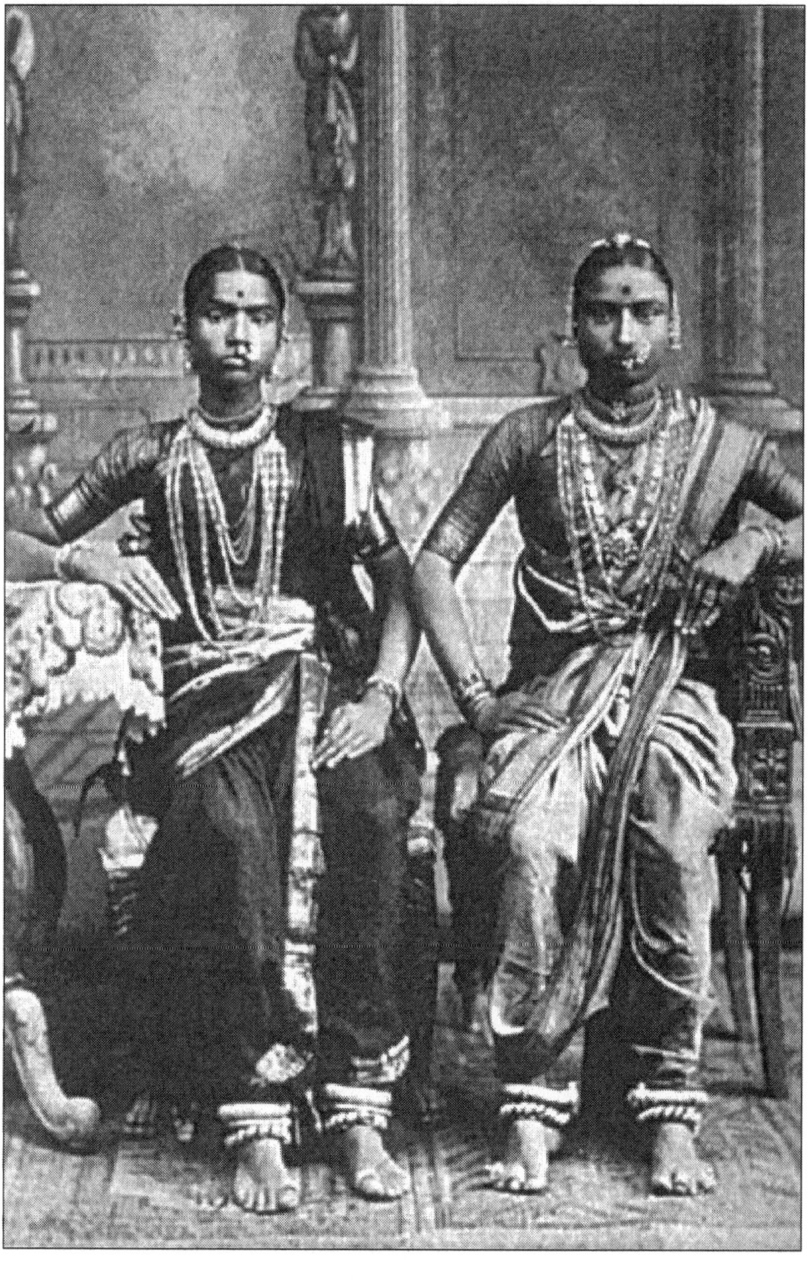

PLATE 4.4: A Photograph of Two Devadasis in Tamil Nadu in the 1920s
Source: https://commons.wikimedia.org/wiki/File:Devadasi_1920s.JPG (accessed 26 July 2016). Public domain image in India.
Photo courtesy of Anurima Banerji.

effeminacy, and venereal disease. Colonial officials harboured strong apprehensions about the effects of these 'disorders' on the military. To promote heterosexual behaviour, discourage same-sex relations, and ostensibly protect them from infirmity, the army allowed soldiers to consort with women who offered them a (paid) sexual outlet—women who may have been prostitutes, dancers, casual lovers, or non-marital partners. (The men often attended nautch parties and visited brothels for the purpose of sexual gratification.) Believing that heterosexual performance augmented patriarchal power, the army sanctioned these relations, but predictably made the women exclusively responsible for ensuring the soldiers' sexual hygiene.

The Indian version of the CDA, patterned on the earlier 1864 Act that took force in England, mandated the setting up of 'Lock Hospitals' in *lal bazaars* (red-light districts) where 'prostitutes' (in the legal code there was no way of distinguishing them from other classes of women) were required to register and submit to an intrusive physical exam, to let doctors and bureaucrats confirm they were free of any debilitating ailments—not for their own welfare, but so they would not run the risk of infecting their male partners, though this aim was obscured by paternalistic rhetoric. The failure or refusal to register at a hospital, notify the authorities upon change of residence, or follow any of the other protocols could result in a woman's arrest:

> XIV. Any WOMAN registered under this Act SHALL, ON RECEIVING NOTICE from any such officer as the local Government shall from time to time appoint in this behalf, PROCEED TO the certified HOSPITAL named in such notice and place herself there for medical treatment.
>
> If after the notice is delivered to her, she neglects or refuses to proceed to the said Hospital within the time specified in the said notice, an offer of Police shall apprehend her and convey her with all practical speed to such Hospital, and place her there for medical treatment.
>
> XV. Whenever any such WOMAN AFFECTED WITH contagions DISEASE places herself or is placed as aforesaid in a certified Hospital for medical treatment, she SHALL BE DETAINED there for that purpose by such medical officer of the Hospital . . . until discharged by him by writing under his hand.
>
> Medical treatment, lodging, clothing, and food shall be provided gratis for every such woman during her detention in the Hospital.[33]

Officially, the women under supervision were given a bill of clean health, or, upon discovery of illness, forced to stay in a certified Lock Hospital on quarantined until they had been treated successfully. The intent of this programme, catalysed by moral panic, was supposedly to prevent the supposedly hapless soldiers from succumbing to the temptations of native women and jeopardizing their health, potentially placing at risk the entire military machine that drove Britain's imperial ambitions.[34]

The women, in turn, deeply resented this whole process and sought to outwit their state tormentors. Veena Oldenburg's fascinating archival research on Lucknow's tawaifs, for instance, unearthed the ways they undermined the colonial fantasy of control through elaborate stratagems devised to circumscribe the strict protocols established by state regulations:

> These new challenges provoked these women to intensify their struggle to keep out an intrusive civic authority that taxed their incomes and inspected their bodies. Characteristically they responded by keeping two sets of books on their income, bribing the local da'i, or nurse, to avoid bodily inspections, bribing local policemen to avoid arrests for selling liquor to the soldiers, or publicly refusing to pay taxes even when threatened with imprisonment.[35]

Sustained feminist agitation in Britain and India led to the law's eventual repeal in 1888.[36] However, it was soon replaced by the 1890 Cantonments Act, which disappointingly introduced similar measures under another guise. It gave the government power to put in place mechanisms for the 'prevention of the spread of infections or contagious disorders within a Cantonment, and the appointment and regulation of hospitals', without specifically attaching such rules to measures for controlling prostitution.[37] Clearly, the new policy undermined the provisions of the CDA's repeal. The report of the committee appointed to examine the rules at play regarding prostitution and the treatment of venereal disease in the Indian army found that despite the formal abolition of the CDA, the 'looser' 1890 regulations were being flouted in at least ten army cantonments and that such practices continued de facto as they were from the time of the CDA's instatement, despite de jure changes. The new rules, the committee noted, 'have in effect been used, if not to set up, at least to assist in maintaining, a system of periodical examination of prostitutes, which is practically compulsory . . . and with the effect practically of licensing those who are pronounced to be physically fit'.[38]

While certain classes of dancers not directly involved in, or 'suspected of', prostitution could have avoided the perils posed by the CDA and its successor, they were still tangled up in a moral discourse that excessively eroticized the nautch and had to confront the quandaries that arose as a consequence of this association, given the broader scrutiny they faced with the heightened legal focus on sexualized female bodies. Perhaps this paranoia surrounding venereal disease, and the apprehension surrounding the putative purity of the soldier—the very agent charged with advancing imperial power—engendered the atmosphere that led to hysteria around the dance (presented as a practice that overlapped with sex work), culminating in the anti-nautch movement, which commenced its campaign in the 1880s and led to the gradual dissolution of temple performance and other types of dance entertainment as legitimate vocations.[39]

In negotiating this blurry line between the permissible and impermissible, women framed and vilified as prostitutes/nautch girls lost a great deal of social prestige, like hijras, and contended with the precipitous decline of their vocation. These were the conditions of imperial life: colonial law enforced its 'normal' rules of conduct, and the women's actions outside these bounds were cast as decidedly 'abnormal', pernicious, and prurient. The rigour and aesthetic of their dance now represented, instead, anarchic and shambolic movement. To the imperial voyeur, the native prostitute and dancer debased themselves and flouted social propriety, perturbing the social and legal order as they participated in a libidinous spectacle of moral disarray, extolling all that was exotic, erotic, and dangerous.[40] *Queer.*

Indian Penal Code

The final group targeted for their queer activities were subjects deemed as sexually perverse for committing 'unnatural offences', listed under Section 377 of the Indian Penal Code as follows:

> OF UNNATURAL OFFENCES.
> 377. Whoever voluntarily has carnal intercourse against the order of nature with any man, woman, or animal, shall be punished with transportation for life, or with imprisonment of either description for a term which may extend to ten years, and shall also be liable to fine.
>
> *Explanation*: Penetration is sufficient to constitute the carnal intercourse necessary to the offence described in this section [emphasis and capitals in original].[41]

The laconic language of the law implicitly assumes a male sexed subject, with its focus on 'penetration'; notably, consent holds no significance at all, and the parties involved could be punished for committing acts 'against the order of nature'; it gravely equates acts of voluntary sex and rape. Curiously, 'penetration' is 'sufficient' as proof of a legal violation, but it would seem to leave open and equivocate on the subject of non-penetrative sex. And although, technically speaking, lesbian activity could have been targeted under these tenets, in actuality the code was applied exclusively to men accused of engaging in bestiality or homosexual acts.[42] This group also included hijras (who, let us recall, were described in the CTA not as intersex or women, but as impotent and thus effeminate biological males who dressed 'like' women)—bringing us back full circle to the discursive and material correlations between transgender performance, dance, sexual deviance, and abnormal movement.

The case of *Queen Empress v. Khairati* (1884) served to corroborate that these dynamics were indeed ideologically intertwined. In that case, an individual named Khairati was tried under Section 377 after being picked up for 'singing in women's clothes among the women of a certain family'—though s/he was not a 'eunuch in the literal sense'—and undergoing a medical exam, the results of which prompted the authorities to suspect s/he was a 'habitual catamite' who had been a 'subject of sodomy'.[43] Khairati escaped conviction, only because there was no substantial evidence pointing to his indulgence in sex with an accomplice, or any witness accounts, and the status of the bodily marks were arguable at best. The required proof of 'penetration' was thus missing. In the aftermath of this verdict, a commentary on this case in *Mayne's Criminal Law* qualified the limits of the Section's applicability:

> A conviction under this section [377] cannot be sustained, when the charge neither stated time nor place, nor pointed to any person with whom the offence was committed, and when the evidence merely proved that the accused went about in woman's clothes, and bore upon his person the physical signs of habitual sodomy. As the Court pointed out, the evidence was at the very least defective in not making out that any offence had been committed within the jurisdiction of the Court.[44]

Despite these legal constraints, the law makes it perfectly clear that both 'going about in women's clothes' and 'sodomy' are morally reprehensible, injudicious, and trespass dominant imperial norms.

Although it tersely targeted the aforementioned 'unnatural offences', in reality only a handful of cases came to court under Section 377 in the Raj era. Anjali Arondekar, in her superb analysis of the law, found just three cases brought up for prosecution before the turn of the twentieth century, observing that 'sodomy in colonial India became naturalized as a frequent phenomenon . . . and yet one sparsely documented in the official archive'.[45] But what the law proscribes often reveals what proliferates in social life, whether as a recurring phenomenon or marginal event—even when the empirical evidence of such performances are unavailable, elusive, missing. This may be because, as Gayatri Gopinath puts it, many queer practices existed under the radar and evaded the imperial 'logics of recognition and visibility'.[46]

However, the IPC was not the first to identify sodomy as a criminal act; a precedent for Section 377 appears to have been embedded in the 1845 Articles of War Act, implemented prior to the Raj at the time of East India Company rule. In that text, Article 32 lists as eligible for punishment '[a]ny Officer who shall behave in a manner unbecoming the character of an Officer', while Article 43 specifically mentions those '[w]ho shall be guilty of any other *disgraceful conduct*, being of a cruel, indecent, or unnatural kind'.[47] Punishment included suspension, fines through garnishing of wages, or dismissal from the service. Article 132 declares that an officer or soldier who is convicted by a general court martial '[o]f an unnatural crime' is guilty of an offence 'punishable by Imprisonment not exceeding 7 years', with or without hard labour.

This 'unnatural crime' is to be understood in context, implicitly indexing homosexuality, as it appears among a list of sexual offences similarly condemned. What is notable here is that a moral equivalence is established between indictments for 'unnatural acts' and acts of 'culpable Homicide not amounting to wilful murder'; arson; rape; kidnapping children; and 'intentionally wounding, maiming, or otherwise doing corporal injury to any person'.[48] Listing sodomy in this spectrum of criminal acts magnified its allegedly inherent perversity. Whether the IPC Section 377 modelled itself or took note of the mention of 'unnatural crimes' in this Act is not fully known, but it seems plausible, given the British preoccupations with native sexualities and the deviant behaviours of the colonized.

While the laws criminalized such 'unnatural' behaviours, the unspoken predicate here was that the commission of such acts necessitated the identification of an 'unnatural subject' at its core. That is, the law presumed the unnatural act itself was not possible without the pre-existence of an aberrant actor—a wilful agent initiating the offence, or abetting it.[49] While this postulate is not declared verbatim in the text, one can infer this on the basis of the colonial dispositifs that generated these laws, which are discussed at length in the 'scientific' discourse on sodomy and homosexuality found in medical, psychological, and sociological literature of the day.[50]

Victorian thought pathologized same-sex relations, since these enactments challenged social roles prescribed according to physiological sex characteristics. The homosexual was constituted as a pervert whose sexual desires were antithetical to the definition of masculinity as necessarily heteronormative. As such, the male 'homosexual' underwent devaluation through feminization, categorized as less than male due to his refusal to establish his masculinity by engaging in intercourse with a biologically proper woman. This medical discourse, added to dominant Christian beliefs in sodomy as a sin, singled out homosexual men for scrutiny and scorn.[51] Those committing 'unnatural acts' were positioned as abject, depraved, iniquitous. *Queer.*

Conclusion

Upon further analysis, we can discern that there was a deeper meaning to queered bodies under the British Raj. For the imperial apparatus saw India as a queer body itself; in this metonymy both were sites of disease, contamination, impurity, abnormality, and forbidden sexuality, and thus the colonizer appropriated the right to dominate the colonized by justifying its intrusions as a political imperative.

The laws examined here expose how the idea of abnormal movement—as embodied by hijras, dancers, and homosexuals—was central to the formation of the 'queer' imaginary and the queer politics of the Raj. Imperial legal doctrines ensconced a set of oppositions identifying the Western colonizer as a guardian of morality and transmitter of civilization, and classified India as a site of primitive savagery. '[T]he distillation of essential ideas about the Orient—its sensuality, its tendency to despotism, its backwardness' served the function of legitimating Western rule, a phenomenon recorded in the systems and institutions of imperial jurisprudence.[52]

The colonial law of this time inscribed a system of formal, centralized norms, replacing the different written and customary practices that had until then reigned in specific regions and communities across the subcontinent. It produced new taxonomies and identities through procedures of signification that had not existed formally prior to the colonial encounter. It imposed a regime of discipline and punishment that was transnational in character, with the Raj bringing legal doctrines rooted in English law to India, which served as an exotic laboratory where an exacting science of punishment was brought from the domain of the civilized to the primitivized. Finally, the law produced new discourses of movement—it sought to regulate or criminalize forms of mobility, the insurgent movements of and between dancing bodies, the bodies of eunuchs and prostitutes, tribal bodies, and gender non-conformists. And though these subjects existed on the peripheries of imperial life, they were discursively centred in imperial legal acts—named only to be excluded. The law had to be invoked with full force for this congregation of volatile bodies to be tamed.

And yet, what is the entity that moves with the greatest force here? It is the law; it arrogates to itself an exceptional capacity for mobility that supersedes the combined force of the dancing body, the hijra body, the sexually perverse body, bodies committing unnatural acts. Colonial law thus appears as one such exemplar of a moving space—an instrument that seizes authority over foreign territory, and over the subjects which make up its populace. It claims for itself the right to movement across borders, to encroach upon and occupy the terrain of the colonized, the terrain of difference, to articulate the power of the norm, announce its ability to insinuate itself in the practice of everyday life. The bodies of the colonized and criminalized were, thus, not the only ones to produce a 'moving space' through their (purportedly) renegade actions; the law as a mobile space sought to capture within its realm and jurisdiction those bodies performing aberrantly in a bid to exert over them the normative principles of colonial command. This legal complex gathered together, on arbitrary grounds, a variety of deviant subjects configured as 'queer', all targeted for traversing the colonial landscape against imperial dictate, for moving abnormally in their bodies, for their unruly choreographies of desire and self.

Notes and References

1. These Oxford English Dictionary (OED) entries include meanings of the word 'queer' from its first appearance in 1390 to the end of the nineteenth century.
2. Judith Butler, *Bodies That Matter: On the Discursive Limits of 'Sex'*, New York: Routledge, 1993.
3. Gayle Rubin, 'Thinking Sex: Notes for a Radical Theory for the Politics of Sexuality', in *Pleasure and Danger: Exploring Female Sexuality*, ed. Carole Vance, Boston: Routledge, 1984, pp. 267–319.
4. Elizabeth Grosz, 'Experiments in Desire: Bodies and Pleasures in Queer Theory', Keynote address, Queer Studies Conference, Toronto, May 1993; see also Robin Wiegman and Elizabeth A. Wilson, eds., *Differences: A Journal of Feminist Cultural Studies*, Queer Theory without Antinormativity Special Issue, vol. 26, no. 1, May 2015.
5. See Gayatri Gopinath, *Impossible Desires: Queer Diasporas and South Asian Public Cultures*, Durham: Duke University Press, 2005; Ruth Vanita, ed., *Queering India: Same-Sex Love and Eroticism in Indian Culture and Society*, New York: Routledge, 2002; Ruth Vanita and Saleem Kidwai, eds., *Same Sex Love in India: Readings from Literature and History*, New York: St. Martin's Press, 2000.
6. See, for instance, Naisargi N. Dave, *Queer Activism in India: A Story in the Anthropology of Ethics*, Durham: Duke University Press, 2012; Geeta Patel, *Lyrical Movements, Historical Hauntings: On Gender, Colonialism, and Desire in Miraji's Urdu Poetry*, Stanford: Stanford University Press, 2002; Rakesh Ratti, ed., *A Lotus of Another Colour*, Boston: Alyson Publications, 1993; Gayatri Reddy, *With Respect to Sex: Negotiating Hijra Identity in South India*, Chicago: University of Chicago Press, 2005.
7. On this history, see especially AIDS Bhedbav Virodhi Andolan (ABVA), *Less than Gay: A Citizen's Report on the Status of Homosexuality in India*, New Delhi: Prince Offset, 1991; Anjali Arondekar, *For the Record: On Sexuality and the Colonial Archive in India*, Durham: Duke University Press, 2009; Suparna Bhaskaran, *Made in India: Decolonizations, Queer Sexualities, Trans/National Projects*, New York: Palgrave Macmillan, 2004. See also Laurence W. Preston, 'A Right to Exist: Eunuchs and the State in Nineteenth-

Century India', *Modern Asian Studies*, vol. 21, no. 2, 1987, pp. 371–87; Supreme Court of India, *National Legal Services Authority v. Union of India and Others*, Opinion by K.S. Radhakrishnan and A.K. Sikrii, 15 April 2014, http://indiankanoon.org/doc/169908548/, accessed 7 May 2016.

8. British colonial rule in India can be divided into two parts: the Company period, which refers to the presence of the East India Company in the country as traders from 1608 and as rulers from 1757 (following their win at the Battle of Plassey); and the Crown period, known as the British Raj, which lasted from 1858 to 1947. See *Imperial Gazetteer of India, volume IV*, Oxford: Oxford University Press, 1909, p. 5.
9. Akhil Reed Amar, *America's Unwritten Constitution: The Precedents and Principles We Live By*, New York: Basic Books, 2012.
10. Ibid., chapter 6; Justice William Douglas, *Griswold v. Connecticut*, 1965, US Supreme Court Opinion, https://www.law.cornell.edu/supremecourt/text/381/479, accessed 4 August 2016.
11. Janaki Nair, *Women and Law in Colonial India: A Social History*, New Delhi: Kali for Women Press, 1996.
12. Vanita and Kidwai, *Same Sex Love in India*, p. 113.
13. ABVA, *Less than Gay*; see also Manil Suri, 'How to be Gay and Indian', *Granta*, 25 June 2013, http://granta.com/how-to-be-gay-and-indian/, accessed 4 August 2016.
14. Bhaskaran, *Made in India*.
15. CTA preamble; see Andrew Lyon, 'Contagious Diseases Act No. XIV of 1868 and Criminal Tribes Act No. XXVII of 1871', in *Law of India, Vol. II: Miscellaneous Laws*, Bombay: Thacker, Vining & Co., 1873, pp. 194–200, 208–15.
16. CTA Part 1, in Lyon, *Law of India*, pp. 2–6.
17. Giorgio Agamben, *Homo Sacer: Sovereign Power and Bare Life*, tr. Daniel Heller-Roazen (from Italian), Palo Alto: Stanford University Press, 1998; Subir Rana, 'Nomadism, Ambulation and the "Empire": Contextualising the Criminal Tribes Act XXVII of 1871', *Transcience*, vol. 2, no. 2, 2011, pp. 1–22.
18. Shoshee Chunder Dutt, *The Wild Tribes of India*, London: T. De La Rue and Co., 1882, especially p. xiii.
19. E.J. Gunthorpe, *Notes on Criminal Tribes Residing in or Frequenting the Bombay, Berar and Central Provinces*, Bombay: Times of India, 1882.
20. Ibid., p. 53.
21. Ibid., p. 49.
22. Ibid., p. 80.
23. CTA 1871, Part I, No. 13, in Lyon, *Law of India*.
24. Vinay Lal, 'Not This, Not That: The Hijras of India and the Cultural Politics of Sexuality', *Social Text*, vol. 61, 1999, pp. 119–40.
25. Michel Foucault, *The History of Sexuality*, tr. Robert Hurley, vol. I, New York: Random House, 1990.
26. CTA 1871, Part II, No. 24 [b], in Lyon, *Law of India*.

27. CTA 1871, in Lyon, 'Contagious Diseases Act No. XIV of 1868', p. 214; capitals in original.
28. According to their self-definitions, the hijra category includes intersex peoples born with ambiguous genitalia, castrated eunuchs, transvestites, and those who express identification with the opposite gender but do not undergo castration (if biologically male). See Serena Nanda, 'The Third Gender', *Manushi*, no. 72, 1992, pp. 9–16; Nanda, *Neither Man nor Woman: Hijras of India*, 2nd edn., Belmont: Wadsworth Publishing, 1999.
29. Kay Jordan, *From Sacred Servant to Profane Prostitute: A History of the Changing Legal Status of the Devadasis in India, 1857–1947*, New Delhi: Manohar, 2003; Kunal M. Parker, 'A Corporation of Superior Prostitutes: Anglo-Indian Legal Conceptions of Temple Dancing Girls, 1800–1914', *Modern Asian Studies*, vol. 32, no. 3, 1998, pp. 559–633.
30. Davesh Soneji, *Unfinished Gestures: Devadasis, Memory, and Modernity in South India*, Oxford: Oxford University Press, 2012, pp. 6–12.
31. An anglicization of *naach*, a colloquial Indian word for dance.
32. *Times of India*, 'The Nautch', 21 August 1882, p. 3; capitals in original.
33. CDA, 1868, in Lyon, 'Contagious Diseases Act No. XIV of 1868', p. 197.
34. Sumanta Banerjee, *Dangerous Outcast: The Prostitute in Nineteenth-Century Bengal*, Calcutta: Seagull Books, 1998.
35. Veena Talwar Oldenburg, 'Lifestyle as Resistance: The Case of the Courtesans of Lucknow', *Feminist Studies*, vol. 16, no. 2, 1990, pp. 260–1.
36. Josephine Butler, *The Constitution Violated: An Essay*, Edinburgh: Edmonston and Douglas, 1871; Philippa Levine, *Prostitution, Race and Politics: Policing Venereal Disease in the British Empire*, London: Routledge, 2003.
37. Government of India Legislative Department, 'Cantonments Act, 1889', in *The Unrepealed General Acts of the Governor General in Council, 1885–1890*, vol. V, 2nd edn., Calcutta: Office of the Superintendent of Government Printing, 1898, p. 333.
38. Secretary of State for India, *Report of the Committee Appointed by the Secretary of State for India to Inquire into the Rules, Regulations, and Practice in the Indian Cantonments and Elsewhere in India, with Regard to Prostitution and to the Treatment of Venereal Disease*, London: H.M. Stationery Office, 1893, p. xxv.
39. Soneji, *Unfinished Gestures*. See also Amrit Srinivasan, 'Reform and Revival: The Devadasi and Her Dance', *Economic and Political Weekly*, vol. 20, no. 44, 2 November 1985, pp. 1869–76; Frédérique Apffel Marglin, *Wives of the God-King: The Rituals of the Devadasis of Puri*, Oxford: Oxford University Press, 1985; Margaret E. Walker, *India's Kathak Dance in Historical Perspective*, New York: Routledge, 2016.
40. Yasmin Jiwani, 'The Exotic, the Erotic, and the Dangerous: South Asian Women in Popular Film, A Colonial Legacy', *Canadian Woman Studies*, vol. 13, no. 1, Fall 1992, pp. 42–6.
41. In John D. Mayne, 'Unnatural Offences', in *Mayne's Criminal Law of India*, 3rd edn., Ch. XVI, Madras: Higginbotham and Co., 1904, p. 177.
42. Significantly, lesbianism was not explicitly mentioned in the Indian Penal Code as the law was primarily aimed at suppressing gay male sex. ABVA,

Less than Gay. Though the terms of Section 377 could theoretically have been extended to cover, at least implicitly, lesbian sex acts, historically there is no evidence that it was used for this purpose in the Raj era. As many scholars have pointed out, lesbians were rendered invisible for the most part under imperial law. This was congruent with the misrecognition and suppression of native female desire prevalent at the time Levine, *Prostitution, Race and Politics*.

43. Arondekar, *For the Record*, p. 68.
44. *Reg. v. Khairati*, 6 All, 204, quoted in Mayne, 'Unnatural Offences', p. 177.
45. Arondekar, *For the Record*, p. 10. Arondekar reveals the following cases were brought to court: *Queen Empress v. Naiada* (Allahabad High Court, 1875–8), *Jiwan v. Empress* (Punjab High Court, 1884), *Queen Empress v. Khairati* (Allahabad High Court, 1884).
46. Gopinath, *Impossible Desires*, p. 16.
47. Legislative Council Calcutta, Act No. XX of 1845, Articles of War, issued 16 September, in *Bombay Times and Journal of Commerce*, Part I, 18 October, p. 687, and Part II, 22 October, p. 695, Calcutta: Fort William, Home Department, 1845; emphasis in original.
48. See Articles 124, 126, 131, 133, 135 in ibid.
49. Foucault, *The History of Sexuality*, vol. I.
50. See, for instance, Isidore Bernadette Lyon and Laurence Waddell, *Medical Jurisprudence for India: With Illustrative Cases*, 3rd edn., Calcutta: Thacker, Spink, & Co., 1904; Carl Westphal, 'Contrary Sexual Feeling', *Archiv für Psychiatrie und Nervenkrankeiten*, vol. 2, 1870, http://www.well.com/~aquarius/westphal.htm, accessed 10 May 2016.
51. ABVA, *Less than Gay*.
52. Edward Said, *Orientalism*, New York: Random House, 1978, p. 204.

PART II

Framed in Spaces: Presence and Representation

5 Performance Sites/Sights

Framing the Women Dancers

URMIMALA SARKAR MUNSI

Introduction

From everyday movement practices to specific dance-related movement activities, bodies occupy, use and create space—and this *spacialization* is deeply gendered due to the multiple social, political and economic influences that construct the logic of occupation of a space by a certain body, in a given time. Such *spacialities* are constructed both by being in the space and by being viewed as an occupant of the space. Dance sculptures, of mortals as well as gods and goddesses on temple walls, and the evidence of extensive presence of dance and dancing bodies in Indian culture from the second century BC have created a spatial association for dancers that has given them a coveted space in the constructed image of independent India. As much as this association was a historical one, it was highlighted to project a certain cultural capital for the independent country by its nationalist leaders. Dancers therefore received privileged treatment compared to other performers, which included a lot of incentives, and also moulded many of them towards uncontested and unquestioning acceptance of the regulatory structures of the authorities who often fixed the space, time and occasion for the dancers to put their art on display.

Dancers, especially women dancers, occupy spaces like prominent prosceniums, specially constructed performance arenas during state ceremonies, festival events, Indian historical, cultural and tourism websites, national advertisements campaigns like 'God's Own Country', 'Incredible India', 'India Shining', and so on. All these spaces are created to allow a certain way of viewing the dancer and her art. Patricia Uberoi writes: 'In many of the genres of representation, however, women are not only visible, they are prominent objects of attention—even of admiration and worship—and one can hardly complain of their invisibility and neglect.'[1] She also goes on to say that it is the correct or incorrect ways of viewing in such spaces that become an important point in the critique of the process, because of the 'social constraining nature of the stereotypical imagery'.[2]

The concept of the marginal space accorded to the female dancer, the extension of such a space to encompass various 'other' marginal cultures differently acknowledged and put on show by the nation state vis-à-vis the Indian state, as well as the inhabiting process by the subjects concerned, are the key threads in this chapter.

In most cases such allotment of rights to inhabit a space in a certain manner is accepted by the citizen subject simply because of the socialization processes that reaffirm, time and again, society's dominant ideologies and beliefs, along with kinship ties and patronage networks within civil society, that have hardwired a citizen subject's idea of 'rights'. Classical dance and its status as a 'high art' is an ideal example of this conundrum—driven, guided and controlled by a stereotype for the aesthetic, the presentation and the expectation, carefully constructed as part of the nation-building process since the nineteenth century. Women dancers play an active role in the perpetuation of that stereotype, often unconsciously, by carrying out the role of cultural agent, throughout and also after their active career.

How does one approach the conceptual frame of 'space' of the woman dancer in relation to her dance? Is it the physical space where the performance takes place? Is it the space that the performance creates in the minds of the audience? Or is it actually the metaphysical idea of the space that is created by the interaction of the values and normative understanding that a performative practice and its practitioner acquire over a certain historical time?

According to Partha Chatterjee, the nationalist response to the colonial condemnation of the treatment of women in India 'was to construct a reformed tradition and defend it on the grounds of modernity. In the process, it created the image of a new woman who was superior to Western women, traditional Indian women and low class women. This new patriarchy invested women with the dubious honor of representing a distinctively modern national culture.'[3] These categories were clearly visible and followed in the realm of dance, where the classical dances became sanctified to be a high form of cultural practice, permitted and appreciated as a learned skill for urban middle- and upper-class women. As a result of the segregation of 'other' practices and the simultaneous emergence of classical dances like Bharatanatyam,[4] Kathak[5] and others, it was mostly the ritual and social dances amongst rural communities (like specific tribes or caste groups) which automatically became the inferior categories, according to the rules of hierarchization of the state agencies.

Dealing with the specific issue of hierarchization, Roma Chatterji has raised an important question with regard to the value and authority of 'the folk arts', asking: 'What are the classificatory schemes within which they come to be recognized to be as having artistic value?'[6] The common practice of categorization that this question refers to is the way in which the folk/classical binary structures exist and continue to justify the space accorded to the practitioners in the respective categories—consciously feeding into the 'social imaginaries'[7] of the larger and universal 'national' vis-à-vis the more specific, multiple 'locals' being principally varied in character and function.

In this chapter I try to establish a connection between the visibility granted to each of the categories created through such hierarchization as mentioned previously by the allotment of specific spaces (and therefore type of audience) to the dances in India today. In my opinion, such specific visibilities result in the formation and continuation of the spaces that the women dancers find themselves occupying. I focus on three different kinds of performance venues and occasions—each a part of the 'embodied practices of the state' and larger than life in terms of its reference to history/memory/spectacle/identity. The chosen representative performances are intentionally situated in spaces with specific references to a particular set of histories and memories, establishing the links between the performance, the space, and a temporal legitimacy. These three spaces are: (1) the much advertised spaces of numerous temple festivals, organized by the Government of India; (2) the Republic Day Parade, organized in New Delhi as the spectacular space for performing one's national identity and citizenship; and (3) the cultural evenings at popular tourist sites and local festivals, organized by respective state governments.

Through the classical genres of dance in India, the 'national culture' is given its identity by bringing together several diverse styles and referring to their significance in terms of the oneness of the Indian nation. Thus the spaces for the performances of such dance presentations are chosen with diligence; they must accord respect to the high cultural capital as also the efficacious history of the said dance 'traditions'. More often than not this respect is intertwined with the religious canon associated with a particular 'classical' dance form. The reference that these dance performances seem to need is a connection with key words like 'history', 'tradition', and 'national culture'.

Such a hierarchically supreme position allocated to the classical dances needs to be seen in contrast to all the regional forms of less fortunate dances that then get categorized as 'folk' or 'ritual' forms. The spaces accorded to these 'other' regional forms become appropriated in a very different fashion in the same agenda of exclusivity and exclusionary practices of the state, where these performances of lesser stature are presented by the nationalist project—in sites specifically designed for larger audiences as spectacles of exotic community/'folk' culture. To just name a few as examples, the dance forms such as Chhau and other mask dances from different parts of India, Tera Taali and Kalbeliya from Rajasthan, Bhangra from Punjab, the drumming traditions of Manipur and Kerala, and the 'exotic' dances of the Nagas are all used as tools to reinforce the belief in the concept of 'unity in diversity' and the undeniable authority and control of the state since independence, on occasions such as the Republic Day Parades, Independence Day Celebrations, opening and closing ceremonies of Commonwealth games, and similar grand, and often spectacular, events.

Another space for the organized display of exotic and unfamiliar cultural traditions is the tourist circuit, where the act of 'gazing' at the 'other' is becoming increasingly popular and is legitimized within the rubric of the current emphasis on global traffic which translates into capital gains for the state and the region. While such displays for tourists may be defended and read as cultural tourism on one hand, the free rein given to private entrepreneurs and local agents in many cases signifies extreme exploitation of women and children on the other.

The agency, awareness, intentionality, and ability to control the dancers' engagements with such spaces are in no way comparable in the three aforementioned sites and sights. While the woman dancer invited to perform at temple festivals by the Ministry of Culture of the Government of India treats such inclusions as trophies, for the nameless woman dancer participating in an Independence Day celebration to honour some dignitaries this may be just one exciting day in a life of drudgery. For the women and children roaming the dunes of the Thar Desert in Rajasthan, performing for tourists and earning on a daily-wage basis, this is an occupation, a means of survival. Hence, each case needs to be discussed separately, against the conceptualization of their significance in relation to the changing context in a global economy (commodification of spaces and bodies), frames of reference (historical/social/political/economic) in postcolonial shifts and their influence on reception (through feminist/ethnographic lenses).

It is extremely important to first locate these performance spaces within the gender discourse. In terms of the dancer's agency in post-independence India, many of the so-called 'modern' performance spaces are hegemonic and arguably masculine in nature. In my opinion these spaces make a show of their control over the dancer's art, communication, and rights by directly establishing the voice of control and of regulation.

Embedding Dance: Sculptural Scenography

The subsuming of the woman dancer within historical sites/sights has been one of the strategies of showcasing Indian heritage. As Anthony Jackson and Jenny Kidd write:

> Visits to the museums and heritage sites have in recent years become (not least in promotional rhetoric) less about the *object* and more about the *experience*: an 'encounter' with the past that is 'brought to life', peppered with the 'events; and advertised through the list of 'What's On'. The increased use of performance has been seen perfectly to exemplify this trend, rendering it subject to criticisms of 'Disneyfication' and 'edutainment'.[8]

The Incredible India website[9] provides lists (and some information) for prominent festivals according to the month. For the Mamallapuram Dance Festival, Tamil Nadu, it says: 'Once the ancient port of the Pallavas, Mamallapuram plays host to a vibrant festival of dance in January/February every year. Exponents of classical dance forms such as Bharat Natyam, Kuchipudi, Kathak and Kathakali from across the country perform against the magnificent backdrop of the Pallava Rock Sculpture along the sea shore.'[10]

The historically implicated sculptural narrative that is commonly given in such festivals as Mamallapuram, Khajuraho or Konark is as important, or even more important, than the content of a particular dance presentation therein (see Plate 5.1). The narrative establishes history and tradition as the principle lens through which to view the site as well as the sight(s), and creates a backdrop almost as an introduction as well as a logic for all that is to be viewed at this site. This narrative, woven with the help of sculpted dance figures, is already there when the dancer enters the space, as the overarching reference and stays on after the dancer finishes her presentation. The timeless and unspecified historical reference takes away the edges of specific rulers' power/time/religion, etc., and creates a presence of an intangible structure of an absent yet powerful patron, who has immortalized his patronage on stone and, therefore, allowed dance and the dancer a space in history and ever after.

This space already needs the dancer to fit in, and becomes even more hegemonic with the reinforcement of the strictures imposed by the modern state in terms of the particular reference to the thematic of the festival. This space also presupposes a reception and fixes the

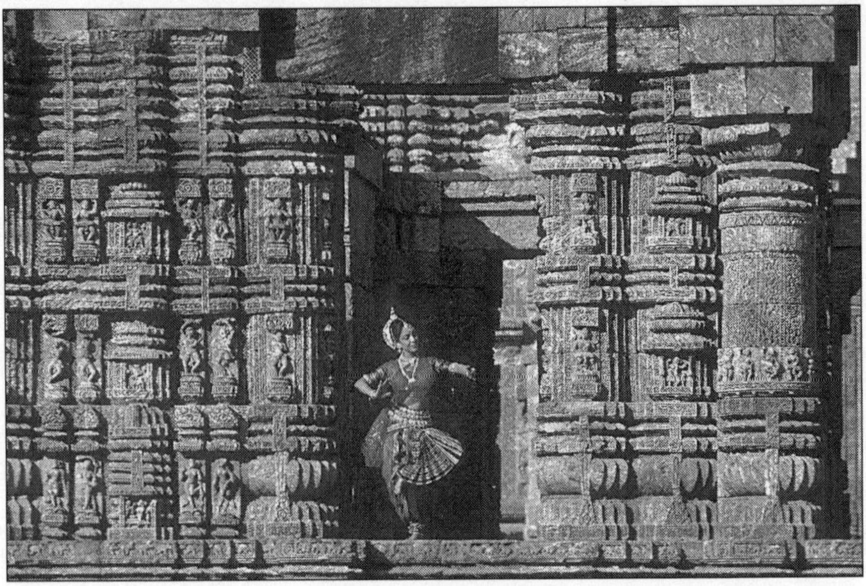

PLATE 5.1: Madhavi Mudgal at Konark Sun Temple, Odisha.
Source: Photo courtesy of Avinash Pasricha.

nature of the gaze that the performance receives. Also important is to note the need to create an aesthetic legitimacy for the female dancer's presence in the public gaze. In this space, even today, the ideal Indian is responsible for carrying forward the tradition and passing it on to the next generation, rather than being invested with the power of changing it. The audience is programmed to be transported to the world of references of continuity of tradition, and reaffirmation of a script being retold while the authority and authenticity of representation in such sites is claimed as by the state's signature and presentation of the event.

Partha Chatterjee, while writing 'The Nation and its Women', mentions 'the new patriarchy' advocated by nationalism, where he says this patriarchy 'conferred upon women the honor of a new social responsibility'.[11] He sees the idea of emancipation of women being associated with the historical goal of sovereign nationhood as the reason behind the creation of a new form of legitimized subordination.[12]

> It served to emphasize with all the force of inspiration, what had in any case become a dominant characteristic of femininity in the new construct of 'woman' standing as a sign of the 'nation', namely, the spiritual qualification of self-sacrifice, benevolence, devotion, religiosity and so on. This spirituality did not, as we have seen, impede the chances of the woman moving out of the physical confines of the home; on the contrary, it facilitated it, making it possible for her to go into the world under conditions that it would not threaten her femininity.[13]

It is this question of Chatterjee's idea of 'going out in the world' that links to my question of space in this present context. For staging a performance of a so-called classical dance, the regularized format contains a reference to the space of origin as the sense of belonging, giving both the dance and the dancer a right to be a part of a version of the nation-state version of history. Hence, classical forms like Bharatanatyam or Odissi have made it a rule to have some format of reference, like an idol, on stage. This, in my opinion, was a way out of the uneasiness that even the dancer herself could not get out of while placing herself in a distinctly public space and in front of the public gaze. My argument is that even when the 'state apparatus' plans a festival, in the current times, the logic behind the use of the material space of the archaeological sites as festival venues lies in the wish to draw out the metaphorical references of these spaces where 'the feminine subject'[14] becomes redefined.

The spaces of the numerous temple festivals organized by the Ministry of Culture and/or Ministry of Tourism, Government of India, reiterate time and again the connections between the disciplined bodies within tradition and the '(willing) obedience coming from inside'[15] the dancer. Here the important notion is the sense of self-discipline generated within the dance community as the model behaviour of the ideal citizen, where the importance of appearing as the image constructed by the state becomes an uncontested given, if one has to belong to the government organized festival circuit. This aesthetic imagination becomes reaffirmed by the constructed historical projection of the space, in which 'the design of the environment is a crucial aspect of a heritage setting because it is utilized not only by performers but also by the visitors themselves'.[16]

Spaces Celebrating Nationhood: Republic Day Parade as a Case Study

The Republic Day Parade—a spectacular space for the nation to showcase its military and cultural might—has emerged as the space for showcasing the ideal state. It further showcases the governed, willing, and obedient citizenry within the masculinity of spectacle as a projection of a certain carefully curated identity of the nation.

In her biography, *Afloat on a Lotus Leaf*, Kapila Vatsyayan's conversation with Jawaharlal Nehru (during her meeting with him before the first Republic Day Parade planning started) is quoted. The biographer, Jyoti Sabharwal, writes: 'On meeting her [Vatsyayan] he said, "Soon, we're going to have our first Republic Day Parade. Don't you think it would be a good idea to have floats on the cultural history of India? Also find out more about the dances and the people of the remote regions of India".'[17]

The parade prioritizes the display of India's army, navy and air force personnel in their finery, along with a moving exhibition of war weaponry, vehicles, ships, aircraft, and even service like dogs, camels, horses, and elephants (see Plate 5.2). Noteworthy are the military bands, constructed very much in continuation of the British tradition, interspersed between the marching groups of military personnel. The audience is used to the overwhelming number of male participants in the Parade, as female contingents are a comparatively new addition and only in last few years are they showcased with pride and as a sign of recent gender-inclusivity in the military services.

Building upon the ideas of aggressive performance of the nation, with the projection of a 'pan Indian cultural reality'[18] framing the social, cultural and political identity, the birthday of the Republic as the 'motherland' is celebrated on 26 January. In addition to the military display, a spectacular performance of inclusivity and obedience, both of the states and the citizens, is used to complete the picture. The ever-present idea of a Hindu motherland, of course, forms the central rhetoric.

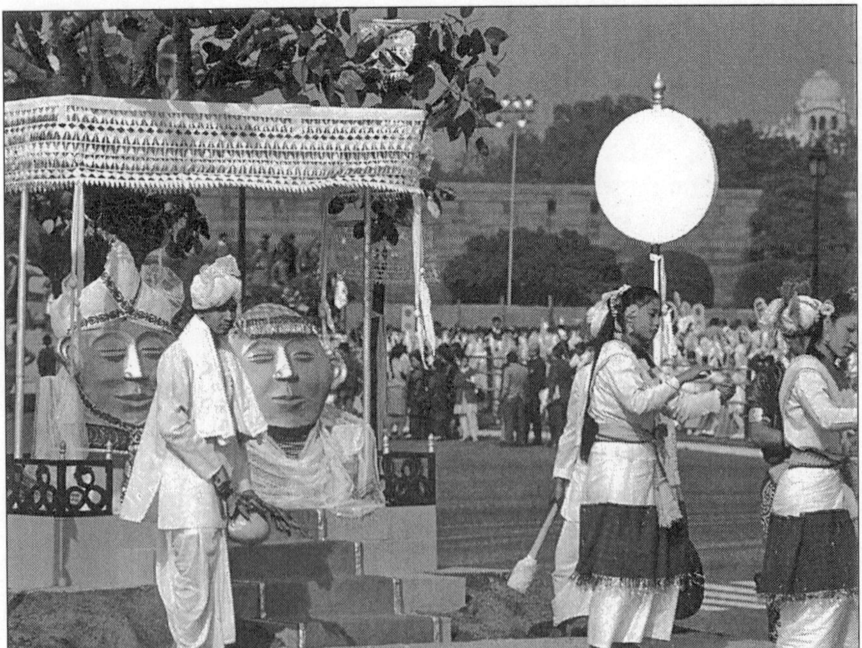

PLATE 5.2: Manipur Tableaux at Republic Day Parade, 2009.
Source: Photo courtesy of Avinash Pasricha.

Such sites are mostly curated ones. In the specific case of the Republic Day Parade, the venue is Rajpath (meaning 'King's Way)[19] chosen specifically for its strategic position,[20] at the historic location of India Gate near the office and residence of the President of India (Rashtrapati Bhavan) and all the principle offices of the Government of India. This site is one of the most beautifully curated spaces for showcasing all that Delhi stands for and, therefore, all the more significant for the spectacular showcasing of the nation's cultural and political power. This single and unified vision of the country, in all its strength framed by the simultaneous references to its history of valour and culture encourages both visitors and audiences to meaningfully decipher what they see according to their own frames of reference. Hence, Royona Mitra views such a site as an 'agent of interpretation'.[21] Taking off from here I would like to build my argument on the construction and interpretation of hierarchized citizen subjects, among whom the principle and visible hierarchies arise out of class, caste, and gender.

The legitimization of gender hierarchy becomes clear in the works of several authors, like Patricia Uberoi, for example, who writes:

> Thus a national identity was constituted through the construction of the ideal Hindu women, and her characteristics derived from a hierarchy of textual authorities: the Vedas, Shastras, epics, puranas, and so on. In the process, obviously, a number of exclusions came into play; (i) of other religions and cultural traditions by the newly emerging Hindu tradition, as already suggested; (ii) of lower caste practices by Brahminical and Kshatriya models [Chakravarti 1989]; (iii) of folk genres by the new genres of the comprador bourgeoisie [Banerjee 1989]; and (iv) of indigenous aesthetic values by those of the colonial power through the psychology of identity with the aggressor [Nandy 1983].[22]

Kumkum Sangari describes the display as that of an 'an assertive state-sponsored display of Indian tradition and culture, especially of the classical, the folk and the tribal, intended as a saleable compensation for the lack of democratizing initiatives on its own part'.[23]

I would like to take this a little further. It seems that the incorporation of certain performative practices commonly used for such in this festivity[24] is also on the basis of the same criteria of social control and disciplined citizenship in similar ways as with temple festivals, working with ideas on sociopolitical practices associated with imposition of control over a social (especially gendered) body. Alexandra Howson mentions D. Lupton's work in social construction of medicine while discussing regulatory and disciplinary methods of imposition of control. While the first is in connection to institutions and populations, the second is associated with 'practices and disciplinary mechanisms in which individuals usually engage . . .'.[25] Howson goes on to explain that the enactment of such obedience generates a sense of discipline that accepts regulatory power and helps in perpetuating a 'liberal governance' in which self-surveillance becomes a part and parcel of daily lives.[26] Howson mentions Foucault's discussion on 'practices of self' to iterate that the individuals do not need to be coerced into such practices, but instead do so as a result of having internalized the disciplinary mechanisms.

One needs to analyse the applicability and plausibility of 'practices of self' as an idea while examining the actions of the male and female participants in the gendered spaces allocated in the Republic Day Parade. The process of curation started with the implementation of the Nehruvian vision of independent India and was later fine-tuned by officers and cultural specialists and planners like Kapila Vatsyayan. The cultural display may be seen as complementary to the military display, but the display itself is not outside the strictly bifurcated male/female binary. Most of the tableaux of the different states and organizations position the male and female bodies to reaffirm the clichéd gendered imagery of the male as warrior/farmer/worker/breadwinner, and the female as housewives/mothers. The aesthetic objectification of passive subjects in such displays of marginal citizens has been discussed by several scholars such as Jyotindra Jain[27] in his essay on the Republic Day Parade.

The celebratory display of the controlled body of the folk and tribal dancers thus constructs a place, even outside the specific space and time of the parade, and relegates the folk and tribal dancers to accept a position of inferiority in the cultural framework of the national image.

Cultural Evenings at Popular Tourist Sites and Local Festivals Organized by State Governments

Cultural tourism in India in its present organized, packaged and performative form is a relatively recent phenomenon. Within tourism studies there have been discussions on the creation of the 'other' cultures and 'ways of life' in order to attract tourists round the year, beyond the so-called perfect and peak tourist seasons. Following Tylor's definition of culture[28] it can be said that culture can be museumized and re-presented both as the way of life of a group of human beings as well as the material and immaterial products that such ways of life produce or incorporate. Tourism strategies utilize such showcasing of 'culture' and in the process use local artistes, especially women, to embody the 'ways of life'.

The Rajasthan government's tourism website[29] describes its year-long plan of celebrating Rajasthan in the following terms:

> Rajasthan has one of the most colorful and vibrant deserts in the world. The great Thar Desert has much to offer through a plethora of celebrations. Festivals and fairs, music and dance, are a part of life in the State as well as in the desert. The yearlong festive fervour and cattle marts turn into delightful fairs. Festivals hold an unusual lure for the Rajasthanis and they have any number of reasons to celebrate. Pageantry is in the form of weddings or rituals, or to promote trade. Each region has their own form of folk entertainment, traditions, dialects adding to the Indian diversity. Some of the fairs are: Pushkar Fair, Desert festival, Elephant Festival and Camel festival. Having attained international repute, they are not to be missed.[30]

Similar advertisements are found all over the internet. The presentation of 'ways of life' may be differentiated into three key forms depending on the way women are used in the scheme of planned events. The first type is the presentation of the 'authentic'[31] way of life, as a part of local festivals such as the Hornbill Festival in Nagaland; the second option, very popular nowadays, is an organized and structured cultural programme for an evening of performance, for two/three hours, like the evening performances and dinner packages organized at government and non-government venues for tourists, which provide employment to a group of musicians, singers and (mostly women) dancers. The third type of performances are loosely planned contracts at smaller sites, where dancers (again largely women) accompany male musicians for a short performance.

The histories of colonial expositions across Europe in the nineteenth and early twentieth centuries, that projected the colonized and conquered subjects as the bodies on display, get replayed in many ways in all such festival spaces, where the clear binary between the viewer as the one with agency and the viewed as the one who is made to believe that this is a way of creating a presence and through that a certain form of agency, gets reproduced as a template in a newly fashioned neo-coloniality. The hierarchy now is not between the white colonizer and the 'native' subject, instead it is between the privileged urban citizen and the 'primitive' other. The colonial expositions in Europe[32] which used such stereotypes to showcase the colonies and their 'uncivilized' and 'primitive' inhabitants, along with animals from the same regions, may not be a term of reference for the tourists who are satisfied to pay for the 'authentic' presence of the different Naga tribes lined up in all their finery and displaying their weapons, headgear and ornaments to greet the visitors at the entrance to the arena of the Hornbill Festival during the inaugural ceremony performance. Arguments for organizing such festivals are many. They have definitely increased tourist footfalls in Nagaland during the winter months. These festivals and the organizational work that goes behind such week-long events are increasing a space for inter-tribe dialogue, and such festivals may be the only occasions during which a Naga child gets to experience her/his own culture. Such festival spaces, hence, are becoming a template for cultural tourism in all Indian states. The Sangai Festival in Manipur and the Hornbill Festival in Nagaland are now events to look forward to for the people of these states who claim both state and people support for these events. The festival space for Hornbill is divided into specific areas for different kinds of performances and audiences. The rock concert draws its own crowd and is one of the most popular events for young people who travel long distances (even from neighbouring states) to enjoy the ambience and the local and invited bands. The stadium with its huge ground hosts traditional games and dances by the different Naga tribes, from morning till early evening. It also is the space where international dignitaries are brought in as special guests to witness the events. This is the most controlled space in the festival with an extremely structured and planned schedule. The planned preparations are visible in the traditional dresses, ornaments and props that become part and parcel of the games, dances, and musical presentations. The other important space is a slightly separate ground where the traditional Naga dormitories[33] are constructed for the Naga tribes. Each of the Naga tribes displays their traditional dresses, weapons, and essential equipment to offer a glimpse of the everyday life to visitors. The 'performance' of life and work, along with the selling of their own traditional food and liquor, has been supported by the elders of the community as they hope such a display to be educative for the young people from the different Naga tribes. This area adjoins a temporary market which sells ornaments, dresses, props, musical instruments, and many other handcrafted artistic and utilitarian products—the products that could recreate the 'Naga-ness' away from Nagaland, for the outsiders when they are back home in their own place of residence. Thus in such festivals the template is to introduce national and international tourists to the ways of life of a state/community/ethnic group through live performances of sports, dance, music, and theatre on one hand, and the performance of what could be taken as representative of the unknown and often exoticized 'other'.

The evening performances as well as the site-specific performances for tourists happen throughout the year. Such 'made easy' performances to experience and 'know' the local culture may use male as well as female performers from the local community, but this creates a specific vulnerability for the woman performer by inviting tourists as participants to such spaces for 'enjoyment' and 'entertainment'. In her book *Staging Tourism: Bodies on Display From Waikiki to Sea World* (1999), Jane

C. Desmond talks about the gendered stereotypes that get continued through the reference and a certain kind of reading of the Hawaiian history, which now is also evident when one looks at the history of tourism in Hawaii. She uses the example of the popular image of the hula girl[34] in comparison to the male performers. Desmond's writing on the use of exotic imagery for a certain white male consumption is also reflected within the tourism circuit which serves a certain form of primitivized entertainment to foreign as well as alienated urban upper-class tourists from within India, projecting women as focal objectified bodies, sometimes tactfully, and sometimes not even bothering to hide the enticement/sexual appeal that the entertainment wants to create. Consumption of embodied 'otherness' as a product that is being 'sold' is privileged on a given hierarchy of power. Desmond writes: 'Live performers not only authenticate these packaged differences: they also offer the possibility of contact with them.'[35] In the Indian context, the growing popularity of staging culture usually is a devised continuation of catering to the colonizer's gaze. The bodies (mostly of women) are staged as the 'authentic', ready and eager to please, often taking away the gendered difference from the male/female gaze of the tourist. The 'power of the ideology of primitivism', as conceptualized by Desmond and many others, becomes evident in the reproductions of referential stereotypes (e.g. dance and performance's dependence on and association with intoxication among the 'native' subject) and gets to be the universal formula of successful tourism strategies. It is what tourism management banks on, as an easy planning tool. The trick is to displace the current time with the help of such stereotypes, to place the 'native' bodies in an imagined time and space whereby the staged 'culture' of the community in view can fit easily into the stereotypically generalized image of the 'other'. Above all, the usual ending of the evening with an open invitation to the audience to experience the dance by dancing along often creates a sense of accessibility in urban tourists, who are otherwise used to seeing performances usually either on proscenium spaces or film screens. Though it would not be fair to project all such spaces to be the same, many of them are really unsafe and exploitative spaces for the performers (especially women), even within the so-called safe space of the government-backed cultural tourism (see also Plate 5.3).

Women Performers and the Threat of the Margins

Scholars of dance studies have continued to discuss the history of dance within the framework of the colonial encounter and nationalist

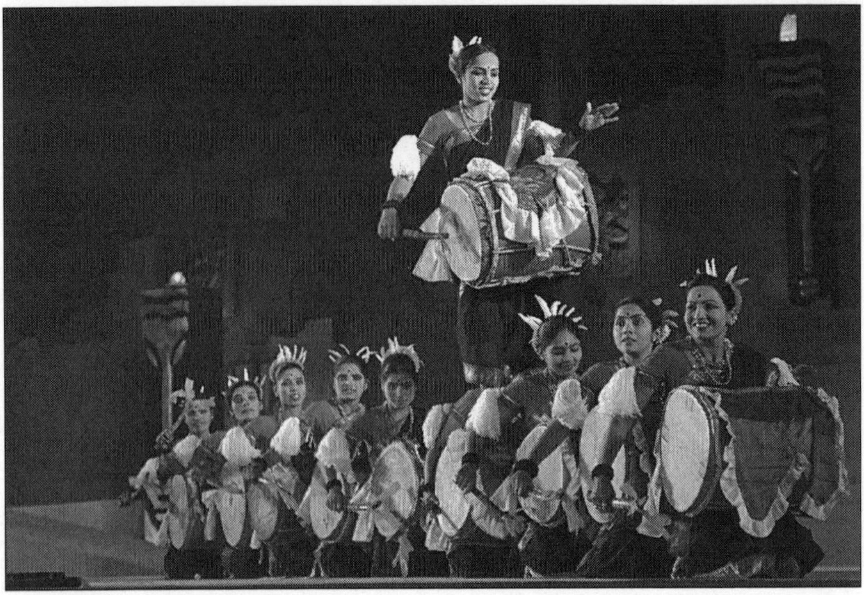

PLATE 5.3: Folk Dance Festival, Talkatora Stadium, New Delhi, 2007.
Source: Photo courtesy of Avinash Pasricha.

strategies for the stereotypes that are at play in the world of dance. India has seen progress over the many post-colonial decades that have passed and also the several changes in regimes of political power that it has gone through. Many of the evolving sociopolitical developments in areas like that of social position of women, display of masculinities, objectification and aestheticization of women and their bodies in media on one hand, and contrasting/contradictory images of women within the tropes of idealized domestic conjugality, are results of the neo-liberal global market on the one hand and the increasingly more conservative fundamentalist propaganda on the other.

In the contemporary India that the dancers inhabit with other citizens, dancers' practices may create and perpetuate a world which Jain had mentioned as a 'frozen space',[36] their realities take them through ever-changing adjustments to the changing world around them. Here I suggest the necessity of looking beyond the post-independence nationalist strategies as the guidelines for analysing sites and spaces accorded to the woman dancer. I acknowledge that these sites/sights are originally a result of the post-independence nationalist endeavours and plans. However, it is also necessary to acknowledge that the logic of choosing to continue with such spaces and thematic framework for the woman dancer, in contemporary India, rests on certain needs of governance and image projection that emerge out of India's global presence and functioning in the 'here and now', in contemporary India, rather than with reference to history or tradition. Here I also suggest that the position of subservience to the mytho-history that becomes a given for a woman dancer as the ideal obedient subject, in comparison to the resistive theatre actress, is what the dancer chooses to project because it ascertains access to state patronage and visibility in the Indian dance scenario worldwide.

The space of the 'other' is being consolidated consistently over the post-independence years by organizations like Zonal Cultural Centres, through allocation of grants and funds, and also by the process of acceptance of allocated positions, by the 'others' themselves. It is a similar situation for almost all marginal community performances. This phenomenon affects a large number of anonymous women dancers (as well as male ones). In classical dances the situation seems to be better, even if marginally, as individual recognition through grants and recognitions are much more in number. The celebratory displays that they find themselves in—like Republic Day Parades, opening of the Commonwealth Games, etc.—hold an anonymity for participants, where a group identity is all that one has, rather than any individual presence. Viewed as an exhibition rather than a performance, the transitory character of such displays do not draw attention to detailed performative elements, but rather constitute a part of the jigsaw puzzle, constituting the colourful image of India.

The performance of 'belonging' by the dancer, or the inclusionary or hierarchizing practices of the state, both refer to the process of the state's constitution of the desired narrative. In both cases the tools are those of embodied practices. In the case of the woman dancer, either a practitioner of one of the privileged classical dance styles or one from the numerous communities who constitute the marginalized 'other', the embodiment of exclusion or inclusion becomes a part of their life as dancers. As against the classical dancer (who is aided by the hierarchical superiority accorded by the state and included completely within the framework of legitimacy of the ideal citizenship) the woman dancer from the peasant or tribal community becomes increasingly marginalized through economy, socio-cultural position, and exclusionary practices of the state.

Notes and References

1. Patricia Uberoi, 'Feminine Identity and National Ethos in Indian Calendar Art', *Economic and Political Weekly*, vol. 25, no. 17, 1990, p. 41.
2. Ibid.
3. Partha Chatterjee, 'Colonialism, Nationalism, and Colonialized Women: The Contest in India', *American Ethnologist*, vol. 16, no. 4, 1989, p. 622.
4. Avanti Meduri discusses the process of classicalization of Bharatanatyam to contextualize the dance and the dancer in the history of Tamil Nadu in 'Bharatha Natyam: What Are You?' *Asian Theatre Journal*, vol. 5, no. 1, 1988, pp. 1–22.
5. Pallabi Chakravorty's book *Bells of Change: Kathak Dance, Women and Modernity in India* (Calcutta: Seagull Press, 2008), discusses, critically, the journey/relationship of colonial nautch dance and restructured classical Kathak through the lenses of nationalism, postcolonialism, transnationalism, and globalization.
6. Roma Chatterji discusses the ways in which some 'tribal dances' have acquired greater visibility than other dance forms in eastern India to analyse different representations of community and social structure in the writings on folk culture, which leads to differential circulation of knowledge about cultures in the public sphere, in her book *Folklore and Performative Arts of Purulia, Bengal*, Indira Gandhi Centre For the Arts, Delhi: Aryan Books, 2009, p. 120.
7. Ibid., p. 121.
8. Anthony Jackson and Jenny Kidd, *Performing Heritage: Research, Practice and Innovation in Museum Theatre and Live Interpretation*, Manchester and New York: Manchester University Press, 2011, p. 1.
9. The Incredible India website (http://incredibleindia.org/index.php/experience-india/fairs-and-festivals [accessed 24 May 2016]) provides a month-wise as well as state-wise calendar of such festivals with specific reference to the historical significance of the festival space in the promotional passage written for each.
10. Incredible India, 'Mamallapuram Dance Festival, Tamil Nadu', http://incredibleindia.org/index.php/main-travel/24-home/528 (accessed 15 July 2016).
11. Partha Chatterjee, 'The Nation and its Women', in *Nation and its Fragments: Colonial and Postcolonial Histories*, in *The Partha Chatterjee Omnibus*, New Delhi: Oxford University Press, 1999, pp. 116–34.
12. Ibid.
13. Ibid., pp. 130–1.
14. Seemanthini Niranjana, *Gender and Space*, London: Sage Publications, 2001, p. 38.
15. Etienne Balibar, 'Subjection and Subjectivation', in *Supposing the Subject*, ed. Joan Kopjec, London and New York: Verso, 1994, p. 9.
16. Akle Groppel-Wegener, 'Creating Heritage Experience through Architecture', in *Performing Heritage: Research, Practice and Innovation in*

Museum Theatre and Live Interpretation, ed. Anthony Jackson and Jenny Kidd, Manchester and New York: Manchester University Press, 2011, p. 39.

17. *The Pioneer*, 'India's First Republic Day Parade', 30 August 2015, http://www.dailypioneer.com/sunday-edition/agenda/books/indias-first-republic-day-parade.html (accessed 15 December 2015).
18. Uberoi, 'Feminine Identity and National Ethos', p. 43.
19. Rajpath is a ceremonial boulevard in New Delhi.
20. Rajpath runs from Rashtrapati Bhavan on Raisina Hill through Vijay Chowk and India Gate to the National Stadium, Delhi.
21. Royona Mitra, in 'Performing Cultural Heritage in "Weaving Paths" by Sonia Sabri Dance Company', *Performing Heritage: Research, Practice and Innovation in Museum Theatre and Live Interpretation*, ed. Anthony Jackson and Jennifer Kid, Manchester: Manchester University Press, 2011, p. 152.
22. Uberoi, 'Feminine Identity and National Ethos', p. 43. Also see Uma Chakravarti, 'Whatever Happened to the Vedic Dasi: Orientalism, Nationalism, and a Script for the Past', in *Recasting Women: Essays in Colonial History*, ed. Kumkum Sangari and Sudesh Vaid, New Delhi: Kali for Women, 1989; Sumanta Banerjee, 'Marginalisation of Women's Popular Culture in Nineteenth Century Bengal', in *Recasting Women: Essays in Colonial History*, ed. Kumkum Sangari and Sudesh Vaid, New Delhi: Kali for Women, 1989; Ashis Nandy, *The Intimate Enemy: Loss and Recovery of Self under Colonialism*, Delhi: Oxford University Press, 1983.
23. Kumkum Sangari, 'Introduction: Representations in History', *Journal of Arts and Ideas*, nos. 17–18, 1989, p. 3. Sangari discusses the state processes of systematic framing of the hierarchization.
24. I have analysed the journey of Chhau from its space within the community to the national and international arena as well as its inclusion in the 'Representative List of Intangible Cultural Heritage of Humanity' by the United Nations Educational, Scientific and Cultural Organization (UNESCO) in my article 'The Changing Stage: Chhau as an Intangible Cultural Heritage', *International Journal of Arts, Culture and Heritage*, vol. 1, 2012, p. 168.
25. Alexandra Howson, *Embodying Gender*, New Delhi: Sage Publications, 2005, p. 23.
26. Ibid.
27. In Jain's critique of the museumization and display of the tribals and villagers in the tableaux and dioramas, he talks about creating a 'frozen space' which isolates them from any 'evolving process' and traces of 'conflict and change'. Jyotindra Jain, 'India's Republic Day Parade: Restoring Identities, Constructing the Nation', in *India's Popular Culture: Iconic Spaces and Fluid Images*, ed. Jyotindra Jain, Mumbai: Marg Publications, 2007, p. 68.
28. E.B. Tylor defines '[c]ulture, or [c]ivilization, in its broad, ethnographic sense' as 'that complex whole which includes knowledge, belief, art,

morals, law, custom, and any other capabilities and habits acquired by man as a member of society'. Tylor, *Primitive Culture*, vol. 1, New York: J. P. Putnam's Sons, 1920, p. 1.

29. http://www.rajasthantourism.gov.in/Attractions/Fairs-Festivals.aspx (accessed 17 September 2015) describes a long list of festivals in the calendar year to attract tourists throughout the year.
30. See http://www.rajasthantourism.gov.in/Attractions/Fairs-Festivals.aspx (accessed 17 September 2015).
31. The quest for the 'authentic' is identified as one of the major incentives for choosing to opt for a cultural tour. The presentation of real life, real food, real people—the real dress, songs and dances—with tangible presence of their bodies as repositories of all that they proclaim as their very own, and finally letting the tourists become a part of that exotic 'other' life for as long as they choose, has become the trendy outings often advertised by both governmental and non-governmental websites.
32. A series of international colonial exhibitions were organized from the late nineteenth century, which were planned in order to generate trade and business amongst the colonial empires such as France, England, etc., to consolidate the economic connections among empires. One of the most noted was the Paris Exposition which is supposed to have sold 33 million tickets. The exhibitions included a number of pavilions as temporary museums as well as display sites for museumized objects as well as human beings from colonized cultures.
33. The dormitories among many Indian tribes have been described as the youth houses, or the common houses, that traditionally were spaces for the youth to spend time and learn different community activities. With the advent of Christianity, many tribes were forced to give up these associations—the youth were seamlessly socialized over and above the realms of the family to basic details of informal education and shared community life.
34. Jane C. Desmond, *Staging Tourism: Bodies on Display from Waikiki to Sea World*, Chicago and London: University of Chicago Press, 1999, p. 12.
35. Ibid., p. xv.
36. Jain, 'India's Republic Day Parade', p. 68.

6 Protesting through Gestures

Maya Rao in Dialogue with Dance and Theatre

BISHNUPRIYA DUTT

Bringing theatre, dance, and music within a common disciplinary rubric in practice is challenging and difficult, however much one argues for their co-existence. Within the larger colonial and postcolonial historical encounter there is the possibility of viewing the dancer and actor as present within a common space, but in contemporary performance it can be a more difficult terrain to navigate. The spaces I refer to are the urban proscenium spaces which seem to be the location both dance and theatre regard as the only performing space allocated for themselves. Usually these few auditoriums located at the centre of the city (Delhi), and are hired on separate days to host the dance or theatre performance while the funding systems, performers' training and background and even the audience are rarely common. Despite the sharing of spaces, the conversation seems frozen in time without any attempt to be innovative (read, experimental) in bringing the genres together or being conscious of each other's work.

Yet, given the shrinking space of both dance and theatre, such dialogues are a priority. These issues assume greater importance and significance in light of the changing scenario of contemporary India where neo-liberal policies and a growing religious revivalism are influencing culture and performance practices.

In Indian common parlance, the dancer is conceived as one who follows the formal structure of her dance style and is proficient in the codification of the existing grammatical structure which determines her

*Presented in February 2013 at the Women Studies Centre, Jadavpur University, Kolkata, for the World Dance Federation colloquium. Ideas and concepts were formulated through teaching the course 'Critical Approaches to Theatre and Performance Studies: Feminism, Gender and Sexuality' (M.Phil optional course) in 2012 and 2013 with Professor Janelle Reinelt.

posture, movement and (the focus of this essay) the 'gesture', codified as 'mudras'. Not being a dance scholar, for me the codified mudras are mnemonics of the classical dances of India and a significant focus area in dance studies which interprets the development of the elaborate gestural language through mudras as an integral part of the dance vocabulary that is often traced back to the *Natyashastra*. Indian dance history acknowledges this codification as further addition and refinement over existing grammars that became part of the reconstruction project of the new nation in the 1950s. Historically, practitioners and researchers, in conjunction, have reiterated the norms of 'aesthetic perfection' and meanings associated to the gestural language—specifically associated with mudras and generally attributed to the presentational format of classical dance genres, that got shaped in the process of canonization within practice and the generation of meaning in classical dance forms.[1] The mudra range has also increased through the dancers' creative interventions and the evolution of the styles, to include a number of nuanced intermediate movements which to the untrained eye are difficult to detect and read. Not only in terms of the performers but also for the audience, it seems that such intricacies of the 'mudras' demand a more complex reading and conditioned reception.

As an argument I would like to read the prioritization of the 'mudras' in classical (Indian) dance genre as a trend feeding into the growing ideals of femininity which is valorized as 'beauty', 'grace', and 'aesthetics'. While creating an ultra-feminine space the dancers are often pitted in competition against each other to prove their feminine normative perfection.

Theatre, for various reasons, cannot adopt the same norms, where the feminine is the contrast to the masculinity of the protagonist as well as a predominant male cast. Moreover, the dichotomy of the body-mind faculty or the realistic acting methods, instead of encouraging the body to be expressive, insists on restrictions and allows impulses only coming from the logic of characterization. As a result, the actress is usually commanded to keep her hands locked at the back, as any movements of the hand, can be misread as artificial. I deliberately use the gendered term 'actress', as the actress codes of using free gestures were the most restricted and controlled. While the actors often are allowed free body movement onstage, the basic actress codes are more restricted.

The actresses, bound by the dominant realistic narratives, follow orders of restraint and control of the body which are not to be exhibited. Translated in theatrical terms, this means holding back the gestures.

The gesture discourse in theatre has been predominantly a male domain. 'Theatre', which was imported to the colonies, came with the nineteenth-century English acting style where the actor revelled in exaggerated postures and gestures. Utpal Dutt, in his article on Sisir Kumar Bhaduri (1889–1959) on the legendary actor's birth centenary year, shows how Bhaduri was an exception in the acting style followed by his contemporaries.[2]

The style which was practised in general, which he refers to, required every articulated speech to be demonstrated by gestures of the hands. Bhaduri, however, used 'gestures' only for effects to create drama and what in theatre history has become the iconic episodes. In writing histories, it is these poses and gestures of the male star which are extolled and described as memorable acting.

Bhaduri's legendary actress Prabhadevi (1903–52), often regarded as one of the most powerful actresses of Bengali theatre, is praised by the connoisseur as being able to sit at one corner of the stage without any apparent body movements and hold her audience captive with speech and delivery. Yet, till date, no historian has written on Prabhadevi's acting or made an assessment of it. The growing nationalist discourse of early twentieth century and the collusion in Bengal between the nationalist movement and the theatre (1905–47) presented the domesticated women as the contrasting figure to the male protagonist, who had no postures or gestures, but stood as the passive sacrificial body. Hence, the actresses who embodied the codes of domestic conjugality had no scope to use their hands to enhance expression and the codification of the mudras was never a preoccupation for them.

The acting of a number of stage actresses of the progressive theatre movement, such as Sova Sen,[3] rarely ever used gestures to illustrate her words or feelings. Her style was unique, where she would stand still while her voice, speech, and intonations expressed every nuance of her role. It was a style which evoked empathy and had an effect on the audience, and the performance was apparently effortless.

It is historically known that the adoption of Brecht's gestus by the new progressive theatre movement in Bengal in the 1960s and the 1970s at the key postcolonial moment was an effective strategy for the male actors in creating subject positions for themselves. The male actor's tool has often been to use gestures to deliberately enhance the illusion of his physical presence as larger than life. The question that remains as a doubt to most contemporary Indian actors is the ways in which the Brechtian gesture/gestus was different from the older acting methods and pronounced actions by hand movement to enhance speech. Joachim Fiebach describes the gestus as 'anthropological mimesis' which is a cluster of gestures.[4] I would like to understand the cluster of gestures as also contradictory to each other. The gestures to be used are not to seem the natural movement of the character but to expose him as the actor/ commentator. Double meanings are expected to be demonstrated. I will come back to this meaning of 'gesture' when I look at the contemporary performances of Maya Rao later in the chapter.

In a sense, the demure attitudinal stance of the woman performer always contradicts the theatrical energy within which she contains her body. The soft, subservient position is always contested by a voice that can reach the end of the theatres. Through her role, the actress often has to position herself against her male counterpart through a dialectical tension of the control of her body and the latent energy which she contains.

The question in this context for both the dancer and the actress is whether these gestures can be used for their potential impact to create an intervention. At what moment do they transgress, and in the process create a critique of their very own formulation and construction? At what point and where do conversations around these begin? How can these conversations be located as impactful and reverberate in both the genres to start a debate befitting contemporary times?

In this context I would like to draw on an example of Sova Sen's acting in selected scenes of a Bengali adaptation of Bertolt Brecht's *Mother Courage* (1987).[5] At the moment when Mother Courage silently breaks down, made into a legend of theatre acting by Helene Weigel, Sova Sen, knowing that her acting style is far more downplayed and apparently milder than Weigel, refused to imitate the well-known gesture of holding her mouth and bending forward almost in slow motion. Sova Sen actually did it the other way round, bending backwards almost in the pose of laughter but her jaws open to let out a silent scream, which can also be mistaken for a laugh. As an argument I would also like to maintain that the dancer in practice finds it more difficult to make such departures, pertaining to gestures, which creates an anticipated break from the expected. In terms of the dancer and her gestures, I would elaborate in the next section on many such gestures of departure of the dancer/actress Maya Rao (Plates 6.1 and 6.2).

For me, contemporary times are the neo-liberal times where both dance and theatre come together within a common space of culture capital. Rejecting the performing arts as simply too elitist is erroneous, though the very notion of civil society where they perform is a contested site today. I would argue that this requires a critique rather than apathy and indifference at its exclusive status.

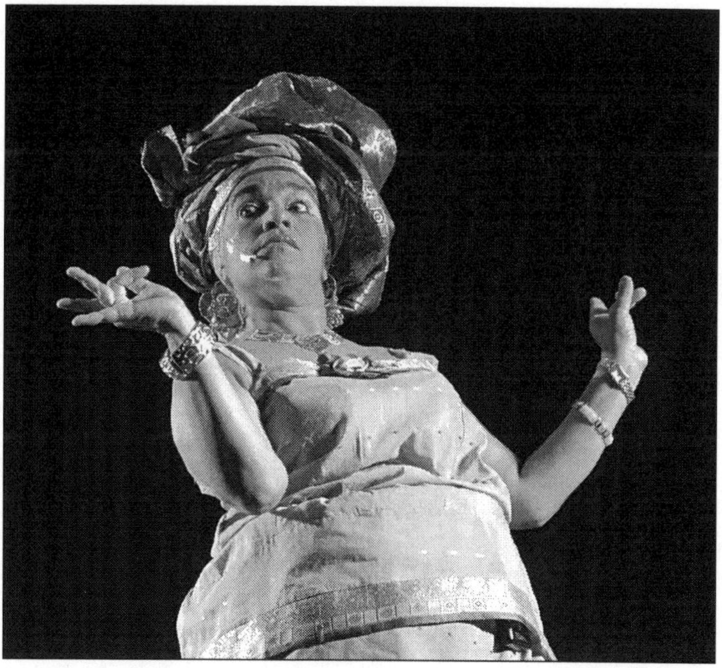

PLATE 6.1: Maya Krishna Rao's Performance brings in References of Kathakali with Theatrical Techniques in *Ravanama*
Source: Photo courtesy of S. Thyagarajan.

The critique of the performing arts as a 'privileged domain' is very true of a postcolonial nation like India, where the classical dance reconstruction projects and institutionalization of theatre were nurtured under the cultural policies in the first phase of postcolonial negotiations of the 1950s and the 1960s. Therefore, not to see it as a part of a 'larger critique of culture and society' would be a misinterpretation.

With the advent of the neo-liberal policies of the state and the increasing networks of production and consumption, thoroughly mediated by global capital, both classical dance and theatre practices have managed to defy the new trends of commercialization and corporatization to a large extent. Here cultural labour and the creative economy will still work with a different logic of meaning generation and representation. By analysing the consequence of the 'event' through the narrative of theatre and performance, I intend to trace alternate trajectories, which that Lara D. Nielsen explains as the 'multiplicities of neoliberal deployments, as they play out in microcosmic and distinctly local modes', of the city space of Delhi.[6]

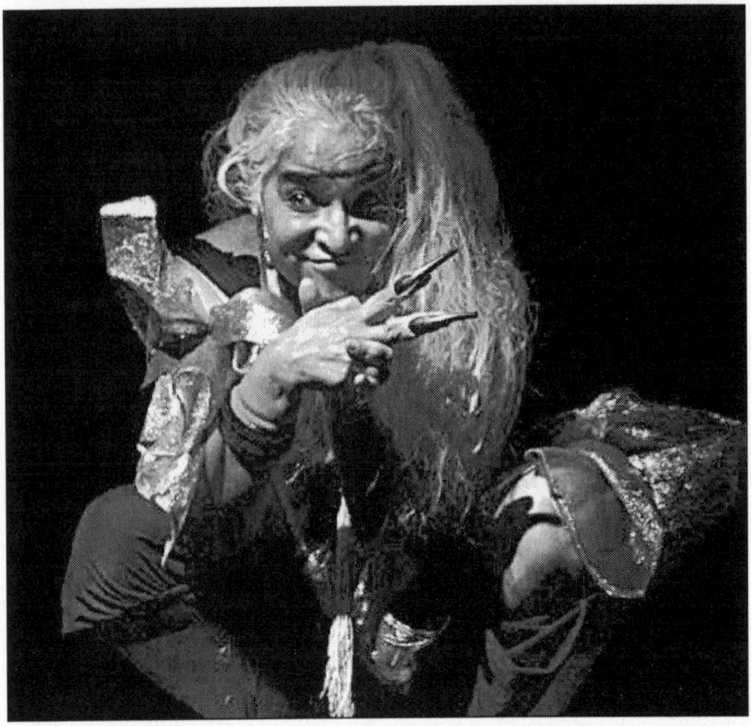

PLATE 6.2: Maya Krishna Rao in *Ravanama*
Source: Photo courtesy of S. Thyagarajan.

Often, dance and theatre performances confined within the proscenium differ from their performance counterparts in the open cityscape which is touted in the world market as one of the new exhibitory spaces narrating the progress of capitalist success. The cityscape is constantly developing and changing and has become a much used scenographic background with enormous deployment of technological apparatus to stage everything from street theatre, dance festivals and music concerts to gay parades and slut walks. These spaces are under very strict surveillance and are important enough to be publicized through widely circulated images as 'safe spaces' to exhibit a range of identity politics, which the state is supposed to promote. It is in that sense the opposite of the older congregational sites. In fact, such alternative spaces are often created to exhibit smaller exclusive communities rather than being larger inclusive spaces. Going against the grain, the performance narratives and representations, hitherto confined behind closed doors of the proscenium, spill out in the public domain by the shift in space and scenography.

The public perception of the few existing proscenium theatres in Delhi has also changed. Increasingly viewed as marginalized spaces which the police and administration cannot cleanse and sanitize so easily, they are a memory of the twentieth century where theatre and dance were still regarded as a domain of the State's cultural vision. The dance space is more often an exclusive space for women both in terms of the performer and the audience. The Delhi theatre in recent times, too, is dominated by what we see as a corpus of women directors who are committed to experimental theatre and are exploring theatrical idioms in conversation with what Anuradha Kapur describes as 'feminist concerns'.[7] I would like to explore the roles of these women directors and locate their performance practice as defying the neo-liberal economy which dominates cultural practice and indirectly becomes a critique of cultural practices that compromise with the neo-liberal economy. Their very presence, Nicholas Ridout valorizes, as:

> passionate amateurs . . . who might participate in and contribute to affective experiences of productive consumption that revive a kind of romantic anti-capitalism. These passionate amateurs are to be found both onstage and off: as fictional figures produced by the labour of the actor; as actors (and other theatrical professionals) working in the production of the play; and, crucially, as spectators for whom the consumption of the theatrical production is itself a form of production, of subjectivities rather than commodities.[8]

Maya Rao's solo performances (see Plate 6.3) can be seen as dialogue with gestures as a key site in the exploration of a new idiom.

The dance-theatre gesture-oriented moments often come together to initiate a critical conversation of an inclusive reading which is very different from the conversation between one dance form with another (be it a classical or 'folk' form). From the perspective of the receiver, who is not versed in dance styles except in an elementary way, the interstices till date had remained only interesting in terms of dance aesthetics. The gesture becomes effective when a dancer like Maya Rao, with her repertoire of Kathakali gestures,[9] starts a theatrical-verbal dialogue with its codification. It is indeed an in-the-face comic dialogue veering between realism and non-realism.

In *A Deep Fried Jam*, for example, Maya consciously or unconsciously uses mudras as a running theme in an otherwise postmodern fragmented performance. If the common theme of *A Deep Fried Jam* is a critique of the new music industry, Maya creates comic encounters with contemporary music, rock and hip hop. She uses a hoarse voice, musical arrangements along with musical scores to create a grotesque soundscape. Her body, clad in knee-length black slacks, T-shirt and jacket, poses and dances to the tunes, but also constantly brings in the so-called

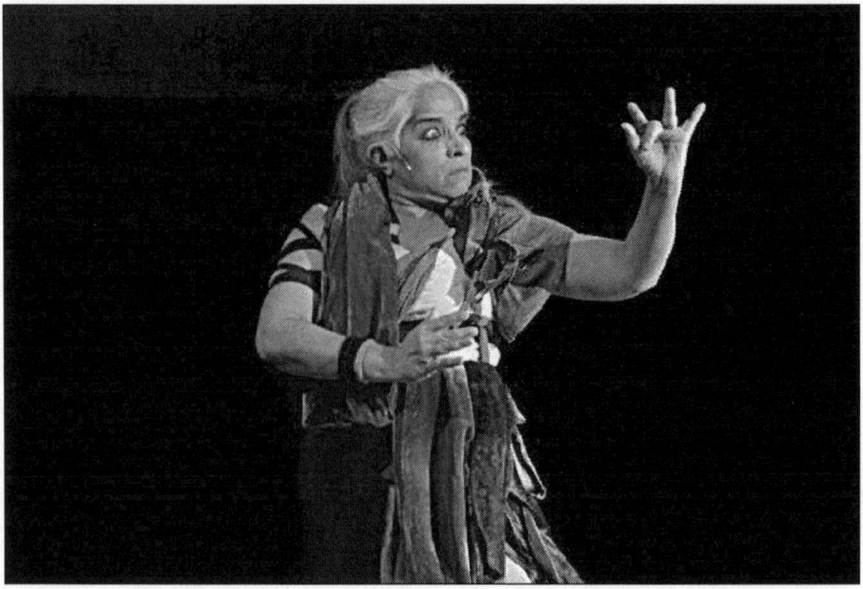

PLATE 6.3: Maya Krishna Rao: Explorations with Gestures and Facial Expressions in *Quality Street*
Source: Photo courtesy of Avinash Pasricha.

Indian dance cultures as a parallel narrative. Maya is not nostalgic about either the dance or the music and her text reflects no sense of loss. It is important to understand her position where both the Western import of a music culture and the so-called Indian dance, vying for attention, focus on the emergence of a hybrid culture which is so celebrated in contemporary India. She moves from dancing to Western music, back into her incongruous stance, always with a gesture.

At one point there is an episode on 'gestures' of Indian dance with a critique. In the costume she looks anything other than an Indian classical dancer. Amidst a stage strewn with wires and cords of the music arrangements lie random props. Most prominent on down stage[10] is a dancing doll dressed in a traditional classical dance costume. Her hands in mudra enhance her dancer status. Maya in the previous episode trying to be the jazz singer in dark glasses is writhing on the floor, when she suddenly turns around and exclaims: 'Actually, I am not a singer; actually, I am a dancer.' She rises from the floor and announces her own dancer identity. She then proceeds with a repertoire of hand gestures or mudras. While demonstrating various mudras she cites the meanings that each gesture can generate: 'the wind blowing', 'scattering flowers', 'scattering flowers on the sacred land', etc. She links her index fingers and asks her audience: 'Would it say anything to you?' She converts her palms into a lotus gesture; she uses the other to become a bee, coming to sit on the flower. She starts imitating the bee sound and her eyes follow the bee in Kathakali style, instantly making her eyes squint, turning the beauty of the mudra into a comic representation.

Maya not only creates a cluster of gestures and converses with appropriate pauses, but also deliberately distances her body, voice, and persona from the pure dance gestures.[11] With appropriate meticulous pauses of absorption and staring at the audience with full frontal eye contact, she comes back to the gestures to denigrate their canonization. The initial self-absorbed look at the gesture and then her own distancing from it, to start a conversation, to return to the gesture is clearly timed and marked out to create, what I would say, is a Brechtian gesture. It brings to its audience a critique of the class, caste, and religious identities which are inherent in the revival processes at play in cultural politics. A multilayered critique emerges combining the serious canonization project of the nation with a Brechtian comic gesture.

In a class comprising students from all over India, the group of students from south India (both Tamil Nadu and Kerala) interpreted the original gesture by Maya Rao—what we assumed came from Kathakali—as a reference to a regimented codification of the classical repertoire as propagated in south Indian cinema culture. The logic they offered was that the use of the mudras in film dancing (in south India) symbolizes the ideal normative femininity imposed as part of the upper-class Brahmanical nation's cultural codes and are very eagerly appropriated by the capital-dominated film industry.

Can we then claim that Maya Rao's performance allows an effective/affective moment of historical critique through Brechtian alienation? In that case, how do we look at this moment of efficacy of a performance culture, which, as is generally argued, cannot negotiate the dogmatism of neo-liberal formations?

Maya's most recent performance, which has received a lot of attention, is in a sense a follow up to *A Deep Fried Jam*; but it also, I would argue, creates strategic inroads to work out new notions of the political-popular-feminist performance strategies in today's context. The *Non-Stop Feel-Good Show* (15 January 2013) has significant connections to her previous themes. In this performance she chooses the media boom in India and the new reality shows, which are gaining popularity.

The music industry as a theme of *A Deep Fried Jam* and media industry as that of *Non-Stop Feel-Good Show* are intricately linked to the neo-liberal markets and its expansion. The private media companies go all out to 'entertain', importing American television ideas, creating Indian versions of them, and along with it, promoting the fashion and cosmetics industry. Maya originally devised her new comic show around these ideas, with a strong comic critique so prominent in her style.

The January 2013 performance also came in the aftermath of the 16 December 2012 rape case in Delhi, when a young woman returning with her friend from watching a movie was picked up by an empty bus and six miscreants. The young woman, who came to be known as 'Nirbhaya', was brutally raped and thrown out of the bus. Widespread protests against sexual violence followed the event creating a charged atmosphere and an unprecedented mobilization in the streets of Delhi. Participating in the protests and after Nirbhaya's passing away on 29 December 2012, in the memorial to celebrate her spirit (31 December 2012), Maya created her now famous *walk*.[12]

In *A Deep Fried Jam*, she had first introduced the idea of walking. At first she mimes walking and running on the sands and evokes memories of Mahatma Gandhi's famous Dandi march, where he walked up to the seashore to manufacture 'salt' against the harsh colonial salt laws. Subsequently, she describes the new cityscape which is demolishing the jamun and other trees with which her childhood is linked, and mimes walking across the city.

Maya employs strategies where we see the walk as a gestural impulse travelling in a complex way. Maya's signature Kathakali gestures carry her from one space to another, opening up conversations which otherwise would have died with one performance (*Deep Fried Jam*), and interesting idioms she discovers as she goes along. *Walk* becomes the final episode of the *Non-Stop Feel-Good Show*, which is a strong critique of Indian media, the corporates, and the State to create a homogenous Indian middle class, culturally representing Hindu traditional values with Western lifestyle. Maya's caricature revolves around an elderly woman (Amma) from Kerala with a strong regional identity which defies all homogeneity. The character stands out by her clothing, strong Malayali accent (a comic device), a middle-class cultural identity, growing impoverization, personifying the uneven development of economic growth and urbanization of contemporary India. Ingrained within Amma's story is the decline and collapse of the last vestiges of Nair matriliny, that had gradually been eroded and delegitimized with colonial and post-independence adoption of a Western practice of a patriarchal nuclear family, and which is finally disappearing with the neo-liberal policies of the state and globalization.

Nivedita Menon, in her book *Seeing Like a Feminist*, almost echoes the collapse of older alternative family system in the opening chapter of her book, indicating how the contemporary scenario does not allow any space to the older feminist engagement with community laws and heterogeneous family structures, marking a fundamental shift in the new forces at play.[13]

If the *Non-Stop Feel-Good Show* is about the media and the aggressive marketing of the cosmetics and fashion industry, it is also aimed at constructing new norms of femininity and feminine bodies. The new normative standards touted are, in a sense, diametrically opposite to what Maya often sees as her Kathakali body being rooted to the ground. It tells the story of contemporary India which is moving towards Western culture, adopting Western clothes and slim bodies to go with it, as is demonstrated so clearly by Hindi cinema and the new generation of the star-heroines who are also the most coveted models in corporate advertising, Maya's performance unravels the incongruity of this trend. Through various mudras used in classical Indian dance to show the dancer-performer transforming herself for her lover or beloved, usually of mythical origin, she shows us how to also look 'feminine' in the normative sense. She dresses in the performance in the most outrageous style and her eyes and gestures belie the text cited for such transformative makeovers.

Then come her comic episodes on the body makeovers. In a gear once identified with the American dedicated jogger, but now a universal costume, Maya Rao comes on stage in white knee-length tights, a short bustier, a red band on her long hair, jogging to pop music. In an American accent she talks about learning to keep herself fit by jogging in the US, where she had moved after her marriage to a man she calls Harinder. She is implying the archaic but still widely practised custom of arranging marriages for young Indian girls, where the non-residential Indian males in the US and other parts of the world are regarded as the most coveted match. Harinder turns out to be a criminal, committing violent crimes, and is sent away. Our heroine moves from Dallas to New York and starts her 'You Yourly, Yoga Institute'. In full view of her audience she turns into the yoga guru by adorning an Indian costume and marking her forehead with vermillion. From the very fashionable, sensual female protagonist, Maya turns back to her Malayali persona. The American accent which she used earlier easily becomes a pronounced Indian (speaking English) accent. She demonstrates yoga movements along with the *rasa* expressions of the *Natyashastra*. *Vibhatsa* (disgust) is the *rasa* which she had perfected as a child, scaring her friends away. Maya now goes through some of the other *asanas* and combines them with *rasa*. Here her skills as a Kathakali dancer, her acting skills (where her tone of narration is very realistic and full of humour), and her gestures often doing just the opposite of her speech or her dance posture, throw up a number of gestures, or, as I had mentioned earlier, a 'cluster of gestures'. The gestures are seemingly unintentional, but never a mere illustration of either her speech or her body movement. They are always contradicting one or the other. While she performs the registers of aesthetic expression of the Indian classical dance repertoire, the gestures are the only indication that this is not really a classical dance recital but an iconic denigration of it through comic acting. The episode ends when she leans back with a jerk and says this is how Shilpa Shetty was kissed by Richard Gere. This is the classic posture of the about-to-be-kissed woman, who falls into the man's arm in total surrender and objectifies herself. The entire spell is broken and the reference to Gere brings us back to the hybrid cultural scenario emerging out of a global world.

Maya Rao anticipates the new emerging market for a yoga-oriented spiritual Indian culture to become a new commodity in the world market, which has since become a reality promoted by the prime minister himself. On 21 June 2015, promoted by the United Nations, the World Yoga Day was celebrated by the global media where the Indian Prime Minister himself sat on the streets of Rajpath (Delhi), leading a group of people to perform yoga. It was telecast worldwide to exhibit a new cultural commodity originating within the Indian tradition.

The performance builds up with two political comic episodes, one mimicking and caricaturizing the Chief Minister of Bengal and her close ties with the Bengali President of India; and the other a host of a cookery show preparing a fish recipe, through which she critiques the then Chief Minister of Gujarat but now the Prime Minister of India. The Kathakali mudras come back with a vengeance while she works with symbolic props, her body, and text. Yet they all work in parallel trajectories. Maya's solo presence on the stage operates at three different levels, running parallel, without any dialogue with each other. We hear pertinent words uttered amidst what may sound like gibberish, heavily accented, a spoken text of 'censorship', 'fish', 'Bay of Bengal', 'industry', 'progress', 'sex worker and clientele'. Her hand gestures are pronounced while she plays and fondles with the key prop she uses in the two scenes—the fish—as if she is trying out two fish recipes, favourites in Gujarat and Calcutta.

The strange costume, very different from Maya's androgynous presence, gives her body a grotesque presence. In the sequence on

Bengal's chief minister, she is a woman as well as a male politician (the President of India), mimicking both and their collaboration in bringing about 'political change' in Bengal, by ushering out any obstacles in the path of neo-liberal progress.[14] One example I would like to cite to bring back a particularly theatrical moment, where Maya uses her Kathakali gesture, is her great political-autocrat caricature of the present Chief Minister of West Bengal. Maya Rao devours the fish with one of her hands clawed, the other hand in the classical dance style creating the most beautiful aesthetic moment of water flowing and a fish drowning and trying to come up to the surface for air only to be caught and physically dismembered to be cooked in the cookery show.

The beautiful mudras never cease and she continues to move from one mudra to another, even while she describes Gujarat as the 'example of shining India' and demonstrates it as an allegory to a 'shining recipe'. She rattles off dismal statistics where the average worker in Gujarat in the Nano factory at Hirapur is paid less than the nation's average, Rs.270 to Rs.332, and how they are deprived of fresh water and nutritious diets on a day-to-day basis. Moreover, there are no hospitals within the vicinity and in times of medical emergency there are no safeguards for the workers. She also highlights the fact that it is easy to throw the ailing worker out and employ fresh workers at a moment's notice. 'The district is also one of the highly polluted areas in India', she claims, but in the most disarming way she looks at her audience with her arms open, her palm and fingers locked in beautiful mudras, and declares that the 'going for us is good'. Conditions to build industry could not have been more congenial where the ruling parties and the industrialists are in nexus to create a free market economy. 'Within seven days all permissions to open factories and build industries are cleared and all we need to do', she directs, 'is get a giant casserole and mix and swirl the fish curry and season it with a pinch of saffron.'[15]

The dialogue delivery and her expression, is one of seduction and mischief, her body often taking on a graceful stance, her costume a short glimmering dress, and her hair tied with a headband and flowers, all of which prevent her from being a beautiful dancer but more like a femme fatale. The content of the speech is horrifying and all her perfect gestures add up to the moment when we realize the truth about neo-liberalism and industrialization.

In the growing atmosphere of active collaboration between neo-liberalism and conservatism in India, where progressive politics and cultural expressions are conspicuous by their absence, Maya's performance stands out not only as a critique and exposure of the cultural symbols which are constructed through the feminine rooted in Hindu iconography, but in her deconstruction of the symbolic representations as Nielsen's emphasis reveals the apparatus that regulate them.[16] Instead of playing into what is seen as Indian identity markers which are easily commodified within the global market, the emphasis on gestures refuses the inclusion and hence is allowed to play with 'deconstructions' to create a range of counter representational symbols in Maya's performance.

Notes and References

1. Sandhya Purecha, *Theory and Practice of Anglika Abhinaya in Bharata Natyam*, Mumbai: Bharatiya Vidya Bhavan, 2003. (This is just one of the numerous research which looks at gestures and other such intricate idioms of Indian classical dance forms. This genre of research is popular amongst practitioner-scholars.)
2. Utpal Dutt, 'Sisir Kumarer Abhinay Prasanga' (About Sisir Kumar's Acting), *Epic Theatre*, vol. 1, no. 6, Calcutta, 1989.
3. Sova Sen (1917–) is one of the leading figures of Bengali progressive amateur theatre. She started her career with the Indian People's Theatre Association (IPTA) in the epoch-making play *Nabanna* (Harvest) (1944) and went on to be the lead actress in the Little Theatre Group and subsequently the People's Little Theatre.
4. Joachim Fiebach, 'A German's Reading of Brecht in 2004: Gestus, Dialectic, Productivity', in *Bertolt Brecht: Performance and Philosophy*, ed. Gad Kaynor and Linda Ben Zvi, Tel Aviv: Tel Aviv University Press, 2005, pp. 53–68.
5. The adaptation *Himmatmai* was directed by Fritz Bennewitz and the performance was staged only once at Gorki Sadan, Calcutta, on 10 February 1987.
6. Lara D. Nielsen, 'Introduction: Heterotopic Transformations, The (Il) Liberal Neoliberal', in *Neoliberalism and Global Theatres: Performance Permutations*, ed. Lara D. Nielsen and Patricia Ybarra, London: Palgrave Macmillan, 2012, p. 8.
7. Anuradha Kapur in a class lecture at the School of Arts and Aesthetics (SAA), Jawaharlal Nehru University (JNU), New Delhi, on 1 March 2012.
8. Nicholas Ridout, *Passionate Amateurs: Theatre, Communism, and Love*, Michigan: University of Michigan Press, 2014, p. 35. See also Nielsen, 'Introduction', p. 2.
9. Kathakali was one of the four dance forms which were given 'classical status' in the first phase (1960s). It's a theatrical stylized form from Kerala depicting narratives from the epics. It has been an area of interest for scholars from performance studies as an authentic Indian theatrical form (Phillip B. Zarrilli, Farley Richmond, Richard Schechner).

10. 'Down stage' refers to the side of the stage that is closest to the audience.
11. *A Deep Fried Jam*, a very popular solo performance by Maya Rao, premiered in 2002, the comic performance of which is very typical of Maya's performance style.
12. Bishnupriya Dutt, 'Performing Resistance with Maya Rao: Trauma and Protest in India', *Contemporary Theatre Review*, vol. 25, no. 3, 2015, pp. 371–85.
13. Nivedita Menon, *Seeing Like a Feminist*, Delhi and London: Zubaan-Penguin, 2012.
14. West Bengal, the eastern state of India, had a left democratic party (Communist Party of India, Marxist) controlling the state legislative assembly from 1977 to 2014.
15. *Non-Stop Feel-Good Show*, 15 January 2013.
16. Nielsen, 'Introduction'.

7 Moving from the Temple to the Studio-Space

Transformation of the Woman Dancer's Labour in Films

PRIYANKA BASU

Introduction

> It is the nature of women to seduce men in this world; for that reason the wise are never unguarded in the company of females.
>
> —(2/213)
>
> One should not marry women who has have reddish hair, redundant parts of the body [such as six fingers], one who is often sick, one without hair or having excessive hair and one who has red eyes.
>
> —Hirday N. Patwari, 'The Status of Women as Depicted by Manu in the *Manusmriti*', *Nirmukta*, 27 August 2011. (3/9)

The *Manusmriti*, a scripture of 2,690 verses divided into 12 chapters and deemed as the manual of Brahminical practices within Hinduism, elaborates at length on the nature and role of women. While servitude, obeisance, conformation, and appeasement towards the man—the brahmin—is the recurrent theme and dominant voice in the manual, the elaboration on the nature/feature of 'bad' women is noteworthy. The two tenets quoted here exemplify: (1) the character of the woman as a seductress; and (2) the list of physical aberrations that segregates the 'bad' woman from the 'good'. Manu's statements on the ideal action and role of a 'pure' brahmin even extend to such warnings as not seeing a woman applying collyrium to her eyes; not seeing a nude woman massaging her body or delivering a child; not seeing a woman having her meal; and not seeing a menstruating woman. Such acts, as is clear from the way they are enumerated in the manual, involve witnessing the actual physical 'excess' in women's action as opposed to their defined and routine roles of chastity, calmness, and bondage. Although, the manual does not seem to indicate who these aberrant women are, the six qualities of bad women—'consuming liquor, association with wicked persons, separation from her husband, rambling around, sleeping for unreasonable hours and dwelling'[1]—hint at the bad woman as the one capable of transacting her body or engaging in sexual gratification. It is, therefore, not unlikely that such aberrant women were engaged in the connected labours of sexual work and performance.[2] Unsurprisingly, then women have also been grouped together with other marginal entities such as low-caste individuals (engaged primarily in manual labour) in the scripture.

The segregation of women into chaste and aberrant and the consequent erasure of their presence in socially visible spaces have now been historically proven. Sandra M. Gilbert and Susan Gubar, in elaborating on this erasure and silence of female creativity, have shown how instead women were idealized as 'the chaste maiden in her passivity'.[3] Elizabeth A. Clark, in writing about women and gender in the study of Christian history, points towards the Gregorian Reforms of the late eleventh and early twelfth centuries which ensured that the Catholic church became a 'women-free space', thus highlighting their demotion.[4] On the other hand, this erasure and silence on the woman subject paved a way for colonial nationalists in the nineteenth century to construct the Vedic age as a golden period of women's presence. It allowed harbingers of cultural nationalism to place the woman subject in complementarity with the ideal of the nation as the mother.[5] This deferment of women's histories, by segregating her into 'good' and 'bad', by expunging her from sociocultural practices/spaces, and, further, by reinstating her in accordance with a nationalist ideal, has urged the writers of feminist histories to venture back and 'trace' the past in written documents. Walter J. Ong justifies this act of tracing by stating how 'the shift from oral to written speech is essentially a shift from sound to visual space'.[6]

The visual space of the written word, as Ong emphasizes, is set in superiority against the oral field: '[W]ords are grounded in oral speech, writing tyrannically locks them into a visual field forever.'[7] Performance, as we know, primarily belongs to the field of the oral; it is ephemeral, difficult to document and hence fragmentarily archived.[8] How do we then place cultural practices of performances as potential archives of rewriting women's histories, especially that of performance histories? Dutt and Sarkar Munsi have shown how the binary between the dramatic text (the domain of the female actor) and the body text (the domain of the woman dancer) was upheld by the colonial discursive practices.[9] The relationship between the written text and performance (body) text being thus underlined, can we then extend this binary towards the understanding of feminine space and cultural labour vis-à-vis performance. It is here that I wish to explore dance and the woman dancer in films and television as functioning between historical stigmatization and the production of new gendered spaces of labour. Within the world of performing arts, dance is fraught between the tension of marginalization and gentrification. The segregation between 'classical' and 'non-classical' dance practices is indicative of this tension, not only in terms of their gendered spaces of practice but also in relation to the cultural labour of the performer. This chapter relooks into the segregation of the classical and the non-classical in order to understand the issues of feminine space and cultural labour. It then discusses the extension of this segregation and the presence of this feminine space in other media such as films and television. Further, it focuses on conceptualizing feminine space within dance by looking into the existing literature and validating it through examples from dance practices in the new media. In conclusion, this essay returns to the segregation between masculine and feminine spaces in order to understand how current dance practices are still informed by historical sensibilities and yet how the popular realm is constructed and construed in relation to its classical counterpart. The following section begins by considering the classicization of Indian dance forms as culturally elevated from the non-classical and how the body text of the woman dancer is carefully reconstructed in order to pronounce this difference.

The Classical and the Non-Classical: Body Text, Feminine Space, and Cultural Labour

The question of colonial modernity in the nineteenth century and the vociferous social reforms in the early twentieth century were crucial in segregating the space of the woman dancer as 'chaste' and 'unclean'. The 'polluted' body of the woman performer, especially those tied with the labour of performance in temples such as the devadasis (in southern India) and maharis (in Orissa), needed to be separated from the ideal of the woman as the representation of the nation. However, much of the stigma against these temple dancers ensued from the stereotype of the woman performer as also engaging in sexual labour within the precincts of the temple. Reformists, therefore, endeavoured to abolish not only the ritual cultural practices that were linked with the initiation of young girls into the dedicatory performance sphere of the temple, but also the cultural worlds of the performances themselves. In the context of the devadasi tradition in India, Amrit Srinivasan, Saskia C. Kersenboom, and Davesh Soneji have indicated that the social status and cultural labour of the devadasis in south India was much more complex than the general stereotype of the 'dancer as prostitute'.[10] In fact, Soneji considers the status of the existent devadasis as strongly informed and influenced by the discontinuities in the process of history writing and infused by an incompleteness. He writes: 'The loose ends of the moralizing projects of colonial and postcolonial modernity, a dance aesthetic that has lost its value, and incipient possibilities of citizenship for *devādasīs* are all emblems of the unfinished pasts of *devādasīs* in South India.'[11]

What was, however, the past social standing of the devadasi from which she came to be drastically removed and relegated to a stigmatized perception? Soneji offers an outline of the social constitution and work of the devadasis as they used to exist. He writes how devadasis:

> [H]ave functioned as courtesans, secular dance artists organized in guilds called *mēlams*, and temple workers, some of whom performed in the public spaces of certain Hindu temples. However these communities have always occupied an ambiguous status in South Indian society. On the one hand, *devādasīs* possessed a degree of social agency in that they were not restricted by the norms of patrifocal kinship. They lived in quasi-matrilineal communities, had nonconjugal sexual relationships with upper caste men, and were literate when most South Indian women were not. On the other hand, records from centers of political power such as the court of Tanjore in Tamil Nadu document the fact that courtesans were commodities regularly bought and sold through the intercession of court. In other contexts, as the concubines, mistresses, or 'second wives' of South Indian elites, they were implicated in a larger world of servitude focussed on the fulfilment of male desire.[12]

It is important how the cultural status and labour of the devadasi as secular artists organized in guilds, as temple workers, and as literate women gets lost under the stamp of prostitution. Perhaps it is here that the separation between cultural/performative labour and sexual labour becomes pronounced and the latter supersedes the former in framing the dichotomous identity of the dancer. While the Madras Devadasis (Prevention of Dedication) Act (1947) criminalized the social, ritual and aesthetic practices of the devadasis, Bharatanatyam emerged as the classicized idiom of Indian dance, purging it of the stigma of temple dancing.[13] The classical dance form under institutional patronage and the guidance of evidently male gurus extricated the dance of the devadasis to shape a new dance which came to be contrasted with the non-classical. The strictures and erectness of posture, gesture, dress code, and positioning on a performance space conceived of as sacred retained only a few vestiges of the cultural practices of the devadasi; the stigma associated with the art of the temple dancer negated and deferred the conceptualization of her cultural/performative labour.

In the case of female musicianship, as Wolf puts it, practitioners are more local and under-represented in relation to their male counterparts:

'Female musicianship is, in some traditions, associated with domesticity; in that realm, women are more "local" in the limited sense of less in the public eye, less geographically expansive in their influence, and so forth.'[14] This connection of domesticity with the respectable and chaste performer can be seen to oppose the fact that certain social environments are detrimental to women; women performers who enjoy a certain mobility, access and itinerancy in relation to respectable domesticity are deemed as 'fallen' and 'public'. As de Bruin writes:

> The social stigma on female performers is perpetuated by the contexts and conditions in which they are presented on stage and the circumstances of their work: this may be the location/neighbourhood where they perform, their lifestyles and modes of travel (including a (semi) nomadic existence), the physical set up of the performance area, ways of costuming and conventional gesture and body language used on the stage.[15]

Both the context of the space and that of labour (or work) are vital to the perception of the woman performer as respectable or 'fallen'. In the case of dance and within the binary of classical *v.* non-classical, the issue of spatiality produces the binary between the 'good' woman dancer and the 'bad' woman dancer; more access to the public space—the predominantly male arena of viewership—exposes the woman dancer to the stigmas of prostitution, thus marginalizing her cultural/performative labour. While the parameters of mentoring in the repertoire of classical dance consciously uphold the realm of the classical as a feminine space, the non-classical or the popular is comparatively threatening due to public gaze. Within this realm of the public gaze, which directly influences the way in which the woman dancer uses her body as text, the demarcation between classical and non-classical comes into play. For example, if we consider the style in which Bharatanatyam is presented—its strict adherence to grammar, the non-excesses of bodily movements, geometrical stiffness of postures, the limitations imposed on the body by tying it down with costume/jewellery/bells—it is clear how, despite the public presence, endorsement and gaze, the woman dancer's body as a veritable text invites an adulation paired with respectability. If we understand this carefully crafted feminine space of the female classical dancer as generating a finished product in the performance, the cultural labour in the process of this production involves a cyclical structure where the mentor (guru), the woman dancer, and the public/audience are the primary actors.

What happens when we try to understand cultural/performative labour in terms of the 'non-classical' or popular dancer? Exposed outside the limits of the proscenium space of classical dance, the non-classical woman performer is faced with more competition from male counterparts and hence 'the way she moves' in dance translates either as 'obscene' or as 'masculine' for the audience.[16] Sanjay Srivastava shows how the voice of the courtesan posed a potential threat to the post-independence project of nationalism and how the innocent child-like voice of Lata Mangeshkar became emblematic of the feminine voice of the nation.[17] This feminine voice was further augmented by her persona of motherhood and her rigid posture onstage as she sang with her head buried in her notebook.[18] Contrary to this ideal feminine national voice was that of Shamshad Begum whose voice was ambiguous, i.e. neither male nor female. Such characteristics of the ideal feminine and the ambiguous relate equally well to the strict dichotomies of classical and non-classical in terms of dance. Despite the dichotomy, however, performative labour in the cultural market results more in competition than in exchange. Lazzarato, in writing about the construction of the cultural labour market, points out how the governing principle of the market is not exchange but competition: 'According to the neo-liberals, only inequality has the capacity to create a dynamics that stimulates the desires, instincts and brains of individuals and incites them to compete with each other.'[19] To understand this in relation to the classical and non-classical binary, we need to understand 'competitiveness' as a common denominator between the two broad domains of dance. I will come back to this issue of competitiveness in a market driven by cultural labourers, like the woman dancer, in the penultimate section of this chapter.

What is therefore the body-text in relation to the feminine space and cultural labour? The body-text might well be defined as the socio-historic processes under the effects of which the female dancer rewrites herself in dance. It is shaped both by the feminine space which the female dancer has come to occupy and the production of cultural/performative labour without which the body-text lacks representation. In the subsequent sections of this chapter, I engage with this relationship among feminine space, cultural labour and body-text vis-à-vis dance as it gets transferred from the liveness of the proscenium performance space to the mediated space of films and television. Following from the example of Bharatanatyam in the aforementioned discussion, the next section looks at the representation of the female classical dancer on popular screen and how the cinematic adaptation of a novel removes the reality of the female dancer from her context and liveness. I discuss the issues of this representation through two texts: *The Guide* (1958), a novel by R.K. Narayan[20] and its cinematic adaptation *Guide* (1965) directed by Vijay Anand.

'Misguided *Guide* and the Shifting Idioms of Devadasi Dance: A Case Study of R.K. Narayan's *The Guide* in its Cinematic Adaptation

'Two Indian Interviews' by Hans Beerman appeared in the summer of 1965,[21] featuring the views of Dr Sarveppalli Radhakrishnan and R. K. Narayan—one of foremost writers of the Indian English novels—in a question-answer format. This was only a couple of months after the cinematic adaptation of Narayan's much discussed novel, *The Guide*, was released in February 1965. The cinematic adaptation titled *Guide* featured Dev Anand and Waheeda Rahman and was directed by Vijay Anand. Narayan, evidently, was not happy with the rendition of his text and summed up his vexation in a much generalized sentence: 'Generally speaking, however, I am sick of movies.' The fact that the novelist was 'the unhappy author' provides us a cue to probing into the relation between the text of the novel and that of the film. However, given the limited scope of this examination I will not elaborate at length on the issues of cinematic adaptations and their 'faithfulness' to the original. Alternately, I choose to focus entirely on the woman dancer in the texts—Rosie/Miss Nalini—hailing from the devadasi practice in Tamil Nadu. I have, therefore, divided this section among the Rosie(s) of the two texts and would conclude by trying to answer a seminal question: was Rosie, the woman dancer, the cause of Narayan's annoyance towards *Guide*, the film; if so, how? By answering this question, which follows from understanding the movement of the devadasi from the space of temple-work to that of the discursive spaces of the novel and then the mediated space of the film, I present this section as an entry point into the concepts of gendered labour, industrial body, and feminine space addressed in the subsequent sections.

Within and Without the Temple: Rosie of the Novel with her Devadasi Past

The Guide centres on the relationships between Rosie, a woman dancer of the devadasi lineage; Marco, her archaeologist husband; and Raju, a railway guide. Beyond the socio-literary qualities of the text, *The Guide* can additionally be understood as a document on the historical processes of marginalizing performance traditions like those of the devadasis. If a reader-responsive criticism can be brought in to understand the text, Rosie can well emerge as the central protagonist of the text, a woman dancer who inhabits several spaces as her dance takes her: from the historic ritual connection with the temple to the urban proscenium spaces of respectable performances. 'The efficacy of the devadasi as a woman and dancer began to converge with the efficacy of the temple as a living centre of religious and social life-political, commercial and cultural.'[22] Srinivasan has further argued and shown how the breakage of the association with the temple leads the devadasi to her economic deprivation apart from the marker of the 'prostitute' preceding the resultant deprivations. Parker has also discussed how the 'crime' of 'dedicating girls to a life of temple-harlotry' was a pure judicial invention.[23] The loss of the temple signifies additionally the loss of the 'divine connection' for the *nitya sumangali* that once generated a wealthy class of patrons for her. If Narayan's novel is to be read as Rosie's case study, one cannot dismiss how she carries forward the traces of this 'divinity' of the past as well as the 'low status' that is continually underlined in metaphors of the serpent—the king cobra—producing repulsions both in her husband Marco and Raju. However, she is also the container of the 'tradition' of the Sadir—the predecessor of 'classical' Bharatanatyam—as Raju encapsulates the evolution of the classicization process in his exclamatory thoughts for Rosie: 'The greatest dancer of the century!'

The process of Sadir to Bharatanatyam is further taken up in the course of the novel after Rosie reveals to Raju her family's past—how her mother devised a different career for her following her schooling, a masters in economics, and her marriage with Marco, the archaeologist. If Rosie signifies the 'loss of the temple', Marco—who publishes *The Cultural History of South Asia* based on excavations at the Mempi Caves—signifies the 'revival'. 'There is', as Gayatri Chakravorty Spivak points out, 'a cultural bond between them in their passion for their cultural labour.'[24] There is a ritual bond between them as well—harking the devadasi way of life—in which Rosie proclaims herself as the 'good housewife' who should eat last. This ritual bond, however, does not sustain itself under the burden of the cultural bond within which each chooses his/her vocation—Marco, that of excavating caves and Rosie, that of excavating 'sacred' literature, thus the two of them forming an archaeology of knowledge. Their paths differ, however, on the question of the hierarchy of knowledge that prompts Marco to declare his vocation as a 'branch of learning' while Rosie's act of dancing is described as 'street-acrobatics'.

Spivak further points out how Rosie 'is not needed in the last phase of the book: the phase of ethnicity over culture' and because 'India is folk kitsch' and 'E.M. Forster had written the "Temple" section' in his *A Passage to India*.[25] But before her quiet exit from the novel before it ends, Rosie has accelerated and produced herself with the acquired name of

'Nalini'[26] as exhibiting a finished product called 'Bharatanatyam'. If Raju guide shifts roles from that of a tourist guide to Rosie's manager, Rosie shifts her idioms of performance. The 'loss of the temple' has ushered in the proscenium and the public for her. The stage is the 'recovery of the temple' where, as she reiterates, 'Lover always means God'. The two are juxtaposed and Rosie/Miss Nalini might conveniently step out of the text now.

Bharat Ek Khoj: Rosie of the Film with her '*Khandani* Devadasi' Past

'If the railway train as a harbinger of progress and class mobility is a cliché of the literature of imperialism, the *nautch* (dance) girl is a cliché of the imagining of British India.'[27] Further on, the nautch or the *naach* (in Hindi) acts as a reference frame in the 1965 film version—*Guide*—where devadasi becomes synonymous with the tawaif[28]and Rosie narrates: '*Meri maa ek khandani devadasi thi*' (My mother came from a family of devadasis), thus almost blatantly suppressing the synonymous tawaif in the sentence.[29] In a flashback Rosie is seen to practise Kathak in her devadasi household, mentored by her mother. Raju's mother, who is 'a good woman', listens to her narrative, thus sympathizing with the *bazari aurat* ('contaminated' woman). The 'contamination' is hinted at more poetically by Raju even as he becomes a manager to the growing Miss Nalini and says, '*Mujhe Rosie mein Nalini aur Nalini mein Rosie ki milavat nazar aati hai*' (I discern a contamination of Nalini in Rosie and vice versa). The cure for contamination is thus no better than *gangajal* (holy water of the Ganges) itself.

However, *gangajal* is only a metaphor in passing. Rosie's contamination is verbally warded off by Raju who harks names of reputed dancers—Uday Shakar, Shanta Rao, Balasaraswati—and their stories of prosperity through dance, which aligns Rosie along with them, since she comes from the *unchi jaati* (high caste). In response to Rosie's belittling of herself enmeshed in her lineage of shame, Raju declares: '*Tumhari jaati kitni unchi hai. Kalakaar bhand nahin hotey hai*' (You belong to such a high caste. High artists are not equal to pantomime performers). *Guide*, the film, is more about the *kalakaar* (artist) in hierarchical contrast with the *bhand* (pantomime performance), just as it is about the binaries of 'high' and 'folk' coexisting. The binary could not have been more visible and pronounced than the snake dance by Rosie who enquires about the *saperan ki basti* (dwelling of gypsy snake charmers) from whom she wishes 'receive' the *naagnritya* (snake dance). Niladri Chatterjee employs the phrase 'corpothetics of nation production'[30] which I choose to use herein in reading Rosie's receiving of the 'folk' mode and shaping it further (as Rosie in the novel had introduced variations in 'The Dancing Feet') in the process of representing the nation. Raju introduces her as 'Kumari Nalini' and describes her as an exponent of Bharatanatyam, Kathak, Kathakali, and folk dance. What follows from this introduction is a series of regional variations of non-classical/folk dance forms from Marathi *lavani* to Kathak and Manipuri in the song 'Piya Tosey Naina Laagey Re'. It is to be noted how Bharatanatyam does not feature anywhere here, apart from a few seconds of a practice session, within the great north-south divide that the film constantly asserts.

The top five films that marked the year 1965 in Bollywood were: *Waqt*, *Jab Jab Phool Khile*, *Himalaya ki God Mein*, *Arzoo*, and *Guide*. While *Jab Jab Phool Khile* and *Arzoo* remained high viewer favourites in representing Kashmir visibly as part of Indian territory, *Guide* attempted the unification of the Indian nation and succeeded at it. One must remember one of the earliest scenes from the film, with the paan-seller's publicity of the betel leaf where each ingredient comes from a different state: betel nut from Bombay, betel leaf from Calcutta, and catechu from Mysore, and Raju sums it up saying, '*Paan na hui, rashtriya ektaa ho gayi*' (This looks less like a paan and more like national unity). While Raju becomes the spiritual machinery in this attempt, Rosie/Nalini becomes the material. She has danced against backgrounds of ruins of temples, fortresses, and the Indian panorama, singing '*Kaaton se kheech key yeh aanchal/ Tod ke bandhan bandhoon payal*' (I shall disentangle my *aanchal* from the thorns/I will wear my bells breaking all hindrances). Bernadette Sweeney, in writing about the performing body and the space it occupies, shows how 'performance meets architecture in our perception of the body'.[31] She cites two examples:

> The use of public outdoor space as performance space where the architecture, designed for a different purpose, becomes inherent to the performance.
>
> The reading of architectural models, where performance facilitates architecture as, effectively, we corporealize the space in our imagined inhabitation of it.[32]

In transposing Rosie, an inherently south Indian protagonist by virtue of her devadasi lineage, to the architectural backdrop of a north Indian milieu, the film helps in erasing the connection that she has with Bharatanatyam. The architecture becomes as inherent to her performing body (representing the idiom of film dance) as she corporealizes it in order to convey the holistic image of the nation dotted with monumental history. Laura Mulvey writes about *fetishistic scopophilia* that draws the 'gaze' of the male viewer to the woman on screen and in the process fragments the female body.[33] Notably, however, Waheeda Rahman is never shown in fragments throughout the film; a potential reason behind such a cinematic motif might be to do with indicating juxtaposition of the woman dancer with the vastness of the cultural heritage that the nation is. Towards the fag end of the film narrative, when Rosie approaches a fasting Raju in Jaipur from London, she pulls off each of her jewels in the scorching heat of the desert, reaching the Swami in as much simplicity as possible. Since Rosie could not have been done away with in the film, as in the novel, she returns as the chaste and the domesticized. She does not need to dance hereafter since cultural India must now merge and be overshadowed by its spiritual/religious self—Swami Raju!

In another interview with R.K. Narayan in 1989, the author clarifies about the setting of his fiction—the Malgudi much familiar to him and beyond which he cannot attempt, given his geographical choices and limitations. Rosie is morphed into this setting while her namesake measures carefree dance steps in the north Indian landscape, both treading the tense terrain of the north-south divide—linguistic, geographical, national. The film could not do away with Rosie in the end, but it did do away with the essence of Malgudi—the author could not have been less 'unhappy' about this bit of 'shifting', 'misguiding'![34] In analysing the break between the novel's text and that of the film, I show how the movement of the woman (devadasi) dancer from the temple to the public perception is central to the understanding of the shifting demands of her cultural labour. By bringing in the case study of a fictional protagonist, Rosie, this section has tried to understand what constitutes her body text as she moves from the written discourse to the mediated space of films. In the following section I further discuss the embodiment of the feminine in mediated spaces by bringing in the concepts of gendered and affective labour vis-à-vis dance.

Spaces of Labour in Dance: From Hyperfemininity to the Manufacture of Industrial Bodies

The representation of the woman dancer as the skilful courtesan has seen a continuity through popular Bollywood films like *Pakeezah* (1972) and *Umrao Jaan* (1981, 2006) on the one hand, and through popular songs in films such as 'Jab pyar kiya to darna kya' in *Mughal-e-Azam* (1960) or 'Salaam-E-Ishq meri jaan' in *Muqaddar Ka Sikandar* (1978), or the more recent 'Maar dala' in *Devdas* (2002). Jhala, following from film historian Rachel Dwyer, underlines how the spectacle of the courtesan's body is presented in combination with the spectacle of the scenery, costume and jewellery.[35] In recreating the past glories of the Persian culture or the Awadhi court, the juxtaposition of cultural artefacts—silver candelabras, Islamic arches, Persian carpets, gushing fountains—with that of the courtesan underlines what we might understand as the hyperfemininity of the virtual body on the audience-consumer. Hyperfemininity can be understood as 'an exaggerated adherence to a feminine gender role as it relates to heterosexual relationships'.[36] Extending this definition of hyperfemininity to the popular onscreen representation of courtesan dance, we can say that dance, here, is enmeshed with the role of the female protagonist in the film. Hyperfeminine roles, as these courtesan films indicate, assert a feminine space within which the cultural labour of the female actor-dancer is held in sharp contrast to masculine portrayals. To bring back the example of the body-text of the dancer Rosie from the previous segment of this chapter, her feminine frame in the cultural labour of dance was used to point the magnanimity of the monumental cultural heritage. Likewise, in courtesan dances (as well as songs) in films, the feminine frame is held against the backdrop of cultural artefacts, but the space is more intimate so as to allow the effects of hyperfemininity (through facial gestures of the female dancer) to be more pronounced on the audience-consumer. Sadanand Menon says, on the production of affect through dance, 'To affect the audience, a certain set of skills, intensity and other factors are needed both in the performance and the content sense.'[37] Not only then would hyperfeminine gestures of the courtesan onscreen concern the intricacies of *abhinaya* (acting) in the dance but also focus on the emotive content of the lyrics, thus achieving a blend to affect the audience. Both the roles of the courtesan as a protagonist of the narrative and as a dancer are important in this sense.

How does hyperfemininity get transformed into manufactured industrial bodies? What changes does this transformation bring into the body text of the dancer vis-à-vis the feminine space and cultural labour? Consider, for example, the item number 'Anarkali disco chali' by Malaika Arora Khan from the film *Housefull 2* (2012). Malaika enters into the screen space dressed in the easily recognizable stereotype of the costume which has now come to be called the '*anarkali* dress'. As her slow-paced movements culminate into the refrain 'Chhod chad ke apni Salim ki gali/Anarkali disco chali' (Abandoning the dwellings of her own Salim /Anarkali ventures out to the disco), she tears open her costume to dance skimpily clad for the rest of the song. The change in appearance is marked by a sudden change in dance gestures—pronounced hip and chest movements and a signature step—with supporting male dancers in the background. The lyrics exhibit this transformation further:

Ek sitamgar ne mujhko deewaron mein chunwaya

Mere dil ki dhadkan pe lakh pehre lagwaya
Mujhko pyari azadi, qaid mein ab nahi rehna
Zulm zalim wahesi ka ab na mujhko hai sehna
Mujhko hip-hop *sikha de*
Beat *ko* top *kara de*
Thoda sa trance *baja de*
Mujhko ek chance *dila de*
Main ghoom loon, main jhoom loon.[38]

[A tyrant had once buried me behind walls
He put guards on my heart pining with love
I love my freedom, and don't want to remain confined
I will not tolerate oppressions any more
Teach me hip-hop
Put the beats on high
Put on some trance music
And let me have a chance
So that I whirl and whirl with it.]

Clearly, the song parodies the earlier popular courtesan dance number, 'Jab pyar kiya to darna kya' from *Mughal-e-Azam* by subverting the popular/mythical love story between Anarkali and Salim, and by allowing the item performer to assert her agency and sexuality in the lyrics quoted here. The item dance, though seemingly hinting at the hyperfemininity of the woman performer as the seductress, has crossed the hyperfeminine paradigm to become what we can understand as a manufactured industrial body under the process of affective labour.

The strategies of affecting the audience through dance performances in market-driven economies are multiple and varied in terms of the 'changing role of affective labor in the capitalist economy'.[39] Hardt explains how the development of Marxian and Freudian frameworks have contributed towards the conceptualization of affective labour as 'desiring production'.[40] He writes: 'On the one hand, affective labour . . . has become firmly embedded as a necessary foundation for capitalist accumulation and patriarchal order. On the other hand, however, the production of affects, subjectivities, and forms of life present an enormous potential for autonomous circuits of valorization, and perhaps liberation.'[41]

This duality of function of affective labour can be seen in the way industrial bodies of item dancers are manufactured in this era of hyperreality. Susan Leigh Foster in explaining the term 'industrial' in relation to Hollywood describes the characteristics of the industrial body:

The industrial body performs primarily on screen in music videos and in dance competitions, where it celebrates the assimilation of many local styles and flavors of dance into a homogeneous affirmation of youth and heterosexuality. The industrial body has acquired, with its expanding popularity, a more extensive training program, one that adapts quickly to new styles in fashion, movement, and activities in popular culture. Schooled in a mishmash of traditions, including hip-hop, Broadway jazz, and occasionally, ballet, gymnastics, tap, and martial arts, the industrial body is most concerned with its appearance from a front defined by the camera's position.[42]

Following from Foster's conceptualization of the industrial body, we can see how the body of the item performer is manufactured in order to transcend the hyperfemininity of the earlier women dancers (like the courtesans). This industrial body foregrounds a 'highly gendered sexiness. Every move endeavours to put forward the sexual vitality of the dancers as an integral part of their identity and as an important motivation for dancing.'[43] The industrial body is not only gendered but also disciplined and conditioned to negate that which is 'not-sexy' onscreen. Although transcending the hyperfemininity of gestures and focusing more on the conditioning of the body to manufacture a finished product for the audience-consumer, the female item performer still underlines a feminine space for the dissemination of affective labour. It is this feminine space which conforms to capitalist accumulation and patriarchal subjugation and valorizes the exposition of the body, thus generating a new body text for the screen. This body-text in a mediated feminine space combines both the text of the song that the item dancer embodies and the actual movements of dance which sells the dancer as a manufactured product. This move from hyperfemininity to the industrial body also asserts the bifurcation of space into feminine and masculine spaces of dance where dancers are expected to execute strict gendered moves. Not only does the heteronormativity of the feminine space of dance occlude female bonding, it also bleaks the possibilities of male inclusion in feminine spaces, e.g. the excess of male dancers aiding the female item dancer and vice versa, or the six- to eight-pack appearance of the male item dancer in exhibiting 'gendered sexiness'.

Conclusions

The town of Tatanagar boasts of a temple dedicated to Bollywood actress Madhuri Dixit who is worshipped as Durga.[44] Madhuri is deemed as one of the best dancers onscreen that Bollywood has ever produced. Storming the Bollywood film scenario in the 1990s and the 2000s, especially with her skill in the classical form of Kathak, Madhuri took a break from films only to make a comeback recently with an item number titled 'Ghaghra' in *Yeh Jawani Hai Deewani* (2013). Despite the prevalent idiom of the Bollywood item dance number, as it is generally viewed,

Madhuri's item number still reflected the hyperfemininity paradigm that she had deftly executed in several dances as the courtesan in earlier films. For the audience-consumer, Madhuri has thus remained locked in the hyperfeminine principle which requires to be reperformed even if it is an item number. It is possibly this hyperfeminine principle and the realization of the dancer-actress as not just an industrial dancer that accords her a space of worship in a temple. The hyperfeminine could produce the exemplary rather than the manufactured industrial body under affective labour which is more capable of simulating gendered sexiness.

This essay began with the historical segregation of women into 'chaste' and 'fallen', especially by virtue of physical excess. It then differentiated between the 'classical' and 'non-classical' paradigms, mainly through the available literature on the devadasis and Bharatanatyam. Following further from the classical and non-classical divide, this study addresses the stereotyped representation of the devadasi and the courtesan in Bollywood, primarily through the case study of *The Guide* and its cinematic adaptation. By elaborating on the concepts of hyperfemininity, affective labour, manufactured industrial body and feminine space, this essay has further tried to show how the present performances of the item number is held in a strict difference of cultural labour with that of the earlier courtesan dances. The passage of cultural labour onto affective labour (in item dance) indicates a transformation in the body text of the woman performer. Additionally, the passage from courtesan aesthetics in Bollywood dance to the item number highlights the performance of manufactured industrial bodies within capitalist economies and patriarchal orders on the one hand, and the valorization of exposition and liberation on the other.

The issues of labour, especially cultural labour in Indian dance practices, remain to be adequately explored in terms of the communities of female practitioners, their social standing, livelihood, performances, and as agents of transactions. To that extent, this chapter has attempted to outline some of the key concepts in relating gender, labour and space within the realm of classical and non-classical dance practices. While Bharatanatyam and Bollywood have remained the two main areas of enquiry in this study, the concepts of feminine space, body text, industrial body, hyperfemininity, and affective labour can be well extended to study dance in relation to other mediated spaces like television and new media, and creative and cultural industries as part of changing global economies.

Notes and References

1. See *Manusmriti*, 9/13, in Patwari, 'Status of Women'.
2. Note how the *Manusmriti* (9/18) debars women from reciting Vedic mantras during *namkarm* and *jatkarm* purely due to their lack of strength, impurity, and falsehood. Patwari, 'Status of Women'.
3. Sandra M. Gilbert and Susan Gubar, *The Madwoman in the Attic: The Woman Writer and the Nineteenth-Century Literary Imagination*, New Haven and London: Yale University Press, 2000, p. 40.
4. Elizabeth A. Clark, 'Women, Gender, and the Study of Christian History', *The American Society of Church History*, vol. 70, no. 3, 2001, pp. 403–4.
5. Uma Chakravarti, 'Whatever Happened to the Vedic *Dasi*: Orientalism, Nationalism and a Script for the Past', in *Recasting Women: Essays in Indian Colonial History*, ed. Kumkum Sangari and Sudesh Vaid, New Brunswick: Rutgers University Press, 1990, pp. 27–87.
6. Walter J. Ong, *Orality and Literacy: The Technologizing of the Word*, London and New York: Routledge, 2002, p. 115.
7. Ibid., p. 11.
8. Peggy Phelan, *Unmarked: The Politics of Performance*, London: Routledge, 1993; Matthew Reason, 'Archive or Memory?: The Detritus of Live Performance', *New Theatre Quarterly*, vol. 19, no. 1, 2003, pp. 82–9.
9. Bishnupriya Dutt and Urmila Sarkar Munsi, *Engendering Performance: Indian Women Performers in Search of an Identity*, New Delhi: Sage Publications, 2010.
10. Amrit Srinivasan, 'Reform and Revival: The Devadasi and Her Dance', *Economic and Political Weekly*, vol. 20, no. 44, 1985, pp. 1869–76; Saskia C. Kersenboom, *Nityasumangali: Devadasi Tradition in South India*, Delhi: Motilal Banarsidass, 1987; Davesh Soneji, *Unfinished Gestures: Devadāsīs, Memory, and Modernity in South India*, Chicago and London: The University of Chicago Press, 2012.
11. Soneji, *Unfinished Gestures*, p. 3.
12. Ibid.
13. See Avanthi Meduri, 'Bharatha Natyam: What Are You?', *Asian Theatre Journal*, vol. 5, no. 1, 1988, pp. 1–22, http://www.jstor.org/stable/1124019 (accessed 18 May 2016); Leela Venkataraman, 'Negotiating the Extremes: dance', *India International Centre Quarterly*, vol. 33, no. 1, 2006, pp. 93–102, http://www.jstor.org/stable/23005939 (accessed 18 May 2016).
14. Richard K. Wolf, ed., *Theorizing the Local: Music, Practice, and Experience in South Asia and Beyond*, Oxford: Oxford University Press, 2009, p. 22.
15. Hanne M. de Bruin, 'Contextualising Women and Performance in India: An Introductory Essay', in *Between Fame and Shame: Performing Women-Women Performers in India*, ed. Heidrun Bruckner, Hanne M. de Bruin and Heike Moser, Wiesbaden: Harrassowitz Verlag, 2011, p. 16.
16. In the case of female practitioners of *Kobigan* (a folk performance form in verse-duelling/musical contest in West Bengal and Bangladesh), the

onus lies on the woman to stand out as exemplary in competition with the male members. This is achieved in two ways: (1) by maintaining a respectability onstage (neatly pinned saree, erect posture, purity of speech) and (2) by exaggerated body movements (jumping, dancing, winking, or laughing aloud with fellow musicians). In the second case, the woman performer is most often deemed by fellow male performers and the audience as an 'unclean' woman.

17. Sanjay Srivastava, *Passionate Modernity: Sexuality, Class and Consumption in India*, New Delhi: Routledge, 2007, pp. 79–115.
18. Ibid., p. 89.
19. See Maurice Lazzarato, 'Construction of Cultural Labour Market', 2006, http://eipcp.net/policies/cci/lazzarato/en (accessed 9 October 2015).
20. R.K. Narayan, *The Guide*, London: Methuen, 1958.
21. Hans Beerman, 'Two Indian Interviews', *Books Abroad*, vol. 39, no. 3, 1965, pp. 290–4.
22. Srinivasan, 'Reform and Revival', p. 1870.
23. Kunal M. Parker, '"A Corporation of Superior Prostitutes": Anglo-Indian Legal Conceptions of Temple Dancing Girls, 1800–1914', *Modern Asian Studies*, vol. 32, no. 3, 1998, pp. 561–2.
24. Gayatri Chakravorty Spivak, 'How to Teach a "Culturally Different" Book', in *Selected Works of Gayatri Chakravorty Spivak*, ed. Donna Landry and Gerald MacLean, New York and London: Routledge, 1996, p. 239.
25. Ibid., p. 240.
26. Note how the word 'Nalini' is carefully chosen since it signifies a lotus, indicating low status by birth.
27. Spivak, 'How to Teach a "Culturally Different" Book', p. 240.
28. For a recent exploration on courtesan culture in India vis-à-vis the kothi performer, see Anna Morcom, *Illicit Worlds of Indian Dance: Cultures of Exclusion*, London: Hurst & Co, 2013. Morcom begins by understanding the representation of the courtesan, her social standing, and the stigma around her in the Bollywood film *Pakeezah* (1972).
29. Angma Dey Jhala, in tracing the journey of the princely *zenana* to cinema, writes: 'Women who had themselves lived in princely zenanas also became film actresses or brought their stories to the big screen.' Prominent examples in this respect are those of Mumtaz Begum, who featured in the 1925 Hindi film *Kulin Kanta*, and Sitara Devi, who became an actress in the 1930s. Angma Dey Jhala, 'From *Zenana* to Cinema: The Impact of Royal Aesthetics in Bollywood Films', in *Popular Culture in a Globalised India*, ed. K. Moti Gokulsing and Wimal Dissanayake, New York: Routledge, 2009, p. 145.
30. Niladri Chatterjee, 'Screening the Nation: *Guide* and the (Re)production of India', in *A Talent for the Particular: Critical Essays on R.K. Narayan*, ed. Raymond-Jean Frontain and Basudeb Chakraborti, Delhi: Worldview Publications, 2012, p. 140.
31. Bernadette Sweeney, 'Performing Body, Performing Space', *Building Material*, no. 8, Spring 2002, p. 30.

32. Ibid.
33. Laura Mulvey, 'Visual Pleasure and Narrative Cinema', *Screen*, vol. 16, no. 3, 1975, pp. 6–18.
34. Stephen R. Graubard and R.K. Narayan, 'An Interview with R.K. Narayan', *Daedalus*, vol. 118, no. 4, 1989, pp. 232–7.
35. Jhala, 'From *Zenana* to Cinema', p. 146.
36. Melannie Matschiner and Sarah K. Murnen, 'Hyperfemininity and Influence', *Psychology of Women Quarterly*, vol. 23, no. 3, 1999, p. 631.
37. Quoted in Joshua Muyiwa, 'Unknotting, Uncrossing', *Ligament*, 2014, http://ligament.in/articles/unknotting-uncrossing (accessed 18 May 2016).
38. See http://www.indicine.com/movies/lyrics/anarkali-disco-chali-lyrics-housefull-2/ (accessed 20 May 2016) for the full lyrics of the song.
39. Michael Hardt, 'Affective Labor', *Boundary 2*, vol. 26, no. 2, 1999, p. 89.
40. Ibid.
41. Ibid., p. 100.
42. Susan Leigh Foster, 'Performing Authenticity and the Gendered Labor of Dance', *Fluid States—Performances of Unknowing*, 4 June 2014, p. 5, http://www.fluidstates.org/article.php?id=57 (accessed 18 May 2016).
43. Ibid., p. 6.
44. On the concept of performative fan-bhakti at the Madhuri Dixit temple, see Shalini Kakar, '"Starring" Madhuri as Durga: The Madhuri Dixit Temple and Performative Fan-Bhakti of Pappu Sardar', *International Journal of Hindu Studies*, vol. 13, no. 3, 2009, pp. 391–416.

PART III

Choreographing the Space: Identity and Creativity

8 Writing her *Dance*, Dancing her *Self*

Auto-Choreographs from Bengal

AISHIKA CHAKRABORTY

> No woman has ever told the whole truth of her life . . . The autobiographies of the most famous women are a series of accounts of outward existence, of petty details, and anecdotes which gives no realisation of real lives. For the great moments of joy and agony they remain strangely silent.
>
> — Isadora Duncan, *My Life*

Concurring with Duncan, I will, nonetheless, decline to shed those 'petty details' and 'anecdotes' as I seek to recapture a dancer's life that comes out 'strangely silent' on the 'great moments of joy and agony'. I return to those unuttered 'half-truths', as bits of those lies, I argue, make up her inmost self as well as guide us into the 'realisation of real lives'. And, without binding and unbinding those long loose yarns, 'How can we know the dancer from the dance?'[1]

Introduction

'If I want to talk about *Navanritya*[2] I have to narrate the entire journey of my life—how I have become a dancer all through my life. I cannot remember a day (though) when I was not dancing.'[3] As a contemporary Indian dancer-choreographer Manjusri Chaki-Sircar (1934–2000) offers the clues herself in her autobiography *Nrityarase Chittamama*.[4] To read her 'story' in tandem with her 'dance' and vice versa, I set out to interweave her autobiography in dialogue with her danced oeuvre. I read her story as a signature of her self in the moving space and as a testimony of a new woman's life who danced out her resistance against the hegemonic mainstream cultural diction. Did she want to suggest, like another legend of modern dance, 'From the first I have only danced my life'?[5] How much of her 'self' did she etch out on paper and how much was left to be represented on stage? If her dance stays with us as a

*The chapter is part of my ongoing project on contemporary dance in Bengal funded by IFA, Bangalore, India.

staged representation of herself, as her 'auto-choreo-graph', to borrow the expression from Ann Cooper Albright, then how do we, her readers and her audience, entangle and disentangle the joined and juxtaposed inscriptions from her multiple and multilayered, written and bodily, texts? An exuberant storyteller, what 'personal' experience did Manjusri hide from her readers and which part of her life did she decide to make 'public'? This essay looks at the 'body' of her 'writing', taking both inscriptions as a discursive site to explore her feminist-resistive politics.

Written during the last years of her life, Manjusri's book was rushed into publication a month after the suicide of her danseuse daughter Ranjabati Sircar (1963–99), a tragedy that numbed all her emotions, killing her before her actual death. Overtaken by a series of personal disasters, the memoir, not surprisingly, suffers from slippages, showing cracks from within and lapses in continuities. Before amnesia took over her remarkable memory, she started recollecting events, losing the threads somewhere in between, and then painfully realizing that her incurable renal disease had damaged her vision beyond repair. While signing out herself from the stage of life, Manjusri hurriedly finished the manuscript. Released in the Calcutta International Book Fair (January 2000) by a lesser-known publisher, the book is slipshod, an inadequate tribute to a stunning dancer-scholar who once proudly personified academic and aesthetic elegance.[6]

Manjusri took a painful exit in June 2000. She left behind a thriving legacy of a contemporary dance movement and a life story wrapped up in ninety-four pages. Where does her story begin and how does it end? In search of an answer, I leaf through her story, stepping backward and forward in time, crossing those critical moments of displacement, the uprooting(s) from home(s), and shifting across borders. I locate her within and against many journeys of other dancers to see how their initials vary from each other. Finally, to read her dance alongside her written text, I study her signature piece, *Tomari Matir Kanya* (Daughter of your Earth) which, among many, stood for what Manjusri wanted to say about herself and about her choreographic politics on a woman's body and women's movements. Overlapping and merging 'the body of her writing with the writing of her body', I explore how dancing can at once 'set up and upset' the various frames of her self and how closely intertwined with its own physical reality is the 'self' of her dance.[7]

Nrityarase Chittamama: Living with Dance

(In Pabna) . . . as a little girl, I appeared in the role of Srimati in (Tagore's) *Pujarini*. A saffron *ghagra* (long flowing skirt) was tailor-made for the last song, '*namo hey namo*' (I worship you my Lord) . . . But at the final act, in a beautifully lit-up stage, my knickers came rolling down to my feet under the *ghagra*. I could not get up to finish the act. Oh, how did I forget, on my way from the school, I tied its strings on the branch of a tree to create a swing.[8]

Maybe one day, for some obvious reasons, I would have to stop dancing by the age of 11–12. This was however not to be. Partition happened and we were forced to relocate in Calcutta. Leaving behind the sprawling house with ten big and five small rooms our family took refuge in a small room in Suren Banerjee Road, Calcutta . . . The Riot broke out shortly after . . . What sustained me to endure through such distress was . . . my dance.[9]

In 1954–55, I got a job of a part time lecturer in (Bengali Literature) in (Calcutta's) South City College. One day, one of my (male) colleagues enquired, 'Are you a professional dancer?' I fumbled, '. . . Yes, I . . . dance'. Another cracked in, 'why are you here? Dance is your actual profession' . . . It seemed that dancing as a professional was despicable indeed . . . Anyway, I lost my job within a few months.[10]

In 1955, I applied for a fellowship in the *Sangeet Natak Akademi* in the *creative* dance category. (In spite of my long training in classical forms) I decided to go beyond the classical . . . My take was on Tagore, which I choreographed far beyond the (run-of-the-mill) *Rabindrik* style!
. . . I could not get the scholarship.[11]

In America, my sponsors wanted me to showcase the pure Indian Classical before the Western audience. In the first half, out of harm's way, I personified the 'veritable Radha'; after the break, I slipped into a contemporary garb fleshing out the radical bodies of Tagore.[12]

(At) the *East West Dance Encounter* (1985) . . . we staged *Tomari Matir Kanya*, a take-off from Tagore's *Chandalika*. The panel . . . roundly disparaged my approach as pre-modern and passé (discarding Tagore dramas as old hat) . . . While Chandralekha and Kumudini Lakhia championed non-literal contemporary form changing and challenging traditional vocabularies of Bharatanatyam and Kathak, my synthesis of several physical traditions did not seem to hold water. Back home, in Kolkata conversely, and the orthodox *Rabindriks* accused me of reckless departure from the nostalgic thirties.[13]

In 1994–95, I was awarded the Sangeet Natak Akademy award, the highest state recognition for my contributions in creative dance.
I had to wait for forty years to achieve that.[14]

I begin by quoting in her 'own' words, some lows and some highs, weaving various patterns of her life moments. To trace her voice and her subjectivity, I shift my attention from her 'body' per se to the historic and gendered identities that shaped her idiom, seeing her embodied politics as an 'invasive repertoire' of her life patterns, flowing through the social, the political and the personal.[15] Weaving her many fractured selves into one continuous whole, through an intra-texted double reading of her life and dance, her autobiography presents a 'daunting progression' of her self across time and space.

Born on 28 August 1934 in Murshidabad, Bengal, Manjusri Chaki-Sircar spent her childhood in Pabna (now in Bangladesh); but she rose to prominence in the 1950s as a 'creative' dancer in post-independence Calcutta. A feminist, an anthropologist and a dancer with her self-invented idiom, her journey meandered through seminal political moments of Indian history, baring open the political tensions of her time, living and getting through the cultural and sexual politics of the new nation. She told many tales in her story; and a host of stories remains untold. Dislocated by the Boundary Commission's Awards, her narrative met an abrupt disjunction when the idyllic village life was marred by a sudden disfigurement in the political map, forcing a mass exodus to 'India' from 'East Pakistan'. Earning independence at the cost of a triply-sliced, riot-stricken nation, her family joined the endless stream of refugees to take shelter in a dingy room in central Calcutta. Riots, mayhem and expatriation—to the girl of 14 this was what freedom meant. Yet partition was a 'saving grace', her book comes unscathed by the melancholic languor over lost lands, as Manjusri geared up to take in the air of the city, crossing over new realms.

Evincing many shades of coloniality and postcoloniality, Manjusri's idiom was evolved from the fickle culture-scape of Bengal before travelling to Africa and America, the artistic encounters that further changed her dance lines. Exposed to a variety of physical traditions, from classical to folk, from the Bolshoi Ballet to Martha Graham's 'Cave of the Heart', from the Third Theatre Movement to the parallel cinemas, Manjusri embodied what we now call 'glocal', written all over her auto-(choreo)-graphs. She gushed about her duet ventures with the maverick singer Debabrata (George) Biswas, evading the buzzing rumour that hogged the duo, tied in a bond of controversies on and off stage. 'Sleepless' after 'watching Uday Shankar's *Kalpana*, Manjusri was silent about her rejection at the audition of Shankar's company for being 'too tall to join the chorus' as she did not write anything about a similar rebuff at Tagore's Visva-Bharati, Santiniketan. These are the rejections that kick-started an untried, alternative third—a dance that arguably signalled a paradigm shift in the proximate dance movements of her time, deviating sharply from the colonial modern, from the 'household' *Rabindrik* and the neo-classical creative.[16] Winning a battle against cancer, the sexagenarian dancer was elated to receive the prestigious Sangeet Natak Akademi Award for her creative dance. Basking in success, she hushed up the quivering defeats of life, distancing her life from her life story (Plate 8.1).

But, then, why should we expect an open and a straight self-representation from a woman assuming her life should run as a seamless narrative? Why must a woman autobiographer always don the status of the 'truth-teller' while writing her story? Why should the romance of

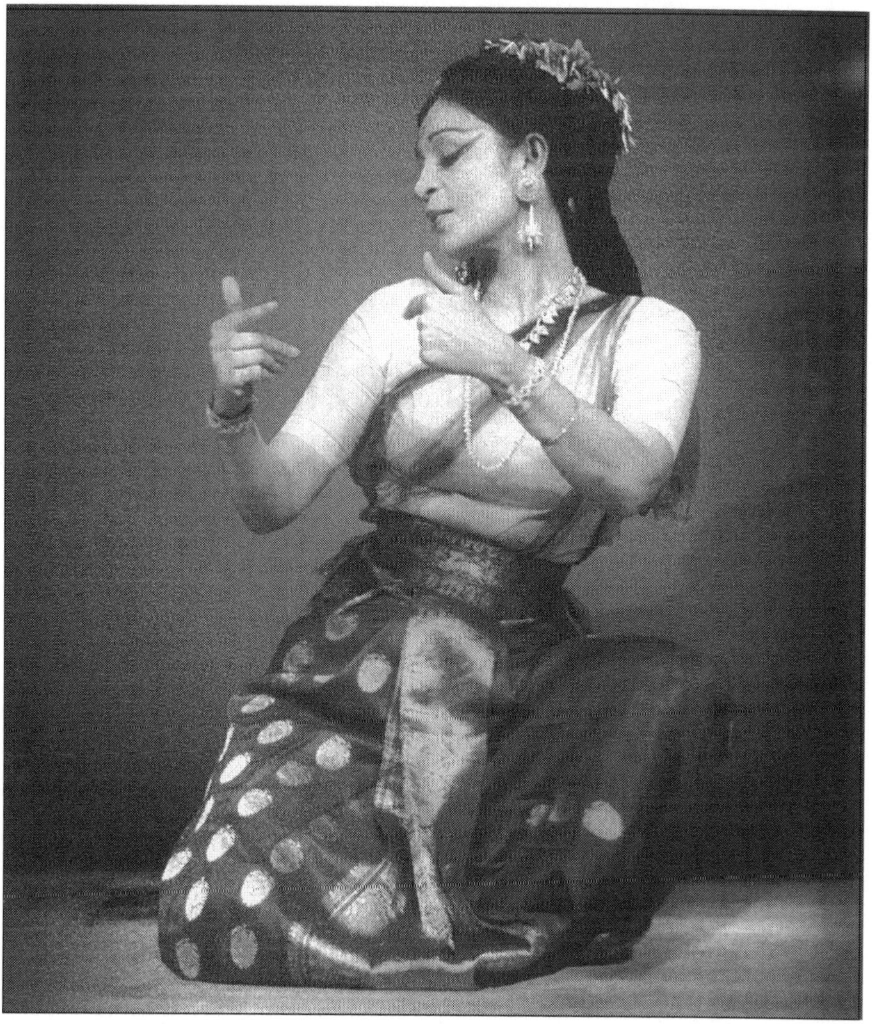

PLATE 8.1: Experimenting with Gestures to Create her Innovative Language of Dance: Manjusri Chaki-Sircar
Source: Courtesy of Dancers' Guild, Kolkata.

an 'authentic' female voice, as Julia Kristeva raised her doubts, remain unmarred by 'lies', not to be interrupted by 'periodic eruptions of the semiotic and the irrational'?[17] Moreover, is there any 'essential, original, coherent autobiographical self'[18] before the moment of self-narrating, before 'making and unmaking of identities'?[19] Judith Butler has already described autobiographical storytelling as a 'performative occasion'.[20] According to Paul Eakin, life story is 'a construct of a construct' and 'a story of a story'.[21]

What happens if even that 'story' is disrupted halfway? How can Manjusri write 'her story' when dialysis started eating into her memory making total recall almost impossible? But then Sidonie Smith quickly reminds us that 'autobiographical narration begins with amnesia and once begun, the fragmentary nature of subjectivity intrudes'.[22] Moreover, the autobiographer has to juggle continuously with the multiplicity of identities—from the bodily to the written, with 'the I before the text, the I of the narrator and the I of the narrated subject'. For the self is not a documentary repository of all experiential history as the very sense of 'self' as 'identity' derives paradoxically from the loss of consciousness.[23] The narrator adjusts, redeploys, resists, and transforms discourses of autobiographical identity; an identity which, according to Benedict Anderson, cannot be 'remembered', but must be 'narrated'.[24]

Speaking Bodies, Scripting Lives

Martha Graham, who once popularized the aphorism that 'movement never lies', defended many half-truths in her life story saying: 'Truth. What is so wonderful about telling the truth? Anyone can tell the truth. It's boring.'[25] Indeed, dancers enjoyed transforming and recreating the 'truth', harking back to the 'forgotten' past, setting the memory down on paper, sometimes transmuting, sometimes suppressing it.

In Bengal, since the late nineteenth century, a plethora of reminiscences had been penned by women writers, the first being authored by a half-literate housewife, Rassundari Devi. Many followed suit, including an 'educated prostitute', Manada Devi; a penniless widow, Nistarini Devi; and the celebrated theatre artist, Binodini Dasi.[26]

Though Bengali dancers were rather late in showing up 'live' on the autobiographical stage, quite a few marked their entries with an emphatic thumping by the next century. Passionately documenting their artistic-aesthetic experiences, their reminiscences charted the historic journey of the middle-class *bhadramahilas*, the 'amateur' performers who took the first steps forward at the inaugural moment of Indian modern dance. By that time, the stage was reclaimed in terms of honour and morality as the colonial elite and administrators joined hands together to cleanse it of the 'undomesticated' dancing girls. In Bengal, as the curtains went up at Jorasanko Private Theatre under the auspices of the Tagores, respectable women made cautious entries as dancers-performers in their home productions. Soon the embarrassed steps ran footloose in open prosceniums and then to the public stage before appearing on celluloid in the most volatile decades of India's cultural history. Writing her journey, from stage to page, Amita Sen was one of the first dancers at Rabindranath Tagore's school in Santiniketan who mapped, in succinct detail, the making of the transcultural and transnational dance language that evolved out of a spontaneous act of emotion into a structured theatrical movement, with changing arrangements of stage, props, and accessories.[27] However, dodging the limelight from herself, Amita zoomed into the persona of Tagore, the dance-maker, who scripted and choreographed the new rhythm of life for the 'new women' of his time, fleshing them out in his modern dance dramas. '*Nataraj* (the Lord of Dance) blessed the poet with the gift of dancing', thus ran Amita's opening lines; with him 'immortal dance was liberated from its fetters'.[28] Trailing her journey from small bit roles in *Natir Puja* to the heroine of *Shapmochan*, she detailed how movements were created by a continuous mixing and mingling of forms as 'Tagore was always eager to import to our *ashram* and teach us whatever impressed him by way of art and beauty'.[29] From the backstage chit-chat to on-stage thrills, Amita's experiential narrative raised many questions: what were the challenges involved in staging the new dance by new women who were suddenly exposed before the public eye? Did conservative society view public dancing by respectable women as a threat to middle-class sexual morality? If the dance triggered a 'new freedom movement' on stage, what were the 'scandals' of that 'freedom'?[30] While Tagore's politics of performance in making the alternative dance idiom remains understudied till date, many such queries remain unanswered too.

'I was not a dancer . . . I did not know anything about *dancing*', thus disclaimed Amala Shankar, the partner of Uday Shankar in his dance and life.[31] But when it came to her 'by chance', she hastened to recompose her nonagenarian frail body; it stayed as an extension of her 'inner soul', as a manifestation of her 'ego'.[32] *Saat Sagarer Pare* (Across Seven Seas), the travelogue written by Amala Nandi, went graphic in describing the incredible journey of a Bengali middle-class girl from Batajore, a small village in East Bengal, to Paris, accompanying her jeweller father, Akhoy Kumar Nandi, to attend the International Colonial Exposition (1931). She made a fortuitous debut as a dancer-cum-drummer in the troupe of the French Oriental dancer Niyota Inyoka. But her 'real' engagement with dance began only after she joined Uday Shankar's Company of Hindu Dancers, embarking on a landmark tour of Europe for eight months. She captured those eight months, describing in depth the seething stillness between the two world wars, the Great Depression, and the rising threats of Fascism. What's more, she experienced the making and unmaking of a brand of Indian modern dance that fulfilled and also outstripped the 'Oriental' imagination of the West, standing in sharp contrast to the Euro-American modernity. Her travelogue trailed the enormously successful dance experiments of Uday Shankar that exposed Indian women to a wider performative space across several geographic borders. Amala's story unravelled the style and repertoire, the challenges and promises thrown open by Shankar and his Almora centre—as an unmediated creative space in colonial India.

And if dance creations can be read as life stories of the dance-makers, how accurate was *Kalpana*, the film made by Uday Shankar (1948) as an auto-imagery of their lives? With running and un-bordered vignette of dance sequences, *Kalpana* screened dream and despair together in a clearly etched 'emotiongraph'.[33] 'The story', maintains Mohan Khokar in his exhaustive study of Shankar's life and dance, 'all too evidently a disguised autobiography of Uday Shankar'[34] not merely archived Shankar's imagination, but also his entire repertoire and his legacy. A blend of 'imagination and reality, of artistry and technique',[35] the movie was a performance of personal memories of Uday and Amala. Purkayastha is right when she says, *Kalpana* remained with us 'as a visual record of his own life and art'.[36]

During her later years, Amala Shankar spoke frank in a rather straightforward confessional narrative, *Shankarnama*, about her love, marriage and break-up with Uday Shankar. She rated Uday to be a romantic freethinker who looked like a demigod on stage and also an artist-polygamous who singlehandedly placed India on the world's dance map. Amala chose to break away from her husband with her two children, but continued to *own* the 'dance capital' of Uday. Even after separation from her husband she held together the ancestry of a century-old repertoire by recreating, repeating, and transmitting across generations the memoirs of Shankar's signature styles. In staging *Ramleela*, *Rhythm of Life*, *Sword Dance* or *Samanya Kshati* (The Minor Loss), Amala continued to make waves, literally, with her arms, sending ripples through her fingers across the frame of time/space. Her student, dance-scholar Urmimala Sarkar Munsi felt that the 'challenge posed by the newness of his open and free form', was ready 'to explore any theme, music or grammar' and cannot be boxed 'within any analysis of performative politics and politics of representation of that time . . .'.[37]

A rather self-congratulatory note came from *Shilpir Atmakatha* (An Artist's Mémoire), authored by Sadhana Bose, the renowned dancer-actress of twentieth-century India.[38] The granddaughter of the iconoclastic Brahmo reformer Keshub Chandra Sen, Sadhana (1914–73) was an iconoclast in her own way. At a time when public performance by women was defamed as a 'trade of prostitutes', wrote her sister Nileena (more popular as the *thumri* singer Naina Devi), all three daughters of barrister Saral C. Sen were self-avowedly 'social rebels'. Sadhana was not only 'exquisitely beautiful'[39] but also 'more mischievous', 'more knowing of the world outside Lily Cottage (their family residence) than her sisters'.[40] In 1930, Sadhana enchanted Tagore with her acting skill in the poet's own work, *Dalia*,[41] while her Manipuri-terpsichorean-gypsy in dance opera, *Alibaba*—directed by her actor-husband Madhu Bose—invited praise from none other than Anna Pavlova. But Sadhana shot to fame as Marjina, an 'overnight sensation' with the release of the film, *Alibaba*, that put her firmly on the map as a dancing star.[42] With a series of blockbusters to her credit, including *Rajnartaki* (Court Dancer), *Kumkum the Dancer*, *Meenakshi*, *Veeshkanya* (The Poison Girl), Sadhana went on to experiment with 'jazz and Latin American rhythms' in a 1952 super hit, *Shin Shinaki Boobla Boo*.

Sadhana never discussed her 'life', in its truest sense, which was evident from its representation. Her story has its visible black holes of absence, as she kept under wraps its underlying tensions. Waxing lyrical about her conjugal romance with Madhu Bose, the actress never spoke about her estrangement as her marriage turned out to be 'the most difficult' causing irreconcilable predicaments at the end. Transgressive of wifely norms of domesticity and dependence, Sadhana chose to live 'independently' opting for a 'childfree' career. By the end of her life she said to have earned 'Himalayan loads of scandals'; but her autobiography did not disclose why and how she earned them.[43]

Diagnosed with throat cancer, Reba Roychowdhury took up her pen to recall her vociferous experience as an activist-performer of the Communist Party of India. 'Those were the heady days', she remembered. 'From 1941 to the end of 1996, there was only work and work.'[44] 'When India was burning with flames of famine, riots and war, we staged *Voice of Bengal* (1944) in the huge ground of Marathi Centenary near the Church Gate Railway Station (Bombay).'[45] Participating in the cultural squad of the Indian People's Theatre Association (IPTA), Reba embodied the discipline, enforced by the party, celebrating creativity amidst austerity, counting hours of rehearsals as an extension of her 'party work'. 'Strict punctuality and rigorous discipline fundamentally changed our attitude towards life.' She detailed her every day:

> By 6 in the morning we queued to have one quarter of bread and one mug of tea. . . . The lunch was served at 10.30 AM sharp. We used to sit in a row to have our rice, *roti*, *dal* (pulses), *bhaji* (vegetable) and *chaas* (yogurt-based drink). For the evening tea we had to stand in a queue once again. Dinner was served at 6 PM.[46]

In between went on rehearsals, learning dance under Shanti Vardhan and fashioning costumes with artists like Chittaprasad.

IPTA enabled educated middle-class women to take up 'communal disciplined living and accorded a respectability and validation' to their activities, 'whereby many women, along with men, chose this form of cultural intervention as the means of communicating discontent or hope or protest'.[47] But, we may ask, were women allowed to question party leadership that 'avoided' gender-based power relations? Did they enjoy 'equal rights' as 'equals of men'? Or did the performance of revolution stop at the very doorstep of home? Though not searching for a complete picture of gender equality, Sarkar Munsi recognizes 'several signs of residue "male" orientation in the structure and function of the Communist movement' and yet acknowledges the 'space' opened and accorded to women by drawing them into public performance for such women who chose to join the mass movement by somewhat neutralizing the conservative bias.[48] A close reading of her life, evidently characterized by political correctness, would reveal that Reba Roychowdhury, a versatile performer otherwise, remained steadfast to the 'Party line' at every *stage*—both in public and in private.

But what happens when a labouring low-class woman, rising to the status of a public celebrity, forges new concepts of 'history and subjectivity' in order to publicize her culturally unsanctioned bodily identity? The recent publication of the autobiography of Calcutta's first Bengali cabaret dancer, Miss Shefali, interrogates the sexual double standard of the 'progressive' elite of Bengal who vouch for 'radical' 'socialist' egalitarianism and yet sternly ban and banish her 'dirty dancing' from the public space of commercial theatre and nightclubs on grounds of obscenity and immorality. Interrogating middle-class *bhadralok*'s political ethics she positions herself—her class, politics, and culture—in opposition to those of her elite readers: '*My* name is Arati Das, (but) *you* know me by the name of Miss Shefali. . . . There was a time when *I* was the reigning queen of Kolkata's nightlife. *I* started my day when *you* dozed off [emphases mine].'[49]

Returning the 'gaze' to her audience, the 'queen' of Calcutta's cabaret moves on to re-establish her links with her city: 'Here is my life; and here goes the cheesy scandal of Kolkata's mid-night leisure and pleasure.'[50]

Eleven-year-old Arati, the youngest daughter of a flat-broke refugee family from Narayangung (Bangladesh), readily accepted the job of a domestic help in an Anglo-Indian family of Calcutta's Chandni Chowk in lieu of 'bread and board'. Soon she was hired for a 'better job' as a cabaret dancer in Firpo's Hotel, with her salary fixed at Rs.700 a month. Holding the bikini blouse the girl broke down on the first night feeling ashamed of her bare body. But when her 'dirty' dancing salvaged her starving family, earning her wealth, property, and even 'respect', how could she keep crying? Shefali remained a spinster, not unsurprisingly, and had to claim aloud in her memoir: 'I am a dancer and not a prostitute.'[51] Bengali *bhadraloks* thought she was both, because she could not be one and not the other. How else could have the transactional exchange of dance transgressed the class/gendered norms of the genteel society?

With a twist in the tale, Shefali stepped out from the night club's ball to hit the stage of theatre, the hotbed of Calcutta culture, transporting her profane cabaret to the sacral space of the Bengali playhouse. This was the time when Calcutta witnessed a steady growth in the alternative (political) theatre drawing crowds in new theatre halls in southern and central parts of the city. But lights started going out in the old playhouses of north Calcutta's Hatibagan-Chitpur theatre *para* (area), now characterized by decrepit halls and seedy commercial entertainment.[52] In one desperate move to win back the audience to the 'theatre of pleasure', Rashbihari Sarkar, the owner of Circarina Theatre, signed up Miss Shefali, the reigning cabaret queen, packaging her erotic numbers in a series of popular bumper hits: *Chowranghee*, *Ashlil* (Obscene), *Asami Hajir* (Produce the Convict), and *Samrat O Sundari* (The King and the Beauty). Huge cut-outs of the cabaret dancer, in garish and skimpy bikini, covered north Calcutta's skyline, causing a kind of visual 'discomfort' to the office-goers in those busy streets. But because of the changing patterns of middle-class consumption these plays also became super hits, making the old Chitpur theatres successfully 'commercial', making them run 'houseful' once again. Miss Shefali, playing her life on stage, saved the commercial theatre, but at the cost of Bengal's most prized possession—its culture, its *kristi* and *sanskriti*.

Hence, 'accidental' fires broke out, 'caused by short circuit', eliminating the 'physical relics' of the old theatres of Calcutta. The moral drive of the state and intelligentsia forced out the immoral commercial theatre and with it, the cabaret dancers from the space of culture and performance, bringing to the surface a fascinating example of how high-minded art pushed down its lowbrow competition, which acquired a new name in the process—*apasanskriti* (decadent culture).[53] Published at a time when the Communist Party was just out of power after three decades of unbroken rule in Bengal, Shefali's subversive testimony vents out her wrath against the hegemony of law and moral policing of the erstwhile ruling elite that once banned her as a sexual outlaw, banishing her dance from the public space.[54]

Returning the body to herself, Manjusri Chaki-Sircar's life story is a record of a different journey, coming out of a different drive. Drawing up an unconventional vocabulary of dance in a distinctly personal/individualist style, she became a 'speaking subject' in the historically and culturally specific discourses of identity and politics. As Floyd Dell looked for 'the Magna Charta of feminism' on the dancing body of Duncan,[55] I look for a similar declaration of faith in Manjusri's moving bodyscapes. I can see how precisely her dancing body emerged as a 'site of struggle', to borrow from Elizabeth Dempster, 'where social and psychological, spatial and the rhythmic conflicts are played out and sometimes reconciled'.[56] But just as Victoria Phillips finds Graham 'uncontrollable' to be 'tapped' within their written texts and suggests to move beyond the 'fossilized patchwork' of life story,[57] I look for a fuller narrative of Manjusri's life by cross-referring to her danced oeuvre, where she repeatedly reiterated her self in her dance.[58]

But then merely the 'visual definition' through her dance does not offer us a straightforward equation of Manjusri's self. In reading Manjusri, one cannot just go along following Victoria Thoms who figuratively interlinked Martha Graham's *Blood Memory*[59] with *Night Journey* (1947) or emulate the way Blondell Cumming's *Chicken Soup* (1981) has been intra-texted by Albright as her auto-choreo-graph. But, following them, I can gather the 'accumulation' of several 'I's[60] that Manjusri repeated and reiterated in a series of dance dramas penned by Tagore, where she found her icons, the extensions of her selves. In constructing and sustaining her 'desired identity' she connects her story with the roles she played on stage, as the fearless court dancer who defied the royal religious order (Srimati in *Natir Puja*); the unloved courtesan, unapologetic of her crime and her love (Shyama, 1939); the warrior princess who claims the space as a physical equal of the hero, changing forever the definition of wife (Chitrangada, 1936); the primordial mother of an untouchable girl (Maya in *Chandalika* [published as a prose play and a dance drama in 1933 and 1938, respectively]); and the queen of the 'land of cards'(Ranibibi in *Tasher Desh* [1933]), who vetoes against the royal patriarchal order. Going inside each of these images—I borrow Albright's observation made in a different context—Manjusri danced some moments of their lives, portraying 'bits and pieces from all these women's lives'.[61] In the last section, I pick up her signature work *Tomari Matir Kanya* (Daughter of your Earth, 1985), where she choreographed an autonomous feminine space of untouchable mother-daughter, who negotiated and contested segregation, exclusion and coercion in defiance of the caste-gendered politics of Brahminic patriarchy. I examine how she autographed her journey in playing the fierce and strong sorcerer mother of a rebellious daughter (performed by her own daughter Ranjabati), weaving a tapestry of body memories accrued over myriad spaces of life, both emotional and geographical.

'Movement Never Lies': *Tomari Matir Kanya* as the Ultimate Autograph

> *Tomari Matir Kanya* comes as a radical interpretation, extrapolating Tagore's indictment against Brahminic Hinduism that religiously guards caste-hierarchy sanctioning untouchability into a feminist critique of the larger patriarchal politics and objectification of the female body. The dance drama hence translated an ancient Jataka story into a collective movement for social advancement.[62]

Evolved out of the Jataka story *Shardulakarnavadan* and the twentieth-century narrative verse *Chandalibhikshuki*, written by the Malayalam poet Kumaranasan, Tagore's prose-play and dance drama *Chandalika* takes a dramatic turn when, on a scorching summer day, Ananda, the Buddhist monk, accepts water from Prakriti, an untouchable Chandala girl. Breaking the taboo of her bodily pollution, she offers water from her 'impure' well, breaching the boundaries of caste and religion. Already charmed by the monk's serene beauty, Prakriti is overwhelmed by Ananda's egalitarian humanism. She falls in love with him and claims Ananda back to consummate her desire, compelling her mother to weave the magic of seduction. Merging Tagore's twin versions, Manjusri took almost three years (1984–7) to build her final dance text *Tomari Matir Kanya* (hereafter *TMK*) that emerges as her discernible signature on the stage of contemporary Indian dance.

As Helene Cixous urges women to resist their silencing by stealing the language of power to write *towards* the difference,[63] Manjusri deviates from the established lingo by writing of and from the body, transforming an ancient tale into her 'own' story, into a feminist text of resistance against Brahminic patriarchy. As Prakriti reaches out to a love proscribed, *TMK* turns into as a saga of collective resistance of the untouchable community against the hegemonic patriarchal order. While Tagore's *Chandalika* locates Prakriti as a solitary woman, put down within her shunned solitary space, Manjusri's choreography puts her at the centre, flanked and fenced by other untouchable girls, hence translating the individual's desire, deviance and rebellion into a collective movement of the oppressed. Prakriti's social marginality and her location at the fringe is more than compensated by the cohesive solidarity of the *chandal* women, the *chandalkanyas*, who always move in a body forming clusters, bonding and relating with each other. In

Manjusri's dance theatre, untouchables occupy and dominate the stage-space while upper-caste flower sellers and curd sellers, and even the Buddhist monk, act as theatrical interventions from outside, intruding and encroaching upon the space, which is 'ostracized', defined as the space of the untouchable. While flower sellers cover the stage with their conceited classical thumping, weaving geometric patterns in circles, triangles and diagonal lines across the stage, the untouchables sinuously flow all over. They roll on the floor, jump at ease, open up arms and throw legs in frontal and sidekicks. Wilfully transgressive of feminine demureness, they slacken the rigidity of structures with open pelvic movements, displaying a range of unrestricted vocabularies. They are shunned by all; but bond together in a synergic binding. They wriggle and huddle together in pain, but rise up in collective defiance against the Brahminic order.

In the story, Prakriti, in love with the monk, persuades her mother, Maya, a Tantrik priestess, to use her magical powers to charm and bring the monk back to her. Maya, after initial procrastination, encounters the ascetic oath of the Buddhist monk with a brutal aggression so as to defeat his sexual abstinence, taking on by extension not merely the religious ascendancy of the Brahminic-Buddhist priesthood but also the patriarchal system as a whole. Deploying her supernatural magic spell, the priestess-mother fiercely fights against Ananda's celibacy, seducing and dragging him to her daughter's desire, till she herself succumbs to her own spell.

But, displacing the romantic love plot from the centre stage, *TMK*, and also Chandalika, establishes the mother-daughter dyadic as the alternate, rather than central, theme of performance. The spatial relationship at the core of the narrative is between the home and the (community) well. The dyad at the centre is the untouchable mother and daughter. The well here becomes the signifier of ostracism of the women living at the bottom of the caste hierarchy and also stands as witness to the liberating moment of the outcaste girl. The two women decide and direct the course of the narrative as their dialogue-dance, though set within the home/well, transcending the private/personal sphere dare to defy the wider caste-gendered politics. Ananda, the monk, both as an ideological intervention and a romantic figure, moves in and out of the narrative, appearing in silhouette or even beyond the wings as an absent performing body. In an unpredictable choreographic move, Manjusri has not shown the only male protagonist on stage, rendering him 'invisible', hence working within/without a phallogocentric universe.

In enacting their roles, the real-life mother-daughter express an instinctive bonding, by clasping, clashing and clinching each other in moments of agony, anguish, and ecstasy (Plate 8.2). While the daughter goes wild in her desperation, hurling herself on the floor, tossing and flinging her limbs violently on stage, the mother stands firm with an uncanny smile on her lips. Surrounded by powerful bhairabis, Maya foregrounds herself as the 'centre', creating, crushing and thwarting thunder, fire, cloudburst and earthquake with her magical power. She invokes her tantra adepts with and against everything that is absurd and inane. When Prakriti jumps against the order in *utplavana* and *ullamphana*, and stretches out of bounds in *Mayurbhanja Chhau*, Maya weaves geometric patterns with classical *sthanaka vedas*, making cordons around her daughter, creating human chains and encircling her with serpentine bodies. Also as a 'performer of motherliness', Manjusri moves in affective synergy with the daughter's body, 'presenting fluidity of emotions and reasoning', observes Esha Niyogi De.[64] 'The non-objectified compassion in a mother witnessing her daughter's agony of

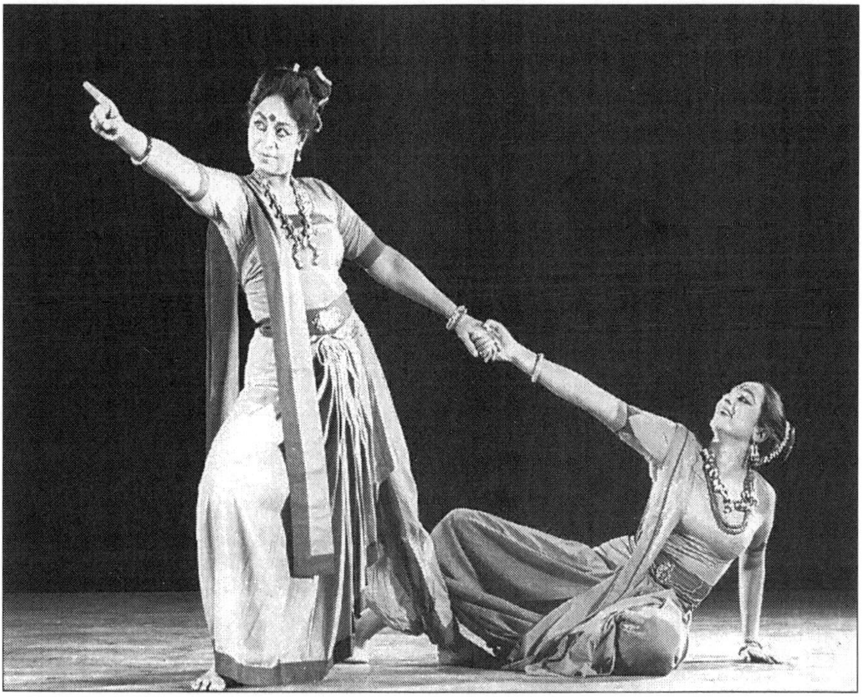

PLATE 8.2: Maya Dragging Prakriti into her World of Magic (Manjusri Chaki-Sircar and Ranjabati Sircar) in *Tomar Matir Kanya*. *Source*: Photo courtesy of Avinash Pasricha.

unrequited love blends' with what Niyogi De calls, 'the non-psychological Sanskrit ethic of *karuna* (empathy)' 'as a self-reneging desire to bond with another.'[65]

My own personal memory can recall how intense was the tussle of emotions between the two and how real their tears and laughter emoted on stage. They danced with and danced against each other, 'following and framing each other' in a mother-daughter dyad where both were engaged in a face-off, one set to complement and challenge the other on stage.[66] Triggering their latent emotions of love and tension, Manjusri and Ranjabati simultaneously brought into play two different ethos, epitomizing two distinctive body politics. Transcending 'real-life' emotions, they were also capable of showing dissimilar signatures to mark out their generations in their own ways. Manjusri's organic dancing body, deeply entrenched in her own 'root', kept expanding and expending her 'cultural capital' amassed within her own 'habitus', unshaken by disparate journeys, migrations, and relocations. Alternatively, her daughter Ranjabati, born in Africa and brought up in America, initials her hybrid and transnational identity, scripting her cultural straddling across frontiers, reclaiming her 'roots', which were not one but many. With difference and concurrence, they complemented each other, not merely as mother-daughter, but also as two genres of feminist performers, writing and representing their bodies in distinctly different styles.

Drawing imageries from the Meitei Maibi ritual of Manipur, and from the Yatmul puberty ritual of New Guinea, Manjusri, the anthropologist-choreographer, creates a human tunnel with her bhairabis making a rite of passage for Prakriti's sexual flowering, initiating her daughter into womanhood (Plate 8.3).[67] In another dramatic collage, the stretched out palms of women create *Sarpabandhani*, a shackle of serpents, symbolizing a polycaphelous snake—a structure defying form of unbridled female sexuality. As her choreographies created new imageries of feminine synergies with the *chandalkanyas*, clustering and moving together as one close-knit collective body, it reflected her alertness in acknowledging 'women's collective role' and their 'power of subversion in a male oriented society'.[68]

Appropriating Tagore to fit into her own cultural experience of postcolonial feminist choreography, Manjusri reshuffled the dominant discourse on gender, culture, and spectatorship. Working outside both the nationalist canon of the sanitized Rabindrik's and Shankar's new-orientalist canon of dance, Manjusri was inspired by 'innovative combination of cosmopolitanism and quotidian practice within bodily thinking by Rabindranath Tagore's dance drama legacy' maintains Esha

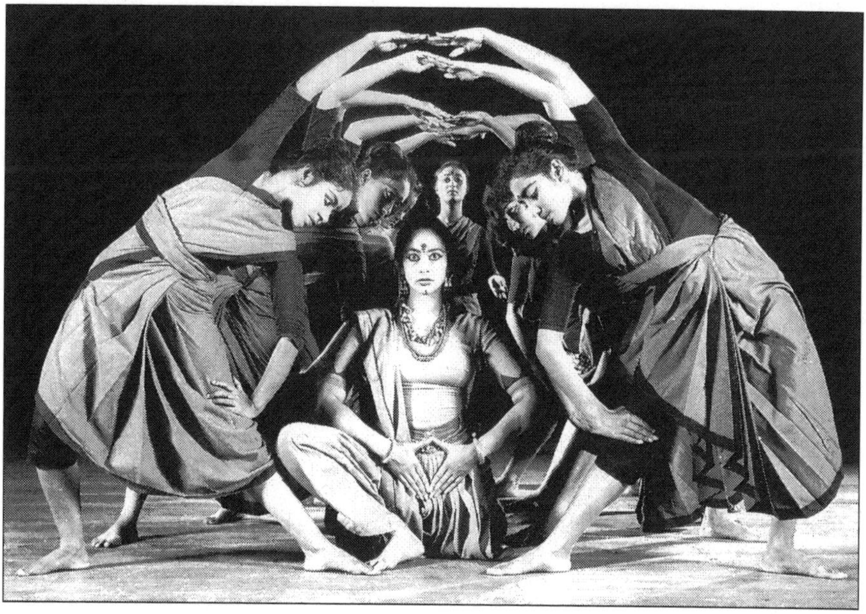

PLATE 8:3: Prakriti Passing through the Tunnel of Puberty in *Tomari Matir Kanya*
Source: Courtesy of Avinash Pasricha.

Niyogi De. As a South Asian contemporary feminist choreographer, she was also able to reassert her indigenous cultural autonomy, resisting not merely the bowdlerizing policies of the mainstream national, but also decolonizing her dance and divesting the dancing body of the inherited and imported legacies of colonialism.

As a narrative of protest, *Chandalika* spawned a complicated story of the mythical emotion into an indictment of caste-gendered violence in contemporary society. 'I saw Chandalika as a saga of transformation', wrote Ranjabati Sircar. 'The death of her mother signifies the beginning of a new life for Prakriti and also the death of old values and beliefs' as 'it liberates her untouchable daughter from her cradle of faith facilitating her movement towards a new world.'[69] Maya's death also signified the end of an illusion, as though freeing her daughter from the injunctions posed by her blood, caste and religion (Plate 8.4).

Curtain Call

Manjusri often expressed her desire to die on stage with Maya, wishing the most glorious death of a performer in her chosen role. But in an irony of fate, her daughter Ranjabati left the stage before her, committing

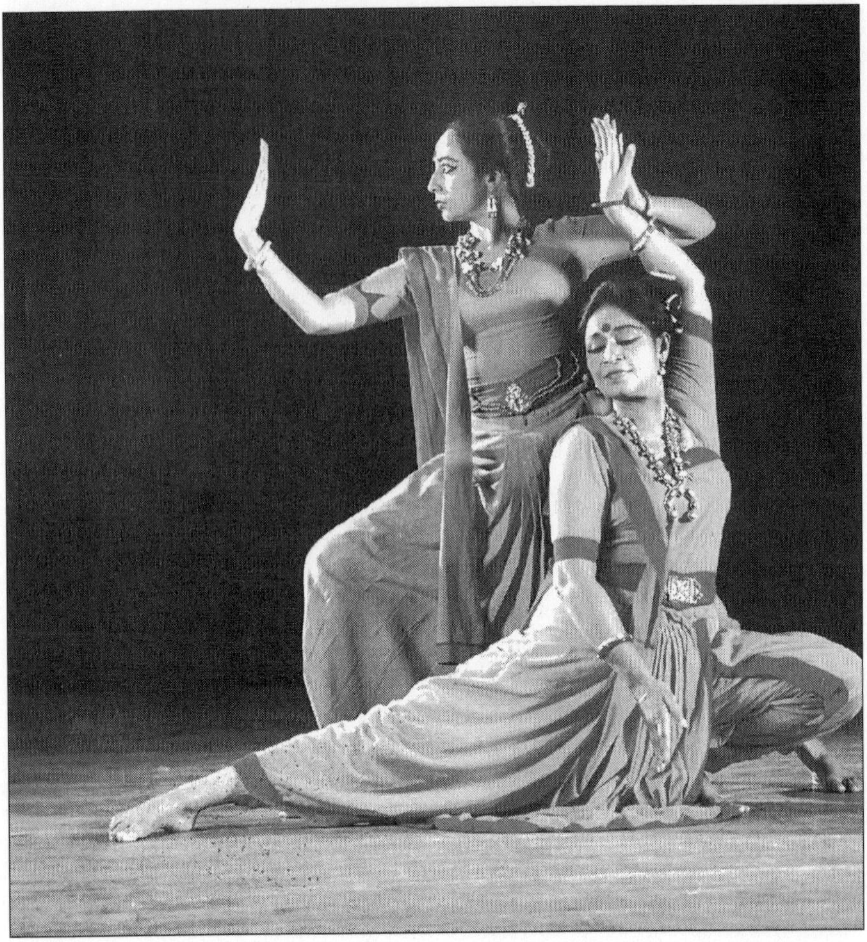

PLATE 8.4: Prakriti (Ranjabati Sircar) Looking at the *Maya Darpan* (Magic-Mirror) while Maya (Manjusri Chaki-Sircar) Brings into Play her Sorcerous Power (*Tomari Matir Kanya*)
Source: Photo courtesy of Avinash Pasricha.

suicide at the age of 36 in October 1999, leaving her as a critically ill and widowed mother to die a lonely death. Manjusri never performed on stage after the death of her daughter. Dancers' Guild staged *TMK*, the dance drama in May 2000, with Jonaki Sarkar and Sadhana Hazra playing the leads as Maya and Prakriti respectively. Weeks before her death, Manjusri, sitting among the audience, watched her signature piece, which she thoughtfully re-choreographed with the new cast, with the eternal faith that 'the show must go on'.

Writing her life on stage as a forbearing woman, unceasingly mothering her wilful yet vulnerable daughter, Manjusri's inscriptions appeared as her natural self-expression, recreating the mother within to stage her lived experience. Immensely proud of her daughter, she once said: 'I have only one child, Ranjabati, who is the greatest blessing. Motherhood is both a pleasure and bondage.'[70] The sudden death of Ranjabati freed her from that 'bondage', robbing her off all pleasures of life. Quickly she pieced together her unfinished life story, which was now drawing to an end, heading towards a virtual termination in the cruellest way. The life story was left scrappy and patchy. But the strength of the feminine writing that has reclaimed her self, through her body and vice versa, celebrates a life that was formidable enough 'to overcome prescription, oppression, silence—to laugh at rules that fix standards'[71]—till it finally succumbed to death.

Notes and References

1. W.B. Yeats, 'Among School Children', http://www.poetryfoundation.org/poems-and-poets/poems/detail/43293 (accessed 18 May 2016).
2. Literally meaning 'New Dance', *Navanritya* was a contemporary dance movement pioneered and christened by Manjusri Chaki-Sircar. A cross-stylization of classical and non-classical dance forms, it is primarily a psycho-physical exercise, which, by exploring the kinaesthetic and philosophical possibilities of the body movement, comes as a social statement by the choreographer, as a feminist resistive intervention, on the dance map of India.
3. Manjusri Chaki-Sircar, *Nrityarase Chittamama*, Kolkata: Miranda, 2000, p. 1.
4. The title of the book, *Nrityarase Chittamama* (literally, 'My heart drenched in dance'), was taken from the song 'Amay kshama hey kshama' (Forgive me my lord), composed by Rabindranath Tagore for his dance drama, arguably his first, *Natir Puja* (Worship of the Courtesan; staged first in 1926 and was made into a film in 1932). An adaptation from the Buddhist literature, *Abadanshatak*, it tells the story of Srimati, a court dancer of Magadha, who embraced Buddhism, going against the royal faith and order. To punish the 'heretic' dancer, the Hindu King, Ajatshatru commanded her to dance before the sacred altar (stupa) of Buddha, thereby to defile its sanctity. Performing protest through her dance, Srimati, however, challenged the hegemonic brahminic order and celebrated her devotion to Lord Buddha by offering her last worship through the spiritual invocation of dance. The protesting body of Srimati was to be silenced forever as she was slaughtered at the very altar of Buddha. Manjusri played the role of Srimati many times on stage and even appeared on celluloid as Srimati in a Bengali film, directed by Devaki Bose in 1961.
5. Isadora Duncan, *My Life*, New York and London: Liveright, 1995, p. 9.

6. Manjusri started her academic journey as a lecturer in Bengali Literature and began her second innings in academics in a different subject on a different trajectory. She earned her Ph.D. in cultural anthropology from the University of Columbia, New York, and authored her first book, *Feminism in a Traditional Society: Women in the Manipur Valley*, in 1984. Focusing on the Lai-Haraoba dance ritual, her work explored the matriarchal social structure of the Meiteis and the socio-ritual status of the Maibis of Manipur. Her postdoctoral work from the University of Connecticut also resulted in one more publication, *Women and Children in a Bengali Village*, co-authored with Ronald P.O. Rohner, in 1988. During the early 1950s, Manjusri successfully ran an all-women's magazine, *Mahila Mahal* (Woman's World) as its organizational secretary.
7. Ann Cooper Albright, 'Auto-Body Stories: Blondell Cummings and Autobiography in Dance', in *Meaning in Motion, New Cultural Studies of Dance*, ed. Jane C. Desmond, Durham and London: Duke University Press, 2003, p. 180.
8. Chaki-Sircar, *Nrityarase Chittamama*, p. 3.
9. Ibid., p. 8.
10. Ibid., p. 21.
11. Ibid., p. 89.
12. Personal communication with Manjusri Chaki-Sircar.
13. Chaki-Sircar, *Nrityarase Chittamama*, pp. 78–9.
14. Ibid., pp. 88–9.
15. Susan Leigh Foster, ed., *Worlding Dance*, New York: Palgrave Macmillan, 2011.
16. Recent dance scholars point to the already and always existing imbalance within the institutional hierarchy of India's performing arts. Entrenched in an unshakable Brahminic tradition and as symptomatic of a new Hindu, high-caste, middle-class identity, the 'Classical' is placed up on the ladder, pushing the contemporary/modern down in the ranking as a heretic insider of a hallowed lineage. In post-independence India, classical dance emerged as the cultural signifier of the new nation, laying its claim to pre-historic antiquity and textual purity. Sangeet Natak Akademi—India's apex body of performing arts—was set up in 1952 along with the new Republic, with an official pledge of 'preserving and promoting the traditional cultural heritage of India's rich performing arts'. Sangeet Natak Akademi, 'Intangible Cultural Heritage', n.d., http://www.sangeetnatak.gov.in/sna/ich.php (accessed 23 September 2016). Simultaneously, under Nehruvian cultural policy, the indigenous folk tradition too assumed an ambassadorial valence along with the 'brand Indian' Classical—to be showcased at every 'India Festival' at an *inter*national level. The creative/modern/eclectic/contemporary dance, which made waves in the decades before independence was gradually pushed to the margin as the centre was taken by the Brahminic classical. *Sruti*, no. 122, November 1994.

17. Sidonie Smith and Julia Watson, eds., *Women, Autobiography, Theory: A Reader*, Wisconsin: University of Wisconsin Press, 1998, p. 19.
18. Sidonie Smith, 'Performativity, Autobiographical Practice, Resistance', in *Women, Autobiography, Theory: A Reader*, ed. Sidonie Smith and Julia Watson, Wisconsin: University of Wisconsin Press, 1998, p. 108.
19. Ibid., p. 114.
20. Judith Butler, *Gender Trouble: Feminism and the Subversion of Identity*, New York: Routledge, 1990.
21. Paul Eakin, *Touching the World: Reference in Autobiography*, Princeton: Princeton University Press, 1993, pp. 102, 120.
22. Smith, 'Performativity, Autobiographical Practice, Resistance', p. 109.
23. Ibid., p. 108.
24. Benedict Anderson, *Imagined Communities: Reflections on the Origin and Spread of Nationalism*, London: Verso, 1991, p. 204.
25. Cited in Victoria Phillips, 'Martha Graham's Gilded Cage: *Blood Memory—An Autobiography* (1991)', *Dance Research Journal*, vol. 45, no. 2, August 2013, p. 65.
26. Rasasundari Dasi's autobiography *Amar Jeeban* (My Life) was the first published autobiography in Bengali to come out in 1876. *Sikshita Patitar Atmacharit* (The Autobiography of an Educated Prostitute, 1932) was claimed to have been authored by a prostitute, Manada Devi, who had also been a student of Bethune School, Calcutta. Nistarini Devi's mémoire *Sekele Katha* (Tales of the Bygone Days, 1913) was a telling description of the penury and exploitation faced by a propertyless Hindu widow; and theatre actress Binodini Dasi's memoirs—*Amar Katha* (My Story, 1912) and *Amar Abhinetri Jeeban* (My Life as an Actress, 1924–5)—were frank descriptions of patriarchal power politics that permeated even the stage of performance, depriving an actress of her rightful claim and honour.
27. Amita Sen, *Shantiniketane Ashramkanya*, Calcutta: Tagore Research Institute, 1977; idem, *Sirisha, Bakula, Amer Mukul*, Calcutta: Nabapatra Prakashan, 2000.
28. Amita Sen, 'Introduction', in *Joy in All Work*, Calcutta: Book Font Publications, 1999.
29. Ibid., p. 53.
30. Martha Nussbaum, 'Tagore, Dewey, and the Imminent Demise of Liberal Education', paper submitted for a conference on Tagore's Philosophy of Education, in memory of Amita Sen, Kolkata, 29–30 March 2006, p. 9.
31. Amala Shankar, *Saat Sagarer Pare*, Calcutta: A. Mukherjee and Co., 2007, p. 92.
32. Personal communication with Amala Shankar, interviewed by the author, 7 February 2015.
33. Mohan Khokar, *His Dance, His Life: A Portrait of Uday Shankar*, New Delhi: Himalayan Books, 1983, p. 119.
34. Ibid., p. 117.
35. Ibid., p. 119.

36. Prarthana Purkayastha, *Indian Modern Dance, Feminism and Transnationalism*, London: Palgrave Macmillan, 2014, p. 78.
37. Bishnupriya Dutt and Urmimala Sarkar Munsi, *Engendering Performance: Indian Women Performers in Search of an Identity*, New Delhi: Sage Publications, 2010, p. 223.
38. Sadhana Bose, *Shilpir Atmakatha*, ed. Debjit Bandyopadhyay, Kolkata: Pratibhas, 2012.
39. Vidya Rao, *Heart to Heart: Remembering Nainaji*, Noida: Harper Collins, 2011, p. 43.
40. Ibid., p. 49.
41. Madhu Bose, *Amar Jeeban*, ed. Debjit Bandyopadhyay, Kolkata: Pratibhas, 2012, pp. 126–7; Bose, *Shilpir Atmakatha*, pp. 26–7.
42. Bose, *Shilpir Atmakatha*, pp. 20, 33.
43. Introduction, in Bose, *Shilpir Atmakatha*.
44. Introduction, in Reba Roychowdhury, *Jeebaner Tane Shilper Tane*, Calcutta: Thema, 1999.
45. Ibid., p. 13.
46. Ibid., p. 14.
47. Dutt and Sarkar Munsi, *Engendering Performance*, p. 227.
48. Ibid.
49. Introduction, in Miss Shefali, *Sandhyarater Shefali*, Kolkata: Ananda Publishers, 2015.
50. Ibid.
51. Ibid., p. 42.
52. Saikat Majumdar, 'The Ashes of Pleasure: How the Curtains Came Down on Calcutta's Professional Theatre', *The Caravan*, 1 September 2014, http://www.caravanmagazine.in/arts/ashes-pleasure (accessed 1 May 2015).
53. Ibid.
54. Sonali Makhija in her case study of the bar dancers of Bombay discusses how with her initiating gaze and sexuality a bar dancer negates the traditional, passive dancer. Though the articulation of the female desire through the gaze is consciously constructed within the male gaze itself, the bar dancer is still able to contest the male gaze, as much as she performs it. The bar dancer, unlike the traditional dancer (assumed by the State), exacts a response to her 'initiation', challenging the notion of dance as merely a spectacle. See Sonali Makhija, 'Bar Dancers, Morality and Indian Law', *Economic and Political Weekly*, vol. 45, no. 39, 2010, pp. 19–23.
55. Cited in Elizabeth Francis, 'From Event to Monument: Modernism, Feminism and Isadora Duncan', *American Studies*, vol. 35, no. 1, 1994, pp. 35–6.
56. Elizabeth Dempster, 'Women Writing the Body: Let's Watch a Little How She Dances', in *Grafts: Feminist Cultural Criticism*, ed. Susan Sheridan, London and New York: Verso, 1988, p. 43.
57. Phillips, 'Martha Graham's Gilded Cage', p. 77.

58. Albright, 'Auto-Body Stories', p. 188.
59. Martha Graham, *Blood Memory*, New York: Doubleday, 1991.
60. Victoria Thoms, 'Martha Graham's Haunting Body: Autobiography at the Intersection of Writing and Dancing', *Dance Research Journal*, vol. 40, no. 1, Summer 2008, p. 9.
61. Albright, 'Auto-Body Stories', p. 194.
62. 'In Search of Protest in Tagore: A New Production of 'Chandalika', *Point Counterpoint*, no. 36, 10 July 1985.
63. See Laura Alexander, 'Helene Cixous and the Rhetoric of Feminine Desire: Re-writing the Medusa', 2004, http://english.arts.cornell.edu/publications/mode/documents/alexander.doc (accessed 18 May 2016).
64. Esha Niyogi De, *Empire, Media and the Autonomous Woman: A Feminist Critique of Postcolonial Thought*, New Delhi: Oxford University Press, 2011, p. 158.
65. Ibid.
66. Esha Niyogi De makes an interesting observation in this context. She argues that 'the performance of mother-daughter synergy is at odds' not only with Hindu societal reality where daughters are presented as 'dowry burdens or at least pieces of property' to be transacted through marriage, but also with some Western feminist theorists like Julia Kristeva who considers motherly bonds as invariably compromising of the 'consecrated' representations of femininity. In *TMK*, the dancer duo's assertive performance of their real/staged relation and their mutual bonding also culminates, De argues, in the staging of collective birthing which comprises a dialectical *bricolage* of indigenous and liberal European notions of the self'. Niyogi De, *Empire, Media and the Autonomous Woman*, p. 158.
67. In an interview to Leela Venkataraman in *Sruti* (November 1994), Manjusri delineated the intellectual-corporeal influences that went into the making of *TMK*: 'My travel and long stays abroad . . . amidst different cultures made me more aware of my own roots', more curious 'in a comparative study of . . . rituals, religion and performing arts'. She detailed further: 'My experience in the field, among women's dance associations of the Ijaw tribe of the Niger Delta (Nigeria), and subsequently in Manipur and rural Bengal . . . gave me interesting materials for choreography and for the analysis of human behaviour in dance.' Manjusri Chaki-Sircar, 'The Sircars and their Navanritya', *Sruti*, no. 122, November 1994.
68. Ibid.
69. Aishika Chakraborty, ed., *Ranjabati, A Dancer and her World: Selected Writings of Ranjabati Sircar*, Calcutta: Thema, 2008, p. 80.
70. Vishnupriya Sengupta, 'Dance is an Expression of a Personal Ideology', *The Asian Age*, Calcutta, 3 December 1995.
71. Alexander, 'Helene Cixous and the Rhetoric of Feminine Desire'.

9 Bharatanatyam and Butoh

An Emerging Gendered Conversation through Site-Specific Dance in Chennai and Singapore

NIRMALA SESHADRI

Born in Singapore, I began learning Bharatanatyam at age 7. This was not a matter of choice; my parents were of the strong view that it was through learning art forms such as Bharatanatyam and Carnatic music that their children would discover and maintain cultural connections with India. I would later come to realize that this was the case with many parents who belonged to the Indian diaspora in various parts of the world. Dance scholar Janet O'Shea refers to this as 'the diasporic demand for cultural symbols'.[1] It was much later, at the age of 17, that my passion for the form was awakened by the realization that the *abhinaya* (expressive) aspect of the form had much to offer me by way of non-verbal tools for communicating complex emotions and experiences that I could not verbally convey as a young Indian girl growing up in a traditional family in multicultural Singapore. There was a clear dichotomy between my personal and public spheres. My classical dance form became a means of bridging my worlds and lending tangibility to the many questions and observations that arose within me.

During 1992–4 and again between 1999 and 2009, I based myself in Chennai for over a decade to learn, teach, choreograph, and perform in India, while I maintained my connection with Singapore. It was around 1996 that I began to think beyond the framework of the Bharatanatyam *margam*. While I was immersed in the practice of the form, I had also begun to feel that it accentuated my place in the Indian ethnic box in Singapore.[2] Also, be it Singapore or Chennai, I found that the dance

*The author wishes to thank Urmimala Sarkar Munsi, Suparna Banerjee, and Shobha Avadhani for their critical inputs. The author is also grateful to Neewin Hershall for his wholehearted involvement and contribution, and his acknowledgement of his views that have been represented.

form was colluding with my orthodox upbringing to impose restrictions on me as a woman vis-à-vis my thoughts and expression. On or off stage, I was burdened by the expectation, placed by various sections of society, to perform the role of the virtuous Indian woman and typical Bharatanatyam dancer. Cross-cultural and interdisciplinary choreographic work became a means of stepping out of this rigid frame to connect to a wider sense of self/identity and community.

Moving away from the normative representation began with the project *Outcaste Eternal.*[3] Following this work, I stopped dancing for three years and delved into writing on the arts. I was grappling with what it meant to have tested the boundaries. In 2003, a new work emerged—*Crossroads: Journeys and Transformations through Life and Dance*—a revisitation of the Bharatanatyam repertoire.

This practice-led research chapter engages with history, performance aesthetics, and presentation as it outlines the process by which a structured and codified form such as Bharatanatyam (the practice and performance of which is largely indoor and proscenium-based) was drawn into an outdoor space of improvisation and sensorial perception through Butoh, sculpture, poetry, music, and site-specificity.[4] Two choreographic works serve as key points of reference—the site-specific works titled *Crossroads: Journeys and Transformations through Life and Dance* (2003–8) (hereafter *Crossroads*) and *I Carry Your Heart* (2015). The works were choreographed and premiered in Chennai and Singapore respectively. Through the description of a creative process that opened up into a space of collaboration and cultural hybridization.[5] This essay explores how the choreographic process that interweaves sites and the dance forms (Bharatanatyam and Butoh) challenges the traditional ideas of the gendered body and provides the ground for the emergence of new contemporary expression in the Singapore milieu.

In this essay, I adopt the analytical lens of body[6] as I examine the intercultural, interdisciplinary, and place/space[7] dialogue that facilitated a shift from an embodied habitus into a fluid and hybridized concept of identity. Drawing on auto-ethnographic as well as ethnographic perspectives, I demonstrate that this intersecting space of Bharatanatyam, Butoh, and site-specificity offers scope for questioning the conventional notions of the body that are embedded in a classical dance form such as Bharatanatyam, as well as in 'erasing cultural differences between "us" and "them"[8] to create hybrid spaces that hold immense possibilities for autonomy, re-contextualization and change with respect to the present-day female Bharatanatyam dancer.

The Dancing Body and its City/Site

The two choreographic works mentioned earlier are linked to the concept of the gendered body and its relationship with city/site.

Scholar Elizabeth Grosz draws a clear link between the body and the city in which it dwells: 'The city is the site for the body's cultural saturation . . . the place where the body is representationally reexplored, transformed, contested, reinscribed. In turn, the body (as cultural product) transforms, reinscribes the urban landscape according to its changing . . . needs.'[9]

Crossroads involved destabilizing the conflation of body and site vis-à-vis the classical dance form Bharatanatyam and the south Indian city of Chennai.[10] Regardless of geographical location, when the transfigured classical form of Bharatanatyam is learnt, the dancer is also being groomed to become a carrier and custodian of a certain culture. For the present-day Bharatanatyam dancer this means embodying some of the *sringara-* (eroticism-) focused themes and texts of the hereditary devadasi's repertoire in an acceptable format, while also propagating the post-revival sanitized version of the form that has bhakti (religious devotion) as its focus.[11]

A collaborative and interdisciplinary duet that hinged on the Bharatanatyam repertoire, *Crossroads* sought to test the boundaries imposed on the practitioner of the dance form. While the roots of my collaborator, the Kalakshetra-trained[12] Neewin Hershall, lie in Kerala and mine are that of an Indian immigrant in Singapore, both of us had shifted to Chennai in the early 1990s to further our training in Bharatanatyam. *Crossroads* began as a desire on both our parts to present the Bharatanatyam *margam* as it had been expected of us. However, we gradually began to question the normative representation, particularly with respect to gender. The production that saw the coming together of Bharatanatyam with music, poetry, film, and visual art was reworked and restaged at various locations in Chennai, including conventional spaces such as Kalakshetra, the Madras Music Academy and Sri Krishna Gana Sabha. It was also staged in other cities and towns in south India and presented for the final time in 2008 in Singapore at the Lee Foundation Theatre.

I Carry Your Heart, an interdisciplinary and cross-cultural performance work, was created and presented at the National University Hospital Heart Centre, Singapore, in February 2015. The 50-minute piece saw the coming together of dance, sculpture, poetry, and music. In creating this site-specific piece, Hershall and I worked through Bharatanatyam and the memory of *Crossroads*, as well as the dance theatre form Butoh as we responded to the stone sculptures at the Sculpture Garden created by Singapore's celebrated multidisciplinary artist Tan Swie Hian. Tan's Sculpture Garden is based on the poem 'I Carry Your Heart With Me' written by American poet E.E. Cummings. The work drew us from the structure and codification of Bharatanatyam into a space of improvisation and sensorial perception. It was a journey through dance, life, and love, one that carried the notions of release and rejuvenation as its leitmotifs. The work also featured French Butoh artist Syv Bruzeau with live music by three Singaporean instrumentalists that blended Indian music (flute by Vishnu Veluri) with Chinese instruments such as the pipa (by Samuel Wong) and guzheng (by Johnny Chia). Hershall and I provided the vocals through song and vocal percussion.

Challenging Traditional Notions of the Body

In revisiting *Crossroads* at this juncture, I am reminded of the day I stepped into the studio and told Hershall that we needed to explore the concept of unpredictability in relation to the *margam*. Gender became an area for investigation as we reflected on the ideas of symmetry and androgyny.[13]

Grosz talks of 'challenging traditional notions of the body so that we can abandon the oppositions by which the body has usually been understood'.[14] The 'male-female binary' that Grosz refers to in this context is what formed the crux of our exploration in Crossroads.

Dance scholar Urmimala Sarkar Munsi emphasizes that 'the past history has shown us time and again that locating the female body within the historically derived public domain of the patriarchal society has silenced any bodily activities or at least muted them in and through classical dance'.[15] Questioning the dance tradition can be an uphill and impossible task, for as Sarkar Munsi points out, the body is trained according to the norms and values of the overarching systems of socialization:

> They train it according to the rules of rightness, social correctness, and the expectations of the families and teachers. In the process, most of the awareness, is shaped and structured according to the perspective of the 'socially acceptable' viewership, many a times completely suppressing much of the instinctive expressions, by schooling these bodies through rigorous training. In other words, even before a mind starts any form of questioning, the bodily values of right and wrong are so deeply embedded in the minds and the bodies of these dancers, that the comfort zone of expressivity remains structured by these value systems all their lives.[16]

The *Abhinaya Darpana* by Nandikesvara, one of the key texts of Bharatanatyam states: 'It is understood that the Danseuse (*nartaki*) should be very lovely, young, with full round breasts, self-confident, charming, agreeable, dexterous in handling the critical passages . . . with wide-open eyes . . . adorned with costly jewels, with a charming lotus-face, neither very stout nor very thin, nor very tall nor very short.'[17]

Believed to have been written around the thirteenth century CE, the *Abhinaya Darpana* serves as a reference point in Bharatanatyam training even in the present day. Passages such as the one quoted here point clearly to the fact that the female dancer's body has been made the subject of the male gaze. There appears to be a greater emphasis on the physicality of a dancer as opposed to the actual dance.

As a female dancer who was trained to portray the nayika or heroine in love who is the central character in Bharatanatyam portrayals, I desperately needed to bring about a shift in my own representation, be it through physical appearance, movements, expressions or themes. Literary scholar A.K. Ramanujan highlights the plight of the nayika: '[T]he heroine . . . is relatively helpless vis-à-vis her beloved. She can only wait for him and suffer the torment of his absence. He, in contrast, is free to come or not, to show compassion, if he wishes, and save her life—or let her die of love . . . she is dwarfed by the inherent lack of equality between them.'[18]

As dancers, Hershall and I existed in the Chennai milieu that presented and resulted in various binaries. I had been drawn to training and presenting solo performances at the sabhas in the city. Hershall, on the other hand, was trained at the renowned Bharatanatyam institution, Kalakshetra, where he and other colleagues have told me that they had been discouraged from attending sabha performances. Undoubtedly, this dichotomy is rooted in the famous *bhakti-sringara* debate of the revival era, the perception of the hereditary dancer both as prostitute and nun and the subsequent transfiguration of Sadir into Bharatanatyam which involved the de-eroticization or sanitization of the form.[19]

By the time we began working on *Crossroads* I had been exposed to the work of two key influential and divergent voices in the field—*abhinaya* exponent Kalanidhi Narayanan and contemporary choreographer Chandralekha. While both the Chennai-based stalwarts had their core training in Bharatanatyam, Narayanan believed that bhakti underscored sringara. She says: 'The closeness and intimacy of the love relationship is an allegory for the closeness and intimacy of the devotee and God.'[20] Chandralekha, on the other hand, stressed on the importance of eroticism but rejected the traditional constructs, mythological narratives and bhakti. Strongly opposed to objectification in the solo dance tradition, she has asked the question: 'Is the audience looking at my dance or at my appearance?'[21]

For the first time, in presenting the *margam*, I abandoned the wig that I normally wore to give the impression of the long plait that had come to symbolize the Bharatanatyam dancer, both on and off stage. Given that Hershall and I were focusing on gender and its similarities, I felt it contradictory to accentuate differences that did not exist. In reality, I had very short hair and so decided that I would abandon the wig altogether. After so many decades of enculturation it was hardly easy for me to make that choice. In fact, I carried my wig to the performance venue, just in case I felt uncomfortable without the wig. But I did not. I knew that conceptually it was correct to do away with it. A couple of days after the performance, Hershall and I asked a group of young dancers from Kalakshetra what they felt about the lack of the traditional head gear. Their reply was: 'For the first five minutes it felt strange but after that the dance took over.' Ironically, it was a Chennai-based modern dancer who had commented that I had violated the form by abandoning what she believed was one of its integral aspects.

The first part of the production was presented through film to represent a point in the past. Here, Hershall and I presented short segments of *padams* (musical poems that are depicted by the dancer through *abhinaya*) that represented a yearning for love. Both of us were dressed in traditional garb which in my case as a woman meant that I donned the wig and plait; head jewellery; accessories for the ears, neck, waist and wrists, as well as the conventional stitched silk costume. Hershall's costume was more minimalistic, and as per tradition vis-à-vis male dancers, he was bare-chested. After a 10-minute video clip, we entered the stage and for most of the live *margam* performance we wore understated dance practice outfits—Hershall was dressed in a cotton dhoti while I was in a short cotton practice saree. In the very first staging, Hershall performed bare-chested in the live performance as well. However, in subsequent stagings of the work I requested that he wear a vest as a means of introducing some symmetry in representation. Initially Hershall was uncomfortable at the thought and told me that it went against convention. It was then that I suggested to Hershall that I might be required to present myself in a similar way. He then agreed to the vest and eventually appeared comfortable wearing it. In the final piece *thillana* we attempted to represent the ideas of oneness, freedom and release from structure and form. For the first staging at Bharatiya Vidya Bhavan Auditorium (Chennai), both of us were dressed in jeans and a t-shirt as we both felt that this outfit would succeed in conveying the idea of gender neutrality. In later performances, we formalized the costume for this segment by dressing in identical grey silk *patiala salwar*s and a sleeveless top.

Dance scholar Janet O'Shea writes: 'Bharata Natyam's repertoire consists largely of songs written between the seventeenth and twentieth centuries. The poems of love and religious devotion that form the basis of the Bharata Natyam canon emerged from the musical and literary traditions of previous centuries.'[22]

In line with the typical Bharatanatyam repertoire, *Crossroads* was centred on the themes of yearning, separation, meeting, and parting. If the songs in the repertoire generally portray the devotee's yearning for union with the divine, *Crossroads* sought to also address the angle of the interpersonal relationships between human beings.

Hershall and I moved in silence at the start, closely mirroring each other's movements to demonstrate the awareness and yearning to connect with the other, to explore points of similarity. In the first *jathi* of the *varnam*, we opened with an *ardhaneeswara*[23] pose in which our bodies were intertwined, following which we explored the idea of a gender continuum, each of us shifting between the male and female binary. Except for the opening section on film and during our solo *abhinaya* pieces in which Hershall and I portrayed maleness and femaleness respectively, the rest of the work did not subscribe to stereotypical gendering. In the *thillana*, we attempted to project a sense of androgyny not only through costumes, as mentioned earlier, but through our movements which were at times equally strong and vigorous and at other times fluid and languid. Unlike the usual *thillana* that concludes with a verse in praise of a particular deity, here we included instead instrumental interludes that offered scope for free improvised movement. *Thillana* was the celebration of the synergy between two artists immersed in a form that is ephemeral and in contact with visual art, an art form that is more permanent. The production had its geometrical underpinnings progressing from the notion of two individuals as points that connect to form a line, and gradually culminating in the idea of a circle that symbolizes freedom from form and structure.

Perhaps the most dramatic shift took place in my solo, the *ashtapadi*.[24] In 2006 we were preparing to perform the work at Sri Krishna Gana Sabha in Chennai. By then I found I had lost interest in the original choreography of this piece. If I was myself so bored, how would I engage my audience? I re-examined the piece and decided to rework it. After all, I was depicting Radha and Krishna in a post-coital moment. I felt the strong need to include my own experience as a woman and to allow for the expressions to be less stylized, to depict an everyday reality. Instead of restricting my *abhinaya* to focus on the face and hand gestures alone, I extended it to include the rest of my body. Radha in this verse has been referred to as the *Swadhinapatika*[25] nayika, one who is in command of her lover. I, therefore, introduced body positions and movements that I felt would convey this stance in a sexual connotation. Since Radha was seeking to prolong the moment and have Krishna indulge her in various ways, I interpreted the verse to be the interim between two sexual climaxes and this was represented through bodily *abhinaya*. In retrospect, the reworking of this *ashtapadi* opened the doors to kinaesthetic exploration that choreographer and scholar Susan Leigh Foster describes as 'drawing upon and engaging with prevailing senses of the body and of subjectivity in a given historical moment'.[26]

Sarkar Munsi highlights the complexities of kinaesthetic exploration in the context of classical Indian dance and specifically the female dancer: 'The reality of her [female classical dancer] everyday life is put aside, as she reclaims her tradition through her body and performance—entering into an imaginary realm of a world that begins and ends with the performance itself, and does not have anything to do with the everyday reality of the body.'[27]

Chennai, as the location in which *Crossroads* was conceptualized, created and staged a few times, offered both resistance as well as support. The work received significant support and appreciation from dance colleagues, some respected dance gurus, the media and organizers. Following our performance at the Madras Music Academy, Bharatanatyam dance exponent and guru Professor C.V. Chandrasekhar was greatly appreciative of the concept and rigour. Newspapers in Chennai and elsewhere described the work as 'unique', 'innovative' and 'an attempt to move away from the stereotypical way of presenting the *margam*'.[28] However it was also felt that while 'the simple practice attire and Nirmala's short hair gave a rare informality to the performance . . . some may find Bharatanatyam in sleeveless tops (in the last piece) unacceptable'.[29] The main resistance to the work came when the shifts took place in the *ashtapadi*. We were told that some in the audience appeared visibly uncomfortable by the rendition. One of my main musicians commented that this version was 'too erotic'. These comments did not lead me to revert to the older version. In fact, Hershall and I felt even more convinced that this was the way forward for the *ashtapadi* within the context of *Crossroads*.

Today, we both believe that even in its resistance to our work, Chennai offered us tremendous impetus to challenge the boundaries of our form. It provided us a critical mix of people who understood the form well enough to recognize the departures we were making and a niche group of individuals who appeared ready for change and so gave us their implicit support. Also, the presence of individuals such as Chandralekha and film historian Vasanthi Sankaranarayanan (who gave us critical inputs during the creative process) inspired us to dare to challenge the boundaries. When all is said and done, Hershall believes that with respect to Bharatnatyam 'change happens in Chennai first'.[30]

The 2008 stagings of *Crossroads* in Pondicherry and Singapore were fraught with tensions caused partly by the physical and emotional transitions that I was undergoing as a mature female dancer. With differences that were accentuated by perimenopause, the attempt to represent gender symmetry within the framework of *Crossroads* seemed futile. At this stage, we laid the production to rest.

Site-Specificity: New Meanings and Interpretations

By 2014, the city/site shifted—both Hershall and I were now based in Singapore. I had begun embodying Butoh through ethnographic field research and working through my bodily memory of Bharatanatyam while Hershall was starting to feel curious about Butoh. By this time, six years after our last staging of *Crossroads*, we felt a deep urge to work together again. In the meantime, my mentor and friend—Singaporean multidisciplinary artist Tan Swie Hian—had taken me to view the stone sculpture garden he had created at the National University Hospital in Singapore. On experiencing the location, I immediately felt inspired to create a work there. As Hershall and I furthered our conversation, we decided we would create our new work at Tan's garden.

In *I Carry Your Heart*, not only had the country and city shifted, the performance location shifted from a conventional indoor theatre space to an outdoor and public space. Creating the work involved working in this space regularly for about three months and responding to it. Sometimes it was just Hershall and myself, while at other times we would be joined by Bruzeau and our musicians.

Bharatanatyam provided a base and broad structure and served as a memory thread both to our classical dance form as well as to *Crossroads*. We worked with fragmented sections of *Crossroads* while also responding to the site that contained the four sculptures, two of which were constructed in pools of water. At the first sculpture that Tan had created to symbolize the coming together of two hearts, we focused on Bharatanatyam, reworking *jathi* and *abhinaya* sections from *Crossroads*. Instead of a recorded track, we were accompanied by live flute with Hershall and me reciting the *jathis* as we moved. This marked a departure from the Bharatanatyam *margam* where a member of the orchestra recites the rhythmic syllables. As we moved towards the second sculpture that depicted multiple hearts, the form shifted to include Butoh. In this segment that was inspired by the notions of freedom and inclusivity reflected in the *thillana* of *Crossroads*, we were joined by Bruzeau. Even as we worked through Butoh, we allowed for traces of Bharatanatyam to enter the space through fragmented utilization of facial expressions, hand gestures and rhythmic passages.

Butoh artist and teacher Marie Gabrielle Rotie describes the form as a means of 'stepping inwards into your inner space'.[31] Butoh gave us tools to respond from within to one another and to our environment. It freed us from the pursuit of perfection, a fundamental aspect of our Bharatanatyam training, to experience an evolving form where we 'learn to be happy with what is unfinished and imperfect'.[32] According to Rotie: 'Butoh is not a style that can be taught as such . . . [it is a series of] open-ended investigations.'[33] It is the very antithesis of Bharatanatyam. *I Carry Your Heart* existed in the interstices of both forms. I would say that this intersection of Bharatanatyam and Butoh reflects the very essence of 'Ma' or 'the space between' through which 'Butoh-ka [Butoh dancers] awaken self-reflexive moments in themselves and their audiences' (Rotie).[34] Hence the interweaving of antithetical dance forms with site (that comprises audience) was the hallmark of this work.

Being a public venue, we were always in the presence of an audience—patients, visitors and staff, many of whom would pause to watch us at work. I was initially self-conscious, although after a couple of sessions I found myself ignoring the viewers. Soon, however, I became comfortable with their presence and felt they became part of the site that inspired and drove the process. Dance scholar Victoria Hunter highlights the pivotal role that the audience plays in site-specific work: 'Site-specific performance . . . actively encourages the audience's participation with both the site and the performance. The audience becomes actively engaged in the construction of meanings and interpretation.'[35]

Throughout our creative process we worked kinaesthetically to locate ourselves and our dance in the site. We did not restrict the audience movement but instead responded and improvised as we went along. Also, we welcomed close proximity with no restrictions on photography or videography. Instead, we allowed for these aspects to inspire our responses. Pooja Makhijani, an audience member, described her experience thus: 'The audience was encouraged to follow the performers as they traversed the Sculpture Garden and responded to the carved works and reflecting pools. At one point, my friend and I found ourselves *literally* in the center of the performance, with the dancers' undulating limbs just centimeters from our bodies. It made for an unforgettable viewing experience!'[36]

In discussing psychoanalyst D.W. Winnicott's notion of 'potential space', theatre scholar Cathy Turner suggests that site-specific performance 'plays at the edges of the frame, exploring the boundaries of potential space' and, therefore, it 'frequently makes surprise inevitable, while foregrounding our relationship with a wider environment'.[37] Makhijani's words reflect the moment in the performance when Hershall and I, on completing the first segment, moved towards the second sculpture in the slow ash walk of Butoh. When rehearsing we had sat on a stone bench in front of the second sculpture to spend a few minutes responding to Bruzeau's movements. However, on reaching the bench we found four audience members seated there. This led to the spontaneous creation of an entirely new segment with us positioned and moving very differently from what had emerged during our rehearsals. Also, these audience members appeared extremely at ease and began to respond to our movements (Plate 9.1).

I must confess, however, that the *ashtapadi* in this work was fragmented and tame when compared to what I had presented in *Crossroads*. Somehow the outdoor public space did not offer me the necessary distance from the viewer and, therefore, a sort of privacy that the proscenium stage

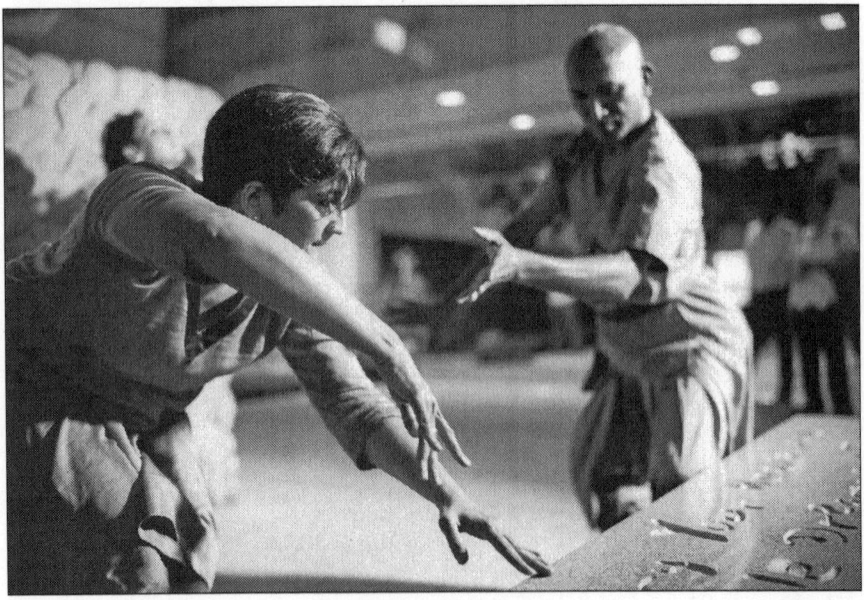

PLATE 9.1: *I Carry Your Heart* by Nirmala Seshadri and Neewin Hershall, expressed through Butoh and Bharatanatyam with inspiration from the National University Hospital Heart Centre Sculpture Garden created by Tan Swie Hian. *Source*: Courtesy of Jeff Low (Style Revisited).

had offered in *Crossroads*. But here I sang my *ashtapadi* while Hershall recited *Bho Shambho*. There was definitely something empowering in this act of singing for oneself.

While we did not consciously strive to project androgyny, Butoh inherently allowed for the understatement of gender and we were free to move as gender-neutral bodies in space. Our costumes, designed by Tan, were fairly casual and inspired by one of my everyday outfits. Just as in *Crossroads*, here, too, we focused on yearning, separation, meeting, and parting which were also the leitmotifs of Cumming's poem on which the sculptures were based.

Tan, who attended both nights of the performance, described the segment in which Hershall and I part ways:

> A never-before-seen piece in an ethereal garden laden with a multitude of hearts whose strings are being stricken in their meandering through the dancers' journey. The first and second stones are well crafted by your movements aesthetically tightening up by degrees the viewers' emotions and when the little brook of pipa starts gurgling, the emotional tension built up in the audiences' hearts starts to burst flowing towards the third and fourth stones. Amidst the light glittering on the ripples you are making in the ponds, tears are welling up in all the eyes surrounding your smiles.[38]

One audience member described it as being 'healing, meditative and peaceful—in a communal sort of a way'. Another viewer shared that it has led her into viewing hospitals very differently—as spaces of healing.[39] Dance critic Stephanie Burridge has written: 'The group reminded us of the empowering spirit of dance that can be a transformative force.'[40]

In creating *Crossroads*, the traditional Bharatanatyam *margam* had been reinterpreted in the very site in which the dance form had been reinvented in the 1930s and 1940s. The collaboration challenged the stereotypical representations of the body that engages with Bharatanatyam and began the shift of the body from its embodied habitus. The same bodies entered a new space of collaboration, site-specificity and hybridization through Butoh. Butoh offered us the necessary investigative tools to situate ourselves within the new site. The site-specific work, with its interdisciplinary and cross-cultural elements, also brought the audience into direct and close engagement with the creative process. The interweaving of the various elements resulted in what Foster describes as a 'procedure of self-location' that 'entails a recalibration of internal and external sensings of one's whereabouts'[41] leading to the creation of new contemporary expression in the context of Singapore. I believe that the intersection of Bharatanatyam, Butoh and this site-specific work holds immense potential in opening up that liminal 'third space', a space of infinite possibilities.

Conclusion

The final scene of *I Carry Your Heart* underscored the multiple criss-crossings—of the body, dance forms, site(s), cities, the senses and gender, as well as the distance that our artistic experience had traversed since *Crossroads*.

Hershall and I have just completed a segment that portrays union. It is a combination of sorts, of fragments of both our solos in *Crossroads*—my *ashtapadi* that shows Radha addressing Krishna in a post-coital moment. Hershall draws from his piece *Bho Shambho* that depicts the devotee's union with the concept of Shiva. *Sringara* and bhakti, male and female are interwoven in the central space of the courtyard at the National University Hospital Sculpture Garden. The musicians are seated in close proximity and we are ensconced in the presence of the audience who stand all around. I sing my *ashtapadi* in fragments, while Hershall recites text and *jathis* from his piece. The musicians provide subtle support. The segment ends with both our bodies in gentle contact.

The pipa and guzheng begin to play an old Chinese melody that conjures a poignant scene of lovers parting. It is slow, allowing Hershall and me to linger in our pose. We gradually part in a repeated and circular Bharatanatyam-esque movement. As we freeze to gaze at the other, I see Hershall's eyes fill with tears as I move away first, towards the wooden platform that separates two square pools of water. There is the inevitability of separation and yet the yearning to move forward on our respective journeys. I move towards the water, placing one foot in and gradually immersing myself in it. It is as though I am entering another time and another space, with my movement completely guided by the music, water, sculpture. I am aware of Hershall's presence in the other pool and of the fact that some in the audience might be more drawn to his younger, male, svelte body and its movements. Yet it hardly matters anymore.

All the dances analysed demonstrate the quest for the artistic subjectivity and identity that gets broadened through the hybridization of dance forms, travels and human interactions. A new aesthetic sensibility has emerged out of a sense of freedom from structure, codification, stereotypical notions of beauty and perfection and, finally, a deep feeling of release from gendered cultural representation and the burden of cultural custodianship.

Notes and References

1. Janet O'Shea, *At Home in the World: Bharata Natyam on the Global Stage*, Middletown, Connecticut: Wesleyan University Press, 2007, p. 55.
2. 'In Singapore, the state manages cultural diversity in reductionist terms. The CMIO [Chinese-Malay-Indian-Others] model cognitively streamlines society into four ethnic groups . . . While the CMIO model is in tune with the demands of mass society and global consumerism, it influences ethnic stereotyping in Singapore.' See Laurence Wai-Teng Leong, 'Commodifying Ethnicity: State and Ethnic Tourism in Singapore', in *Tourism, Ethnicity, and the State in Asian and Pacific Societies*, ed. Michel Picard and Robert Everett Wood, Honolulu, Hawaii: University of Hawaii Press, 1997, pp. 92–3.
3. A dance theatre production which premiered in Singapore in 1999. It was based on the true story of the sexual revenge that a young woman wreaked on the patriarchal Namboodri brahmin community in Kerala (south India) in the early 1900s.
4. Victoria Hunter, '"Moving Sites": Transformation and Re-location in Site-specific Dance Performance', *Contemporary Theatre Review*, vol. 22, no. 2, 2012, pp. 259–66.
5. Homi K. Bhabha, *The Location of Culture*, London: Routledge, 1994.
6. Elizabeth Grosz, 'Bodies-Cities', in *Places through the Body*, ed. Steve Pile and Heidi Nast, London: Routledge, 1998, pp. 42–51.
7. Cathy Turner, 'Palimpsest or Potential Space?: Finding a Vocabulary for Site-specific Performance', *New Theatre Quarterly*, vol. 20, no. 4, 2004, pp. 373–90.
8. Sondra Horton Fraleigh, *Dancing into Darkness: Butoh, Zen, and Japan*, Pittsburgh: University of Pittsburgh Press, 1999, p. 2.
9. Grosz, 'Bodies-Cities', p. 47.
10. Referred to as the cultural capital of India, it is also a key hub for Bharatanatyam.
11. Scholar Davesh Soneji describes the devadasis, who practised their dance form Sadir between the sixteenth and twentieth centuries, as 'temple servants' and 'secular courtesans'. Davesh Soneji, *Bharatanatyam: A Reader*, New Delhi: Oxford University Press, 2010, p. xiii. They were later expunged from the scene because of 'a female sexuality that was exercised outside the acceptable borders of middle class and upper caste womanhood'. Teresa Hubel, 'The High Cost of Dancing: When the Indian Women's Movement Went After the Devadasis', in *Bharatanatyam: A Reader*, ed. Davesh Soneji, Delhi: Oxford University Press, 2010, p. 173. The devadasi was a 'prostitute' to the reformers whose aim it was to eject her, while the revivalists projected her as a 'nun' and sought to 'incarnate her afresh'. Amrit Srinivasan, 'The Hindu Temple-Dancer: Prostitute or Nun?', *The Cambridge Journal of Anthropology*, vol. 8, no. 1, 1983, p. 96. Their transfigured dance was subsequently 'sanitized' of its erotic content to render it more palatable to the higher castes and classes of society.

'Bhakti' (devotion) is the central spirit of *abhinaya* (the expressive aspect of the dance form) and is conveyed through representation of eroticism or *sringara*, sexual union being the key metaphor for the ultimate divine union. While one set of people believes firmly in the portrayal of bhakti through erotic expression or *sringara*, another group believes that bhakti should be represented through supplication to a deity. This has been a point of intellectual and philosophical debate for many decades now. Anne-Marie Gaston, *Bharata Natyam: From Temple to Theatre*, New Delhi: Manohar, 2005, p. 87. The central figures in the *bhakti-sringara* discussion of the revival period were dancers T. Balasaraswati and Rukmini Devi, the former by virtue of being a performer who belonged to the devadasi lineage, and the latter for having founded the leading arts institution, Kalakshetra, and having significantly influenced the revival of the form. While both viewed bhakti as being central to the dance, Balasaraswati firmly believed in the portrayal of bhakti through *sringara*; for Rukmini Devi, bhakti was to be portrayed through surrender to the deity, devoid of sexuality.

12. See note 10, this chapter.
13. Nirmala Seshadri, 'Challenging Patriarchy through Dance', 2011, http://www.twu.edu/downloads/dance/seshadrPaper_Final_(3).pdf, accessed 22 July 2016.
14. Grosz, 'Bodies-Cities', p. 42.
15. Urmimala Sarkar Munsi, '"Century of Negotiations": The Changing Sphere of the Woman Dancer in India', in *Beyond the Private World: Indian Women in Public Sphere*, ed. Subrata Bagchi, Delhi: Primus Books, 2014, p. 308.
16. Ibid., p. 307.
17. Nandikesvara, *The Mirror of Gesture, Being the Abhinaya Darpana of Nandikesvara*, tr. Ananda Coomaraswamy and Gopala Kristnayya Duggirala, Cambridge: Harvard University Press, 1917, pp. 15–16. The original text dates back to thirteenth century CE.
18. A.K. Ramanujan, Velcheru Narayana Rao and David Shulman, eds. and trs., *When God is a Customer: Telugu Courtesan Songs by Kṣetrayya and Others*, Berkeley: University of California Press, 1994, p. 14.
19. See note 11, this chapter.
20. Kalanidhi Narayanan, *Aspects of Abhinaya*, Madras: Alliance Co., 1994, p. 26.
21. In Rustom Bharucha, *Chandralekha: Woman, Dance, Resistance*, New Delhi: Indus, 1995, p. 50.
22. O'Shea, *At Home in the World*, p. 26.
23. The Hindu god Shiva depicted as half male and half female.
24. Song from the *Gita Govinda*, a poem that was composed by the twelfth-century poet Jayadeva to depict the love between Krishna and his lover Radha.
25. Part of the *ashtanayika* or eight-fold classification of heroines in love.

26. Susan Leigh Foster, *Choreographing Empathy: Kinesthesia in Performance*, London: Routledge, 2011, p. 2.
27. Sarkar Munsi, 'Century of Negotiations', p. 308.
28. 'A Unique Performance', *City Express*, Chennai, 19 August 2003; 'When Past met Present', *The Hindu (Metroplus)*, Chennai, 26 October 2005.
29. 'When Past met Present', *The Hindu*.
30. Interview with Marie-Gabrielle Rotie, Christchurch Square, East London, 6 March 2013.
31. Ibid.
32. Nario Goda, in Fraleigh, *Dancing into Darkness*, p. 176.
33. Interview with Marie-Gabrielle Rotie, Christchurch Square, East London, 6 March 2013.
34. Ibid.
35. Victoria Hunter, 'Experiencing Space: The Implications for Site-Specific Dance Performance', in *Contemporary Choreography: A Critical Reader*, ed. Jo Butterworth and Liesbeth Wildschut, 2012, p. 411.
36. Notabilia, 'I Carry Your Heart by Nirmala Seshadri and Neewin Hershall', 12 February 2015, https://notabilia.wordpress.com/2015/02/12/i-carry-your-heart-by-nirmala-seshadri-and-neewin-hershall/, 12 February 2015.
37. Cathy Turner, 'Palimpsest or Potential Space?: Finding a Vocabulary for Site-Specific Performance', *New Theatre Quarterly*, vol. 20, no. 4, 2004, p. 382.
38. Tan Swie Hian in an email to Nirmala Seshadri, 13 February 2015.
39. Personal Conversation between Mrina Avadhani and Nirmala Seshadri, 12 February 2015, National University Hospital Heart Centre, Singapore.
40. Stephanie Burridge, 'Scene in Singapore: February 2015, CriticalDance, 2 March 2015, http://criticaldance.org/scene-in-singapore-february-2015/ (accessed 22 July 2016).
41. Foster, *Choreographing Empathy*, p. 73.

10 Chandralekha

Breaking Free to Counter the Nationalist Narrative in Dance

SADANAND MENON

Central to the two decades and more of reflection, interrogation, provocation, and creation in contemporary dance by Chandralekha has been the question: 'Where does the body begin . . . and end?'

Although Chandralekha stopped performing through much of the 1960s and 1970s (after a flourishing career as a solo Bharatanatyam dancer in the 1950s), by the time she re-engaged with group productions in the 1980s, her position and statement on the 'politics of the body' were well in place. She was unequivocal that the body of the dancer was not simply an instrument for amusing people. She found society in its present form unacceptable and was constantly, as she said, 'indignant' about it. Her quest, through her work with the body, was to effect a change in the consciousness of people. Rustom Bharucha, in his biographical work *Chandralekha*, writes: 'Not only has she broken new ground in the "language" of dance [especially Bharatanatyam], she has resisted the norms of "Indian womanhood" by rejecting the institutions of family, marriage, and motherhood. Resplendently, yet consciously, she remains her own woman. Inevitably, the very exceptionality of Chandra makes it difficult for any writer to categorize her.'[1]

The eminent Telugu poet and historian Arudra would even describe her work 'as a manifesto for an emancipatory politics of the body'[2] (Plate 10.1). Chandralekha (or 'Chandra', as everyone called her) was in search of locating the area of freedom in the body through dance. From her background[3] in the stylized Bharatanatyam form, with its specific moulding of the body in idealized terms, she recognized the need to enable the contemporary dancer's body to evolve from being individuated or personalized, to being universalized and humanized. She would constantly persuade the fifty-odd dancers she worked with during her twenty-odd years as a choreographer to be simultaneously conscious of the source of energy in their body as well as confront the physical and social difficulty they might face in tapping into it. For her, the dancer was someone who did not merely aestheticize the body, but also stimulated the imagination by politicizing it.

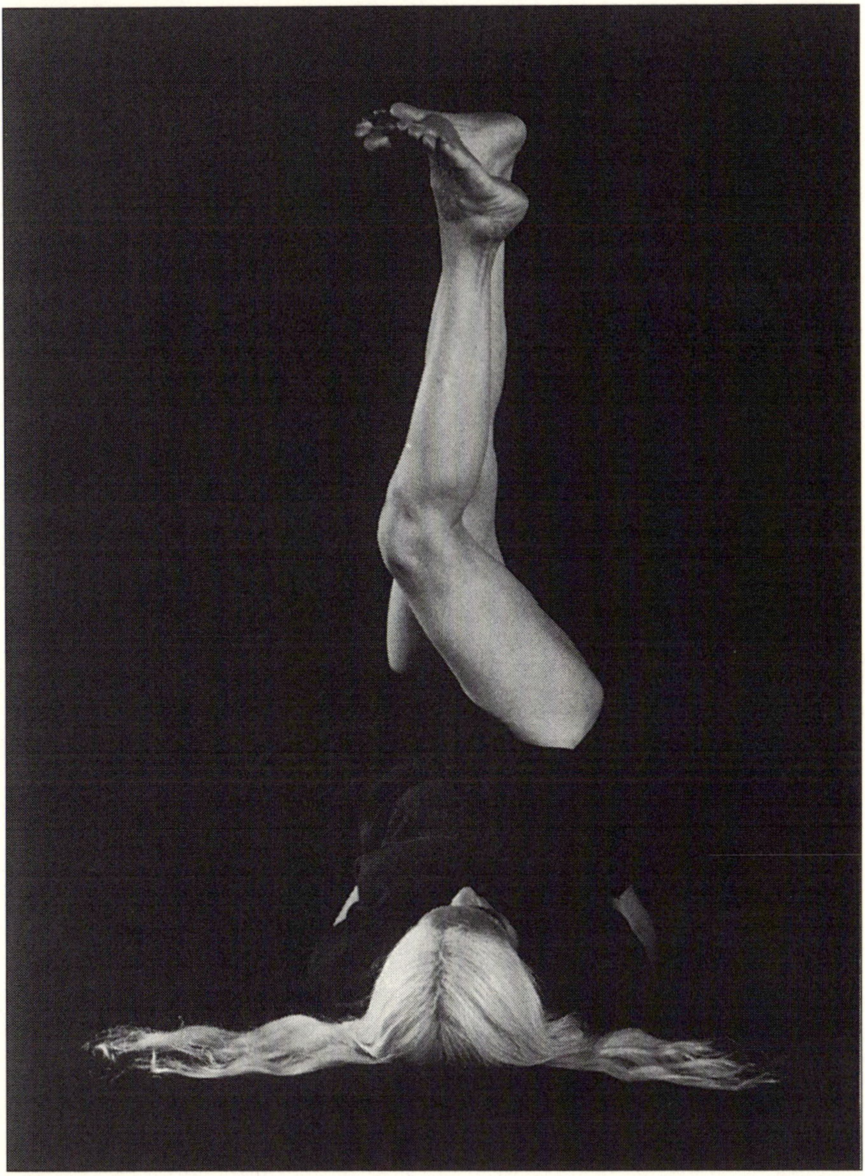

PLATE 10.1: Chandralekha performing the opening 'Sakambhari' sequence in *Sri*
Source: Courtesy of Bernd Merzenisch.

It was with *Angika* (1985) that Chandra, then aged 57, burst into the national artistic imagination, proclaiming the need for reintegrating the diverse Indian physical traditions and exploring new and contemporary directions for dance in India. Highlighting the link between dance and daily physical culture as well as nature, the inspired work highlighted the essential unity of all physical disciplines and proposed a non-narrative, universal, and non-sublimated content for the dance. In the process, one of her critical arguments was against the ongoing de-physicalization of the body in our times through rapid mechanization and the grotesque dilution of body-awareness in the classical dance forms here.

By 2006, when she passed away, her ten full-length productions, several shorter works, scores of lecture-demonstrations, workshops, and collaborations at many prestigious platforms in India and abroad, had posed a volley of crucial questions to the dance world and her vision became the yardstick by which new and contemporary dance from India was being measured. Interestingly, this continues even today, a full decade after her passing away.

Her productions—*Angika*, *Lilavati*, *Prana*, *Sri*, *Yantra*, *Mahakal*, *Raga*, *Sloka*, and *Sharira*—are classic examples of how Indian dance can be modern on its own terms without borrowing from the West (see Plate 10.2).

Chandra's work constitutes an appeal to reappraise the formal beauty and geometric integrity of the classical Bharatanatyam form in an entirely new proscenium space, while being a critique of its mechanically interpreted narrative content. Her critique of the corralling of the dance within the confines of narrow Brahminical religiosity made her consciously search for and foreground a broader, more abstract and non-mythological content. The cumulative direction of her search has been to return to the basics of the body and its energies within changing time/space dynamics.

What can the human body, enveloped in space, yet grappling with the laws of gravity and the relentless passage of time, inspire in us today? How can it be freed of the impositions of caste, religion, and regressive nationalism? Chandra boldly turned away from the decorative, sub-limated and sentimental answers inherent within fossilized—and 'invented'—traditionalism. She returned to simple, yet profound, issues like balance, lightness, slowness, gravity, control, eroticism, sensuality, extension (of breath and spine), and femininity, and amplified them in a complex way to take the cumulative aesthetic resources to a distinctly political plane. She knew that this new expressivity of the body would not fail to engage and move audiences.

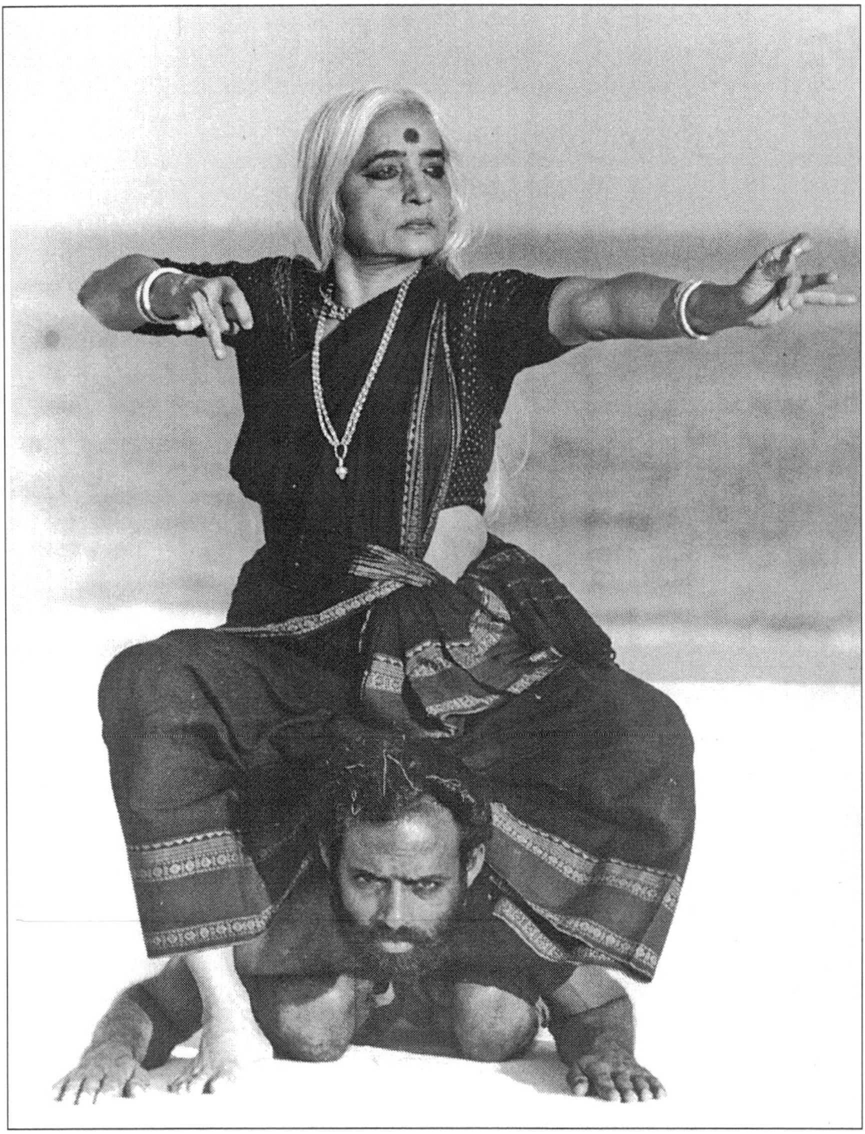

PLATE 10.2: Chandralekha in *Naravahana* Sequence from *Angika*, 1985
Source: Courtesy of Sadanand Menon.

As a subject of constant observation and research, the body keeps transforming our perceptions of time and space. Chandra's intuition and creative insights propose a journey through which we can narrow the distances within our own body and reconnect with our energy centres and our humanism. She was an acute observer of the investment of energy it takes to transform stillness into movement and movement into slowness/stillness and how that affects both the performer and the viewer's consciousness.

In that sense, her process has been akin to the manner in which the abstractions of music or colour are able to reach out and touch our consciousness. It is also, perhaps, the reason why audiences the world over have experienced her work in a physical, sensual, and visceral sense rather than as a spectacle or a piece of entertainment to be consumed.

Among the most important artistic voices from India in the past several decades, Chandralekha's critical aesthetic questioned the reduction of the body to merely something pretty or ornamental or instrumental. She celebrated the intense play between the subtle and the manifest body and its expressions through purity of line and the extension and dilation of the energy field. Her central premise remained the need to recover the unity of the body in fragmenting times and, within that, the indivisibility of sexuality, sensuality, and spirituality.[4]

One of the remarkable challenges Chandra posed, through her work with the physical, visual, kinetic media, was to the nationalist project, within which (for example) the bodies of dancers of reinvented classical forms were commandeered for building a new nationalist and moralist aesthetic. The classical dance forms in India, 'rescued' by the nationalist movement from an earlier history of infamy, suffer from having to bear the burden of such a nationalistic projection and proving their 'Indian-ness' by being Hinduized, tamed, and sanitized of all vestiges of their provenance in militancy[5] and eroticism. They are also used, almost militaristically, to protect the borders of 'disciplinarity'. Though each of the classical forms claims a common descent from the dance of Shiva-Nataraja or the canons of the *Natyashastra*, new conventions of differences between styles and regions were sutured into the presentation of classical dances such as Bharatanatyam, Kuchipudi or Odissi. Such territorial modes of 'sacred' boundaries are a significant way by which the nation state requisitions the body to illustrate its political agenda of 'unity in diversity' and imposes conservative conventions of disciplinary conformism.

The idea of national culture, its space and its function, is built around a social machinery which disciplines and brings in line everyone to an acceptable base of normative behaviour, failing which there is a structure of punishment. We can certainly add to this typology the modern performance space of the proscenium, with its subliminal codes of frontality and one-point perspective. The idea of disciplinarity here would, therefore, sound like a disease, a violent act, which is why, along with Chandra, I too have been an advocate of 'anti-disciplinarity' (see Plate 10.3).

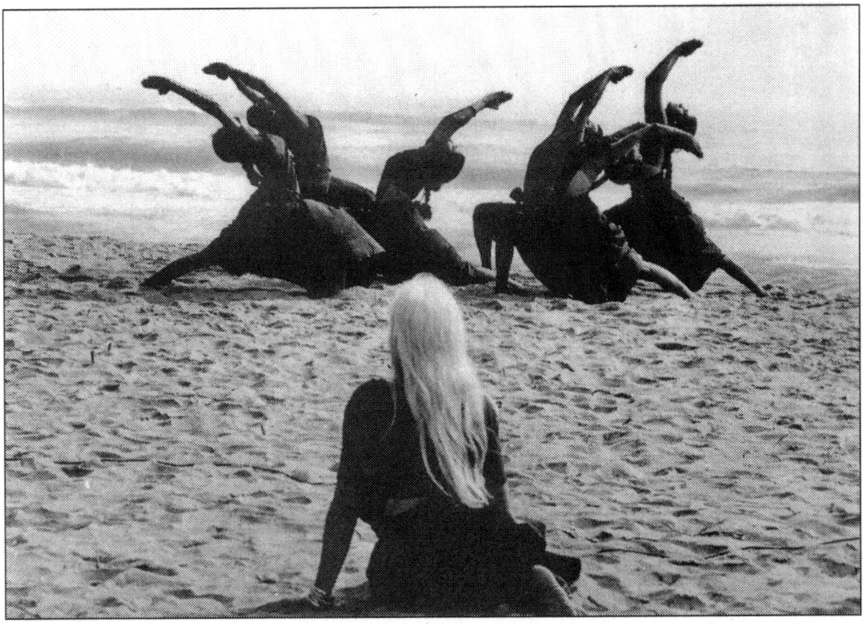

PLATE 10.3: Chandralekha with Dancers, *Namaskar*, 1986
Source: Courtesy of Sadanand Menon.

I had the immense fortune of living and working for over three decades with Chandralekha and Dashrath Patel, both outstanding Indian artists of the twentieth century. They had, in turn, lived for a decade and more with Harindranath Chattopadhyay, one of the founders of iconic and radical pre-independence artists' movements like the Progressive Writers' Association (PWA) and the Indian People's Theatre Association (IPTA). Baba (as we affectionately called him), every day without fail, wrote poems, painted, sketched and sang both classical and radical compositions. He was a *shagird* (pupil) of Ustad Abdul Karim Khan (of the Kirana Gharana), and was but fifteen when admitted to Cambridge and, as a poet, had been proclaimed by Rabindranath Tagore as his successor. He was also an independent elected member of the first Indian Parliament. Chandra did not miss a sunrise or a moonrise, drew *kolams* every day, painted or sketched, danced, cooked, wrote poems or concept notes. Dashrath effortlessly transited from drawing to photography, to graphics, to ceramic, to architecture, to paper collages, to both industrial and craft design. It was a mode of being for them. Never once did they pause to see themselves in disciplinary terms. Their creativity was far too unified to be pigeonholed and, in their expression, one media could not be separated from the other. There was an artistic seamlessness there, which I learnt to describe as true anti-disciplinarity—a sort of, conscious and unconscious, totality. Claiming Chandra's stance as anti-disciplinary, I firmly believe that art and artists—especially dancers—and academics writing on artistic practices need to take care not to fall into the disciplinary trap even if it does provide some advantages of ordering, organizing, and patronage. Its potential to stunt is far greater.

Of course, this is not something that was exclusive to these artists. One can make a long list of artists, writers and scientists in pre-independence India who were similarly versatile. To push the idea further, one just needs to go, say, to a Gond village in Madhya Pradesh. In the everyday life of the tribal community everyone sings, everyone paints and everyone dances. And not one of them calls herself a singer or a painter or a dancer. They are just what they are. Their creativity is not bound by definitions of specializations or disciplines. I believe there is a need for that sense of flow in the creative field, for our forms to feel reinvigorated and more meaningful.

To return to Chandra, her story gives us examples of being simultaneously disciplinary—of preparing the body and the mind for self-awareness as well for being able to connect with one's interiority—and of the anti-disciplinarity that she proudly carried along as her strength, throughout her life.

Chandra's Choreoraphy: An Ongoing Exploratory Process

Chandra herself described her choreography as 'a celebration of the human body'. From *Angika* (1985) till *Sharira* (2002), she choreographed ten pieces, each very different from the other. If one analyses sequentially, it is easy to see how dramatically her approach changed with each production. Certain quests and concerns remained constant in all productions. But, by the time she comes to *Sharira* her working style and format had changed radically. From a large group with some 18 dancers when she started out with *Angika*, *Sharira* had only two performers on stage. Both artists (who continue to perform in the production even after Chandra's passing away) are actually non-dancers. Shaji K. John—associated for a long time with Chandralekha's choreographic explorations—is a Kalaripayattu artist and teacher, and Tishani Doshi is a yoga artist with no dance training at all. Chandra also shifted completely away from her comfort zone with renowned classical Carnatic musicians who had, till then, collaborated in all her productions. In *Sharira*, she intuitively moved to explore the Classical Hindustani Dhrupad style and the acclaimed Gundecha brothers[6] became her new collaborators.

Even right at the beginning of her journey, she had begun positioning herself against the virtuosity of speed in dance performances and constantly spoke against it. Slowness was her antidote to the mindless speeding up which, for Chandra, was merely a quantitative idea. As she and her dancers began getting increasingly adept at slowing down the pace, the effect was often hypnotic. When Henri Cartier-Bresson, perhaps the greatest photographer of the twentieth century and a close friend of Chandra's, saw a rehearsal of *Yantra* in Avignon (France), he had tears in his eyes as he told the dancers, 'Such wonderful slowness; slowness is the only luxury we have left in the world today. Your work will cleanse the eyes of those who see it.'[7]

This is felt even more acutely in *Sharira* because the music and the movement come together organically in an unapologetic excess of slowness. The music does not follow the dance, nor does the dance follow the music. Yet, echoing the physical movement on stage, the dhrupad form is able to elongate and slow down to structures of pace known as *vilambit* (slow) and *ati-vilambit* (very slow). The pace is so reduced that Chandra even remarked gleefully, once, 'Slow, so slow. Now it is possible for the audience to watch and experience this performance with their eyes closed if they want.' Such introspection and experiments with movement were constantly mixed with her social concerns as she steadily left behind the fixed ideas of the dance form she had trained in or had worked with during the beginning of her journey.

New Content

Another of Chandra's primary concerns was around creating new content for the dance. New content does not grow out of thin air. And it does not grow out of newspaper headlines. It also does not grow out of reading a fiction or a non-fiction book. The new content has to come out of the life that you lead yourself. It cannot be manufactured. And the life that you lead yourself has to have a certain resonance for yourself first before it can resonate for anybody else. The core concern for Chandra, in all her works, has been the women's question and, related to it, questions of sexuality, of erotica, of femininity in women—as well as in men—as also what is it that generates *bhava* (emotion/mood) and *rasa* (essence/aesthetic understanding) in the body. A fierce speaker and writer on women's issues, all her work and all her relationships with the dancers she worked with or choreographed were informed by that preoccupation.

A project that Chandra did between 1986 and 1988, soon after she had returned to working with dance and performance, contributed immensely to integrate her feminist concerns with her later choreographic work. It was a set of assignments she executed for the Government of India's Festival of India in the erstwhile Union of Soviet Socialist Republics (USSR). For one, she was the chief choreographer for the inaugural events of the Festival in Moscow, Leningrad and Tashkent,[8] for which she had to coordinate and choreograph over 800 rural and tribal dancers/performers. Finding links and commonalities as well as specific differences between these forms was a valuable experience for her.

Simultaneously, she was also the conceptualizer and visualizer of a massive exhibition on Indian women called *Stree* at the Krimsky Hall in Moscow. She involved a large number of women activists, feminist scholars from the various newly started women's studies departments, artists, musicians, and filmmakers in the exhibition. It's a pity this outstanding exhibition was seen only in Moscow, and that it did not travel back to India; or that it was not presented in India before it travelled out. Once in Moscow, there were severe disagreements between Chandra and her group, who had created the exhibition on one side, and Indian diplomats/bureaucrats there, over the assertion to project Indira Gandhi in a more prominent way. It led to a protest and walk-out by Chandra and her colleagues and the exhibition was quietly allowed to lapse.

However, some of the text panels that Chandra wrote for that exhibition give us a good idea of the conceptual frame of her feminist concerns, her linguistic skills, and her poetic sensibilities, which then also began to inform her dance work.

The exhibition opened with the following panel that Chandra wrote. It was titled, 'A Hymn to Her':[9]

360,000,000 women hold up the Indian earth and sky.
Space-wise they are scattered and clustered in far-flung villages, valleys, hills, forests, cities and towns.
They are bound by age-old customs, diverse languages, traditions, lifestyles, religions.
Time-wise they span thousands of years of history and civilization.
Time lies stratified in their bodies, invisible like strata in stone.
They are old, the youngest of them, and continuous: linked to their prehistory and past in an unbroken way.
They inherited concepts that predate organized religion and consolidated family, concepts not only of equality but of primacy.
They remember—through art, cult, ritual, and imagery—that the female was seen once upon a time, not as a soft and beautiful consort but as a powerful and autonomous woman, at once protector and destroyer, benevolent and fiery.
And though this knowledge is defaced and covered up by time, it shows in the dignity of their bodies, in the poise and presence, the grace and coordination that they bear even as they walk, sit, stand, work.
Today women are distanced from the knowledge and power, which was theirs, which had come to them from female-centred societies.

Today women's image and situation is a hard reality.
Women are caught in cunning and complex social mores.
They are made partners in patriarchy, chained to it legally and morally.
Through sexual division of labour, their space is limited, their mobility and their voices confined.
They have been assigned a secondary role and status in society.
And even as they are deified, their womanhood is robbed of its meaning, its essence.
Today the Indian woman is struggling hard to make connections between timeless concepts and contemporary life.
Today the Indian woman is trying to identify the end of the silken thread from the inert cocoon and draw it out for making meaningful reference points in terms of her life and culture.
It is a search for her identity.
It is a search for her space.
It is a search for her potential to extend,
To transcend particularities,
To generate universal values.

Later in the exhibition another panel called 'A Day in Her Life' reads thus:

She is one of the multitudes,
The classical Indian woman,
The ordinary one—like hundreds, thousands, millions of her kind.
She remains largely invisible in our culture.
She represents the values and ideals of Indian womanhood.
She deserves to be heard.
She deserves recognition.

She rises before the sun rises
It is early, still dark
Only the birds wake with her
Before sprinkling water on her face, on her just awakened eyes,
She sprinkles water on the ground before the house-front—She makes it look auspicious.
The sun is welcome now.

The day begins.
A long day of chores—
water chores
animal chores
milk chores
house chores
children chores
kitchen chores
She moves like a dancer
She works as if she had eight hands.

The tasks are many
The tasks are continuous
how to preserve
how to conserve
how to economise

how to maximise
how to make a little go a long way
It is a familiar sight,
A woman, a mother, a grandmother, bending down, flexing her fingers to pick a grain of rice from the kitchen floor.

All her work, all her concerns are for the small, for the insignificant.
Her work cannot be added up
It is a quality
not a number.
It is an art of living.

In the process of her work, everything changes.
Gently, imperceptibly.
Someone has cold or cough or fever or pain or ache—
she knows at once what to do.

She knows the science of the kitchen.
In the daily food, she adds a piece of ginger, leaves or coriander or mint, a herb, a spice, a seasoning.
From the storehouse of knowledge, she extracts taste and feeling and well-being.
She gives it to all those around her abundantly, unmindful of wearing herself out in the process.

A day in the life of an Indian woman is endless.
It is a drudge without break, without respite, unrelieved, relentless, Difficult to cope with, even with multiple hands.
While men run the world,
She runs life.

The most enduring image in India is of a woman
With abundant and flowing powers.
One who is terrifying and beautiful
One who is awesome
One who is fearless
One who has courage and indignation
who fights forces of darkness and injustice
who upholds values of life
who cannot remain passive and benign
who is roused to ferocity and anger
who wields weapons
who rides on ferocious animals
who annihilates evil
who restores balance.

In our own unbalanced times such women exist, mostly in myth and legend, or as deified goddesses.
Today woman is cut off from her powers.
She has become vulnerable to a thousand evils, she has forgotten to fight. She has become meek.
She suffers injustices and oppression.
She even submits to them.

Today, once again, woman is reaching out.

She cleaves through darkness,
through the inexorable power of Time.
She who knows darkness and terror
in her body
in her mind.

The exhibition highlighted a whole list of achievements of the growing women's movement in India, of which Chandra herself was a part in different ways. Some of those ideas and images, in turn, reflected in her creative process and in her dance work. Across her oeuvre, there are these recurring flashes of unusual, uncommon, unconventional depictions of women, not familiar to the imagery within classical dance narratives and their stereotyped mythological references. Those familiar with Chandra's work remember having been amazed and thrilled with representations of woman as *Naravahana* (woman riding on man) in *Angika*, *Sakambhari* (woman birthing nature and all creation) in *Sri*, *Salabhanjika* (woman as fertility and prosperity) in *Mahakal*, or *Bhayankari* (woman as terrifying, beautiful and autonomous) in *Sharira*. Another favourite concept she used to refer to at feminist and dance forums to challenge the constant valorization of motherhood, was the idea of *Apita-kuchamba* (the goddess with undrunk breasts). Chandra recognized the inherent pro-woman power in these archaic concepts and constantly sought creative ways with which to interrupt her own work with these built-in counters to the mainstream.

On occasion, when she quoted a more religiously identifiable female icon, like 'Dashbhuja' (powerful goddess with ten hands) in *Sri*, she would instantly dissolve the image, de-iconize it and counter it with the depiction of a women's collective that surges forward towards its own independent spiritual destiny. It is interesting that the literary scores of re-quotations of this image from Chandra's work by other choreographers in later years were not sensitive to this iconoclastic process that Chandra subjected the religious images to.

It was a protocol of irreverence she had learnt from her father as well as from Harin Baba. Even before she entered her teens, her father would encourage her to read important texts like, say, the Bible, and even as she went rapturous over it would present her with Robert Ingersoll's agnostic critique of it. Similarly, just as she began getting starry-eyed over the Gita, she would receive a discourse on how it was nothing but a text on Krishna's *atmashlagha* (boastfulness). Critical counter-discourse was, thus, wired into her from an early age. The years spent with Harindranath Chattopadhyay only consolidated this further. Baba's musical and compositional skills were so extraordinary that he could, for example, pick up a bhajan like '*Bin bhojan ke bhagwan . . .*'

(a devotional lament on the deity's distress at not being fed) and at a fever pitch of devotional intensity as he sang the *dhun* (tune), suddenly, with impeccable *laya* (rhythm), transform it to '*Bin bhojan ke bhagwan kahaan, gungaan kahaan . . .*' (How is prayer and devotion possible on an empty stomach?), completely cutting out the deity from it and turning it into a political anthem. Or he could perform what would seem to be a composition of deep spirituality, and for half-an-hour, with head bent and eyes closed and great musicality, transport you into the ecstasy of a seeming Meera Bhajan until, at the very end, everyone would realize with an explosion of laughter that he was actually singing 'God save the Queen'. These were strategies that became second nature to Chandra in her creative work.

The specific location of the body becomes essential within her work, paying attention to the spine, to the idea of the body as a contested site, something that never can be taken as a harmonious whole. She recognized and acknowledged the particular need to historicize things like gait, gesture, posture, the walk, and specificities that mark the bodies in terms of time and space. Her consistent questioning of the idea of the feminine, the way it is perceived, the way it is received, the transgression of space through a specific kind of eroticization of the body in performance also negotiated constantly with her idea of the woman's body as space.

She consciously paid attention to three kinds of physical transformation in her work—self-expressive, representative, and collaborative. In her choreographic scheme, maybe for the first time in the Indian scenario, she deliberately perceived space differently to make a departure from the accepted concepts of lines, by liberally interjecting the diagonal line. Her perception of the horizontal line as the line of time and convention, of the vertical line as the line of history and project, and of the diagonal line as the line of feminist assertion—the line on which the gendered body can cut through and make a new poetical presence—made a difference to the way she used bodies in space in her choreography.

Chandra worked with a very young group of dancers. The age difference between her and them was considerable. She never wanted to run a dance school and she was already in her mid-fifties when she embarked on her new phase of work. Her dancers were typically in their late teens or early twenties. She was extremely patient. She would not push anybody, and worked with anyone who came to her with very different levels of training. She waited for something to reveal itself with respect to the dancer's specific strength, something that made a difference to her self-understanding with respect to the physical process she was going through. Once Chandra spotted the dancer's strong point, she was deft at positioning that within her choreography in a manner that made the individual dancer stand out. As a choreographer, she was protective of her dancers and never exposed their limitations. Even the legendary Pina Bausch commented wonderingly, when she saw Chandra's work for the first time in 1988 in Wuppertal, 'Chandra, unlike in our work in the West where dancers on stage become amorphous and faceless, every one of your dancers registers as an individual'.[10] All that Chandra worked towards was to ensure (without showing it) that the dancers would 'breathe together' on stage and that even those who were not on stage would stay tuned to the pulse from the wings. It created a collectivity from within which each artist stood out.

The impact on the consciousness of her dancers was osmotic. Once a French television team had come to interview and record her work. A rehearsal for *Raga* was on and a few of her dancers were working out on stage. Even as she was talking to Chandra and filming her, the French anchor suddenly shifted the camera and microphone to one of the dancers nearby and said, 'So, madam, what have you learnt by working in Chandralekha's group?' This young girl, a Kalakshetra graduate, was from a highly protected, conservative Tamil family. Very shy by nature, she was also uncomfortable with English. But, at that moment, sitting on the floor, without batting an eyelid, she flung her two legs and arms completely apart in a full split and said, 'I learnt, open body, open mind'. That was the kind of spontaneous impact Chandra had on her dancers.

The event that helped Chandra's return to dance/performance as well as crystallize her ideas was the 'East West Dance Encounter'[11] of 1984, at the National Centre for the Performing Arts (NCPA), Bombay (now Mumbai). Initiated by Georg Lechner of the Max Mueller Bhavan and supported by various organizations, the Dance Encounter turned out to be an event of historical importance, as it facilitated the new choreographies of dancers like Kumidini Lakhia, Mrinalini Sarabhai, Astad Deboo, and Chandra herself, and brought a new vitality to the Indian dance space.

In her landmark paper at the seminar, Chandra laid out her critique of the current landscape of dance as well as her vision of the directions that needed to be taken. She said:

In the prevailing dance situation, there are certain negatives that we have to guard against, and I'm very clear about that.
Spectacular mindlessness
Archaic social values
Faked religiosity
Idealisation leading to mortification of the form

Numbing sentimentality
Literalism, verbalism, dependency on sahitya, on word
Mystification and dollification
Perpetuation of anti-women values.
Rigid standardisation leaving no spaces for exploration
Quantitativeness leading to conspicuous quantity of effects
The easy assimilation into governmental designs for propagating a false image of India, distanced from reality and replete with nostalgia
Distortions of the 'foreign' circuit that squeeze out all essence and convert classical dancers to an item of cultural export
The encroachments of tourism, urbanization, commercialism and packaged entertainment
The cynicism within the solo dance situation and its senseless competitiveness
All this we have to be critical of and guard against.[12]

Chandra worked within this frame that she created for herself—based on the aforementioned observations—and consistently moved away from the narrative form. Storytelling was dropped straight away. By the time she did her fourth work, *Sri*, she had also dispensed with the *nattuvanar*, whom she called 'the male controlling presence on stage'. In the absence of this person on stage maintaining the beats or giving *talam*, the dancing female body became visibly and functionally independent and the dancers learnt to depend more on the music that was composed especially for her work after that time.

It was in *Sri* too that she began exploring pre-Hindu ideas of woman as Sakambhari, first found in an Indus Valley seal, where woman is depicted with her body upside down, with the entire creation emerging from her *yoni* (vagina). The work highlights women in pre-patriarchal societies where they were free. The women's bodies were shown as different, unshackled, adjusted to living and being with nature, and organically inclined towards a balance between male-female co-existence. In the work, Chandra makes radical departures from the Bharatanatyam form and the body it constructs. Working on the idea of the spine as a metaphor for freedom, she excavates new sources for expressivity from a diverse vocabulary of principles of sitting, standing, walking from multiple performative forms across the subcontinent.

Chandra grew up during a time when social movements were strong and many artists, activists, and thinkers in India got formed in it. Feminism had arrived. The political scene was very active. Identity politics was coming up. She acknowledged her responsibility as a human being, a woman, and a conscious dancer. She did not, perhaps, leave a physical legacy—there was no company, no dance school, no students, no archive. Yet her impact was far beyond dance itself. The number of artists, women activists, scholars, and people in the creative community whom she has impacted is legion. She stirred the Indian dance scenario as no one before in recent times had done, and continues to do. She broke free to counter the nationalist narrative in dance. That is her contribution.

Notes and References

1. Chandralekha's politics and her conceptualization of the body in the context of her dance and choreographic work were laid out at the beginning of the landmark biographical work of Rustom Bharucha, titled *Chandralekha: Woman, Dance, Resistance*, New Delhi: Indus (an imprint of HarperCollins), 1995, p. 1.
2. Arudra, 'The Transfiguration of a Traditional Dance: The Academy and the Dance, Events of the First Decade', *Sruti*, vols. 27–8, 1986–7, pp. 17–21.
3. 'It's Bharatanatyam that took me to Madras. . . . I saw different styles; when I was in Madras, I saw Shanta Rao, I saw Tara Chaudhry, I saw Bala Saraswati, I saw all of them and I decided that I would earn the Bala Saraswati style.' *Talking Heads: Chandralekha*, interview of Chandralekha by Sunil Sethi, NDTV, November 2000, https://www.youtube.com/watch?v=T-ClDsz6bi4 (accessed 8 August 2016).
4. Chandra speaks about these three terms—sensuality, sexuality, spirituality—and their connections to the body in *Sharira: Chandralekha's Explorations in Dance*, the documentary film made by Ein Lall, Public Service Broadcasting Trust (PSBT).
5. In her seminal paper 'Militant Origins of Indian Dance', Chandra talks about the grammar and the cognitive system of the community dances in different parts of India that have survived to this day. Chandralekha, 'Militant Origins of Indian Dance', *Social Scientist*, vol. 9, nos. 2–3, 1980, pp. 80–5.
6. The Gundecha brothers are acclaimed exponents of Dhrupad, one of the major traditions of Hindustani classical music.
7. In 1996, when Cartier-Bresson and his photographer wife Martine Franck came to watch Chandralekha rehearse her production of *Yantra* at the Avignon Festival. In my tribute to the great French photographer Henri Cartier-Bresson in the article 'Master of the Moment' in *New Internationalist* (1 October 2004), I wrote that his friendship with Chandralekha dates back to 1950 when both of them were in Tiruvannamalai, Tamil Nadu, during the last days of Ramana Maharshi.
8. The festival was held in July 1987 and it showcased a spectacular choreography by Chandralekha.
9. Unpublished panel by Chandralekha, created specifically for the exhibition Stree (meaning Woman) for the Festival of India in USSR, 1988.
10. Chandralekha was invited with her troupe to Wuppertal by Pina Bausch 1988. In 1994, Tanztheater Wuppertal travelled to India, and Bausch's

choreographic piece *Nelken* or 'Carnations' (first choreographed in 1984) was presented along with Chandralekha's work *Yantra*.

11. East West Dance Encounter (1984), a festival of contemporary explorations in Indian dance, was organized in Bombay by Georg Lechner, the then director of Max Mueller Bhavan. This festival was the occasion where Chandralekha presented her choreographic work *Angika*. This is recognized as a significant event in the history of contemporary choreography in Indian dance.
12. Presentationby Chandralekha at the *East West Dance Encounter*, NCPA, Bombay, 22–9 January 1984 (quoted from the original paper in the 'Chandralekha Archive').

11 The Politics of Space

SAMIK BANDYOPADHYAY

I

In a paper published in 2005, I raised a set of questions:

> Is the dancing body/the dancer's body necessarily a body in free space? To what extent is the performance defined and structured by the space in which the body operates/acts? Can a performance mode be supplanted/transferred from a traditionally conceived/designed/predetermined space in which it has had its origin and in which it has developed over a long stretch of historical time, to a more standardized, universal and hence neutral performance space? Does it not lose in the process the charge and the aura of the original culture in which it has been embedded? Will the dancer practiced/trained in such a performance mode conceived in/for a specific traditional performance space, performing the same gestures and movements, ostensibly in the same manner, in a neutral, universal space, convey the same significance?[1]

Obviously, the context in which I raised the questions lay in the scenario in which the country's major women dancers had defined for themselves performative positions and chosen their performance situations/spaces. They could be put into a number of categories, viz., (1) those who positioned themselves within the accepted classical genres; (2) those who mixed several classical and folk genres, and produced melanges normally around chosen or assigned themes, often for special celebratory occasions; (3) those who addressed the language and symbolic potency of dance to produce creative compositions, often exploring/probing the gendered body; (4) those who unabashedly turned the dance into a text to be read for philosophical, ethical or political messages/statements/credos.

With their artistic choices, they had also fixed their performance spaces; spaces set at different junctures of negotiation, viz., the physical space or 'the stage'; the ambient space or the organizational/presentational matrix that determines the site/location of the performance; and the public space of the audience (ticketed or invited or 'restricted to members'?).[2]

When I raised those questions, I was disturbed by the general indifference of the practising women dancers to the politics of the space/spaces in which they were happily dancing away, and how in their indifference they were allowing the dance experience to be grabbed by a capitalist entertainment industry that would eventually debilitate it to sheer inertia!

The most vulnerable are of course those in the first category who cultivate the aura of the classical only to be closeted into the rules and conventions of a *guru-shishya parampara*, which sets the parameters by which they are judged by a small body of professional critics. Have dancers ever taken into consideration the fact that most Indian languages—the *bhashas*—do not have a word for the classical, or wondered how old the history of the classical as an idea or a regimen is! It is the myth of the classical on which the dancer falls back to turn herself into a diva and her special place on a pedestal, and in the process incarcerates herself in a repertoire in which she has proven her authenticity/traditionality. The lavishly decorated/decked out body becomes more of an iconic showpiece than a dancing body in the protocols determined in collusion by the patronizing/managerial presenter and the target audience of a supposed elite for whom taste for the classical is a marker of class, and the sartorial fashions they display contribute to the public space; all these factors impoverishing the meaningfulness of the performance and curbing any possibility of fresh and original creativity.

Those in the second category are fast falling into the rut of Bollywood extravaganza, with their performance spaces more often than not set in stadiums, makeshift stages in the open, in club spaces that had once provided platforms to the cabaret girls. The audience, ranging from the adolescent to the middle-aged, lap up the kitschy sexuality, the pace and the rhythm and the easy mindlessness.

Those in the third category are a struggling minority, rarely finding the right space for themselves, in the absence of an intelligentsia that is prepared to support and cultivate such an endeavour. The physical performance spaces they find are often the cultural centres of foreign diplomatic institutions in the country or university spaces (more of them available now with the introduction of performance and performing arts studies in the university); the tenuousness of the location standing in the way of a possible development of the ambient or public spaces, in other words, a culture of perceiving the dance as an evolving, changing, growing art.

While those in the fourth category find an immediate public space in an immediately motivated and committed and militant support base of enthusiasts, there is little to assure them that this audience will continue to be with them, for in most cases it is a floating constituency moved by the times more than by the dance.

There is also a tendency in the fourth category to look for an official public space by identifying with and contributing to some governmental or corporate agenda, e.g. in the dancers engaged in the prison projects, where the State offers physical spaces/site for performance, properly and visibly under strict security surveillance, creating in the process an ambient space where the dancer turns into a spokesperson of the State upholding its benevolent public-welfare face, masking its glaring institutionalized injustices, especially in the prison system and the operations of the police machinery. The State-culture interface in this case offers the dancer a comfort which is not just non-judgemental, but also practically non-perceptive, for the prison inmates are considered/treated more as a caged species given a protected space for a limited time than a performing ensemble; something that is more often than not true for the NGO-engineered performances.

With the transactions in the ambient space corroding the construction of meaning in the negotiations between performer and the public space, the physical performance space either closing in on itself or distancing itself in an artificial sacrality (with the first category of dancers), or spilling over with the second category, or finding a precarious balance with the third category or the fourth, it is left to the dancers to rethink and critique their positioning; particularly in view of the fact that both State and Capital are predatorily eyeing the dancer's space, seeking to find ways and means to capture it and cast it into an utterly consumerist, marketable culture industry. The subtle machinations aiming at such a goal are in operation in the politics of spaces in the dance scene in India, with the virtual effacement of a critical intelligence from the print media in place ensuring a silencing of doubts and questioning.

The questions I raised in 2005 come back with greater concern in 2016, calling for caution and wariness on the part of the community of dancers before unknowingly they are turned into neatly packaged export commodities.

II

Set against the agonizing scepticism that runs through the earlier section, the example of Kalakshetra Manipur, led by Heisnam Kanhailal, with the redoubtable Heisnam Sabitri as the lead performer, is a case where 'live theatre', as Kanhailal describes it, restores 'organically' (one of Kanhailal's favourite phrases) the lost continuity between theatre and dance, and relocates the performance in an ambient space, where several cultures are in confrontation (Plates 11.1 and 11.2).

As a matter of fact, Kanhailal was driven to a quest for what he calls

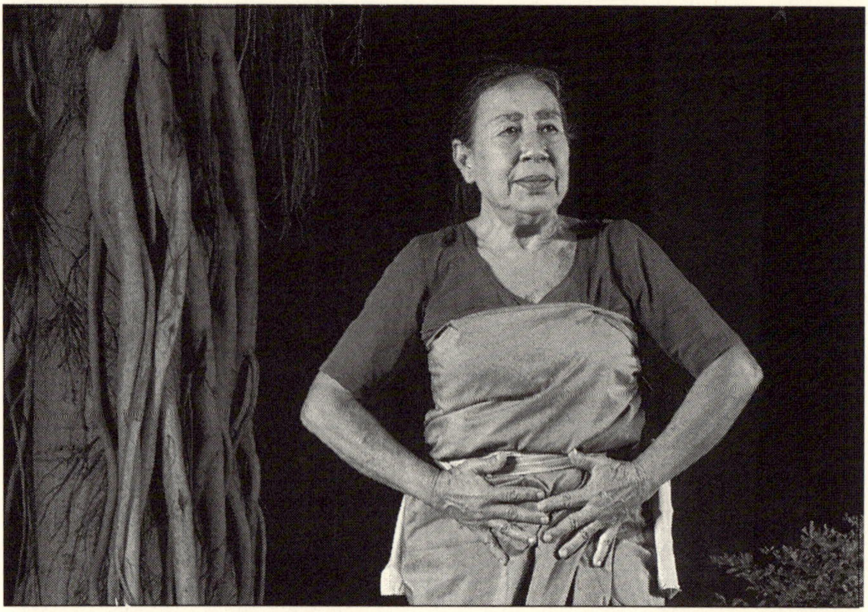

PLATE 11.1: Heisnam Sabitri in *Pebet*, directed by Heishnam Kanhailal. *Source*: Courtesy of Poulami Das.

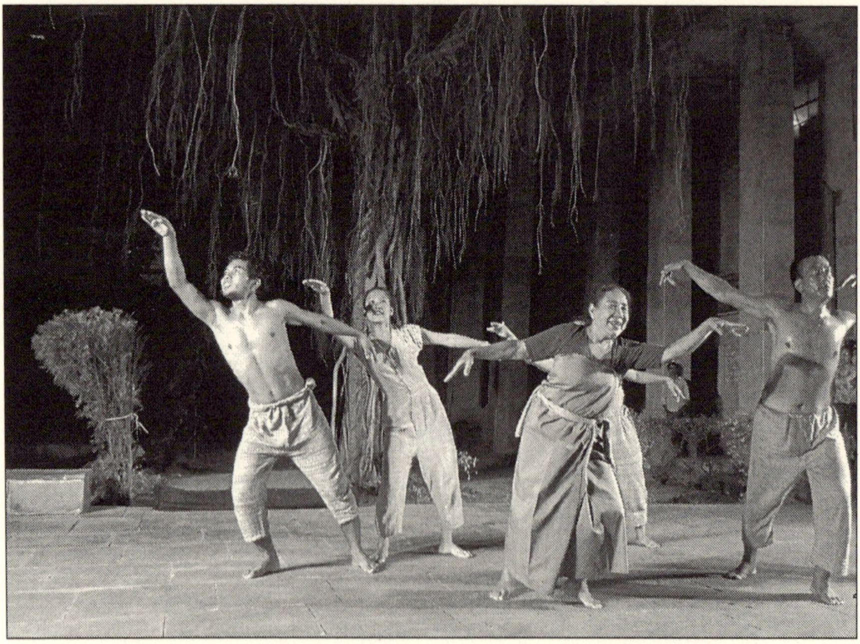

PLATE 11.2: Using Traces of Traditional Gestures from Dance: Heishnam Sabitri in *Pebet*. *Source*: Courtesy of Poulami Das.

his 'new trajectory' by the politics of the clash of cultures being officially camouflaged all the time under the ceremonial pretensions of 'national' festivals and expositions. It was more than personal humiliation for him when he 'had to accept the termination imposed on me by the National School of Drama after three months of training in 1968'.[3] It was a blatant case of ethnic profiling at a 'national' institute showcased by the state ever since its inception. For Kanhailal, it meant alienation from 'the academic and intellectual system of theatre making' and 'the urban and reductive culture'.[4] He needed a little time to 'heal' his 'injured' psyche; before he could

> transform this situation of failure into a real challenge of self-learning. I began to look back afresh at my own Meitei ethnic past—the ancestral past of nature lore and native lore. Bewildered, I wandered into the ethnic jungle of impulses in order to explore the sources of the primeval human nature. The word 'wild' here is not used in its modern pejorative sense, meaning 'out of control,' but in its original sense, i.e. to live a natural life—elemental, pristine or vital. The wild then appears as our wild teacher, wild mentor, wild mother that gives birth to the 'lightening' [i.e. light-emanating] sources of creativity and supports the inner and outer lives of the 'doers' who risk cultural expedition in the wild space of theatre. I was shadowing Nongtham Leima, the 'lightening' lady of the Meitei creation myth, in her home of dark woods to explore an original alternative for an instinctive and subtle form of awareness in reacting to the dominant tension of our time in our localized context. My theatre appeared in its autonomy that the body speaks and vindicates in solidifying the form of social experience with a haunting effect in its best sense.[5]

The trajectory of 'the wild' that Kanhailal sets out for himself is mapped out along several spaces, including the ambient space of the reclamation of an ethnic 'wild', the jungle with its natural nurture, where the body relocates itself in the wary progress through untamed territory; the physical performance location of the *mandapam*, the traditionally conceived/designed extension of the Meitei home into the community, where the private/domestic reaches out to the public in a locational gesture. When the experience of the negotiation with the wild is 'performed'/replicated in the *mandapam*, an enclosure without walls, a mere step beyond the home, the wild is socialized through performance; the dancing/acting body playing out a history, and making history at the same time.

In the rest of India, the performative culture of dance, is 'authoritatively' reconstructed and redefined in an authoritarian space of rigidly defined and scripturally authorized linear/hereditary traditions—*guru-shishya paramparas*, rules, and conventions. It finds itself torn between the two tugs of the safer submission to the 'classical' provenance and absorption in a celebratory/entertainment performance module, and the uncertain terrain of experimental and/or conscientious creativity. Meanwhile, the Manipuri performative culture, through its history of resistance to alien political, religious and gender provocations, has located itself in a position where it can freely draw on the cultural capital of the Maibi at the centre of the elaborate ritual theatre of the Lai Haraoba (Plate 11.3), and the rich history of the series of women's wars—the *Nupilan*.[6]

Drawing on the cultural capital of a performance practice that has never split itself into the categories of theatre, dance, music or even ritual and performance art, the Manipuri dance theatre—as evident in Kanhailal's work, especially in his *Pebet* (1975), *Memoirs of Africa* (1986), *Draupadi* (2000), and *Dakghar* (2006)—all of them with the actress Heisnam Sabitri in the lead role—stitches up the theatre-dance divide even as it marks its own performance space, viz., the intimate arena with the performers and the audience sharing the space even when performing on a proscenium stage (Plate 11.4).[7] Once the performance space is thus 'made', the woman takes the centre stage.

The theatrical role is subtly incorporated/inserted into a dancing body performing The Mother, The Rebel, or One Seeking Emancipation, all with shades of Käthe Kollwitz's monumental figures,[8] the sculpturesque concentration, held in stasis and retained for a while before it breaks forth into movement, often that of stalking in an expansive territorializing dynamic, as if marking and capturing a space to establish her mastery over it. Once the space is occupied/captured, another dynamic comes into play, with words most of the time serving as sounds, setting ideas and thoughts in volition, floating around the dancing body, the dance neither illustrating nor representing them. It is a Manipuri body—a Manipuri woman's body—that engages in yet another women's war, a fresh Nupilan, against the state-crafted agenda of consecrating the Manipuri dancing body into the timid and all too graceful *rasa* dancer inviting the tourist to Manipur from the colourful posters in trains, railway stations and airports, and tourist bureaus. To achieve this emancipation, several rules had to be broken, and it was a pleasant surprise to discover on my recent visit to Imphal that Kanhailal is part of the administration of Jawaharlal Nehru Manipur Dance Academy, which has resolutely over the years resisted the official pressures to standardize and scripturalize a Manipuri dance repertoire, maintained an open and inclusive space for ritual, theatre, storytelling, martial training practices and turned out to be an excellent breeding ground for new choreographers breaking down the artificial barriers between dance and theatre, and liberating the dancer's body in the process from a multitude of constraints.

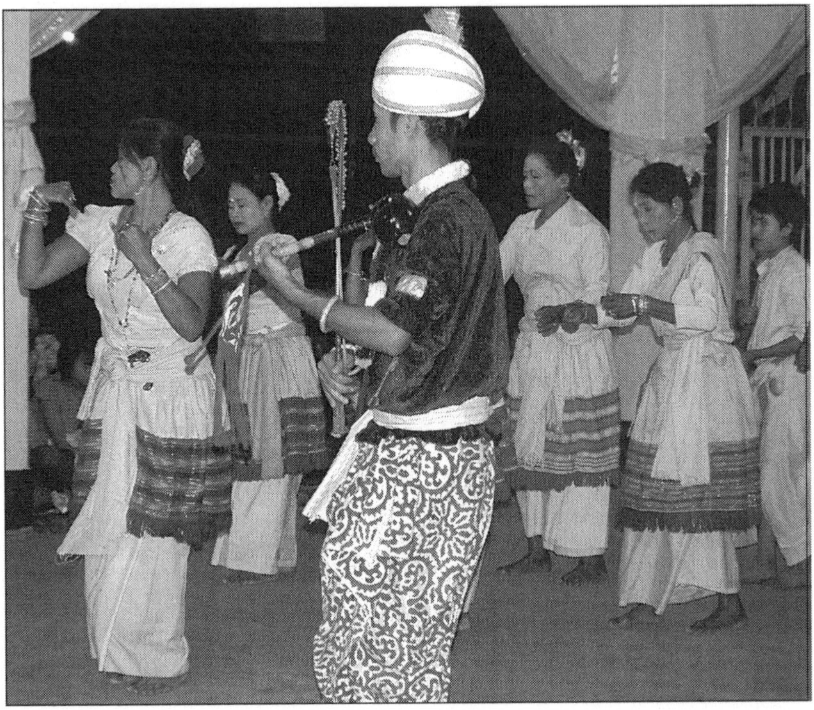

PLATE 11.3: Maibi Women in Ritual Performance Accompanied by a Musician Playing the Pena during the Lai Haraoba Festival in Manipur. *Source*: Photo courtesy of Urmimala Sarkar Munsi.

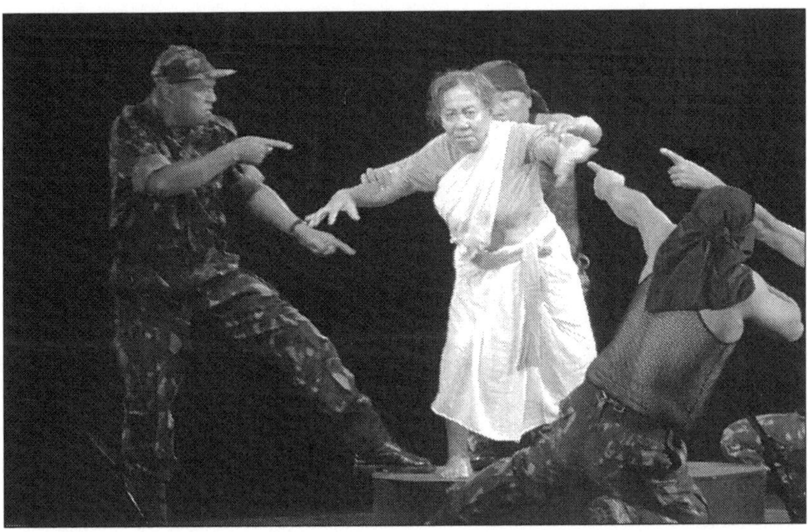

PLATE 11.4: Heisnam Sabitri's Memorable Performance in *Draupadi*, directed by Heishnam Kanhailal. *Source*: Courtesy of Poulami Das.

Notes and References

1. Samik Bandyopadhyay, 'A Plea for Restoring/Conserving Eroding Spaces', in *Time and Space in Asian Context: Contemporary Dance in Asia*, ed. Urmimala Sarkar Munsi, Kolkata: World Dance Alliance–West Bengal, 2005, pp. 85–6.
2. By interrogating the different categories of audience, I am hinting at the politics of charging at a higher rate than legitimate tickets and confining the performance to a more 'exclusive' clientele.
3. C.S. Kanhailal, typescript notes for a projected book, privately circulated.
4. Ibid.
5. Ibid.
6. Saroj Nalini Arambam Parratt and John Parratt, *Collected Papers on the History and Culture of Manipur*, 2010; repr., Imphal: Patriotic Writers' Forum, 2012, pp. 47–63.
7. The performative 'making' of the space through movement and voiced sounds is an essential part of the 'making' of the performance.
8. I am almost sure that neither Kanhailal nor Sabitri have ever been exposed to Kollwitz's imagery.

PART IV

Transformative Space: Empathy and Activism

12 Sitting in My Skin

Kathakali as the Transformative Space—An Interview of Maya Krishna Rao

URMIMALA SARKAR MUNSI

Urmimala Sarkar Munsi (hereafter USM): It is interesting to note that you do not call yourself a dancer, but you acknowledge as your strength your training in Kathakali. Would you like to comment on the process of creating a vocabulary in theatre with specific use of techniques sometimes born in dance and sometimes in theatrical forms—as a pedagogic tool for young practitioners?[1]

Maya Krishna Rao (hereafter MKR): I know very often I am placed as a dancer. Dance is something that I learnt and I can't even call what I do with it now as dance, and which is why I always try and underline this. It is also important to say that I never saw Kathakali as dance. I always saw it as something transformative. I was 6 years old when my mother started taking me to Kathakali class. So, of course, technically I was going to a dance class. But dance was just a word. I was not dancing. I was in another zone where stories got told and we got transformed. That was in childhood. In adolescence, when I was 16 years old, I rejected all that I learnt and went into theatre of Brecht and also other forms. No more Kathakali. But even when I was rejecting it, I was rejecting it as a so-called traditional form and not as a dance form. I have never seen myself as a dancer. That is one thing I would like to say. But it is true that the vocabulary or the terms we use in dance (Kathakali for me) stayed with me as my inspiration for moving and expressing. I came to realize that only when I started teaching theatre, because they asked me to teach acting at the National School of Drama (NSD), and because I had not been to drama school, the only learning I could fall back on for inspiration was Kathakali. So, then I kept dissecting it and looking at it to see what it has given me that I can draw on and abstract from and

*Interview by Urmimala Sarkar Munsi, Delhi, 21 September 2015.

take into a class of actors who want to do plays. In those days and till recently, students have always been from all over the country—though not so many from the North-East, except Assam.

When I was looking at Kathakali as inspiration for teaching acting, I was looking at it through the lens of theatre. But I realize that such a process rearranges one's relationship with the elements of dance, because when one is in a theatre zone, certainly in a kind of space that NSD is, each word from the world of dance starts having very different meanings. For example, if I use the word 'rhythm', it could be interpreted in a way that maybe Stanislavski might have used it. That's a very different notion of rhythm. In dance the word 'rhythm' means specific structures of beats that control or initiate movements. This was the time of realization that I was drawing pure elements of Kathakali dance in my pedagogical structure. And I think this was the first time I was looking at Kathakali as dance. And for me these understandings were hugely inspiring because those were what I took into the classroom.

I had no other way of teaching acting. Because you sit in your body in a certain way, you want to inspire that kind of body in your student, and that kind of body doesn't start where the head leads. A lot of actors, or rather student actors, would come into the classroom with the idea of their head leading them with a certain intelligence. And for me the big challenge was how to get [the students] to sit in another skin in some kind of magical way, and then being led by that skin and the body. And then breaking it down. This was the big challenge. I never knew anything about breath. My teacher never taught me about breathing till I was 45 years old. After that things were never the same anymore. I kept dissecting Kathakali and I would sit alone and move the hand out there in space, and tried to continue moving more and more parts of the body and realized that it isn't just about rhythm, but it's about breath. And then I started realizing that these simple things—like holding my eyes wide in Kathakali—alters and sets in another breathing pattern. All these became the nuts and bolts of imagination for me, because I didn't know any other way to trigger imagination. So, I would not start my day without doing my eye exercises every morning, which is not what you do in a play at NSD. That was the creative and most challenging part. For me the process of how one takes that experience of a Kathakali class and what one gets from it, and finally how one transforms it and gets them [the students] to sit in their own bodies with a sense of amazement. For me, what I got from Kathakali was to sit in my body with a sense of amazement. But that amazement did not come overnight. It came from practising those rhythms every day; it came from doing the *mudras* everyday with Guru ji [my teacher]. It came from all the nitty-gritty of skills that I didn't realize were adding up and imprinting [themselves] on my body over the years. One day, without realizing it, I found myself catching my breath, in a state of self-amazement at the result. So, for [a] long time, I would teach my student this business of how one should wait, telling them, 'If you sit as if you have no energy in your body and you wait, nothing is energized, nothing is ready to open the doors of imagination. You'll keep waiting all afternoon and nothing will happen. So how will you prepare that ground within your body?'

My class became the testing ground. For the first few days and weeks, students would be looking at me [as though to say] 'What is she doing?' Or they would say to me at my face, 'Madam, I don't understand anything.' So, on the first day of my class, I would say, 'I don't want any questions. Just keep doing it and ask questions later. Maybe after the first month or so you can start asking.' I would work with breath and elements like rhythm . . . for them to find their selves (see Plate 12.1).

So when I say that I don't see myself as a dancer, and yet, for me, the vocabulary of dance has become the springboard for improvisation in theatre and for teaching. For me it had to come from a form like Kathakali, which is, if you like, dance theatre. I think that in Kathakali the tension between theatre and dance, the war of imagination is created by that tension between action and dance. That was another thing I was

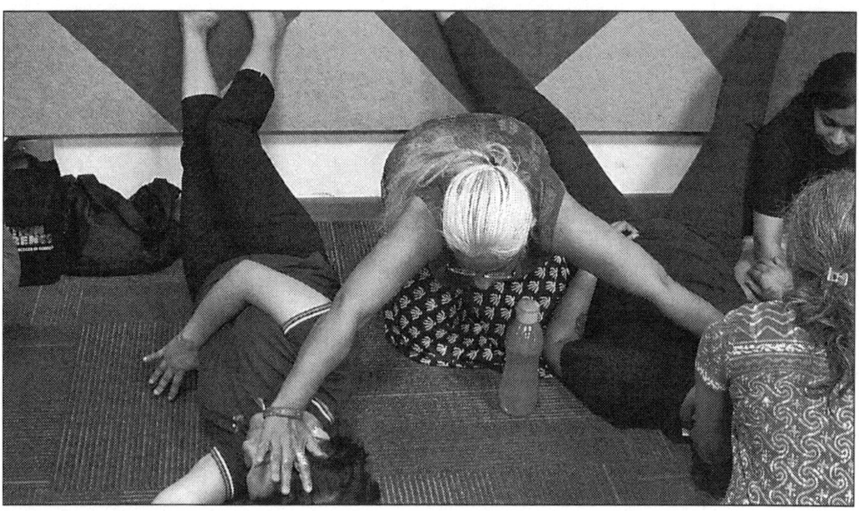

PLATE 12.1: Maya at a TEST (Theatre for Education and Social Transformation) Workshop: With Ruth Ann, Veronica Xavier and Mudita Agarwal.
Source: Courtesy of S. Thyagarajan.

teaching students—this business of anticipation. It is as if something will begin now, but I am in that moment before it. The understanding of anticipation before transformation comes to me from Kathakali. I imagine I am going to use this mudra and imagine being this particular woman character. I take a breath, I half-release that breath, and then I hold on. There is this sense of anticipation, and then you grab her from the air.

Then again, for me Kathakali helps me connect myself (who I am) to where I am. It also creates my space between the audience and me. When a Kathakali performer is looking out, she can see the audience, but that is not all that she sees, she sees even beyond. The Guru teaches us to imagine the flower and then out of that imagination he wants us to construct and communicate the beauty of it. For me there is no imagining the flower; that flower came to be only in that space where I caught it—then it turned into something real for me. Which is why I often teach processes of improvisation by asking students to start from any one gesture and just stick with that gesture and just go on repeating it and go on waiting to see what will emerge next. These are things you learn just from Kathakali—beating the feet on *di-tha-tha-tha-di tha-tha-tha-di tha-tha-tha-di tha-tha-tha* in class in front of the Guru. How many times will you go on repeating the same *tala*? Slowly the fatigue builds up and you cross the threshold. The Guru does not let you stop and your feet are in their own space. One learns to create one's own space of escape. This being both in yourself and out of yourself became what I actually wanted to be able to transfer to them [the students].

USM: We tend to define the different kinds of theatre—dance theatre, physical theatre, etc. In your work you actually bring a lot of elements of these forms, with different definitions, together. Through a range of these forms, how do you challenge yourself and your audience to be involved at different levels?

MKR: That is the result of having trained in Kathakali. I think it is also to do with the fact that when you are in that costume you constantly feel as if you are battling with it—it is so tough to move. The performer has to fight through/with it and does not feel comfortable. I mean, I so enjoyed being in dance class rather than being on stage in a Kathakali costume. But then when I look at those photos later, that's all I ever wanted to do all my life. All I wanted to do was play Ravana endlessly to the end of my life. But when I would actually get into costume and be it, such pressure! How I looked and how I felt inside that costume were two entirely different stories.

USM: When and how did you decide to go into theatre?

MKR: As I turned 17, I said to myself, 'This is it! Now, I'm a modern girl and I have to give up all this classical dancing. I'm only doing Brecht.' We'd only read his poetry. Then we did the play *Mother*. Anu[2] directed it. And I played the mother. It was in Hindi. I was constantly crying because I couldn't voice those words in Hindi but I wouldn't give up. I would come home and read the script over and over, and then go on stage and rehearse it. It was only when I was 29 that I went back to dancing. And then when I was 30, I went off to England. I had just gotten married. I knew I wasn't going to miss my husband as much as I was going to miss Kathakali. I thought, 'Now I'll go away and I won't dance!' So there was only one way I would get over this homesickness in England. It was to do demonstrations and workshops on Kathakali. I think that hiatus made me realize the preciousness of Kathakali.

USM: Would you want to mention some of your works, which you see as political as well as a gendered response from a creative person.

MKR: I taught acting at NSD for a long time. I had to resign from there to able to become a solo performer. My first solo work was after I resigned from NSD in Delhi

Khol Do

The first solo was *Khol Do*. The story is about a father who has lost his daughter who was raped by eight men during the Partition riots. It is a story by Saadat Hassan Manto.[3] The backdrop of Partition lends a political as well as circumstantial reference and a specific purpose to the story. I have always told my students not to accept things as they are and to learn to question everything. I believe that my work is political and I do not want to distinguish between the political and the creative. The changing times and their impact made the process usually different. In *Khol Do*, as it was my first solo, I was still searching for ways to create a performance. I had no idea how to create a performance. The pain of the father for his lost girl was so intense and yet I knew that I could not play her. I've always been clear that I'm not ever going to express suffering on stage. I'm not going to play out a rape. I don't know where it has come from. But I know that I'm not going to sit and clutch my belly and my head and portray pain and suffering. I think that that's also because nothing can ever be greater than the pain which is actually experienced. I, as an artist, have always searched for another route. But, yet, in *Khol Do* the story is about the pain of that girl being raped by eight men. I couldn't go anywhere near that; instead, for me the pain was experienced through the father. And I do think that, having done years of Kathakali, for me the improvisation is, many a times, rooted either in male energy or it is about abstractions, or it is a combination of both. In Manto's story, for me the most pained person is Sirajuddin, the father. The intense suffering and pain that was central to the story had to be routed through the father (Plate 12.2).

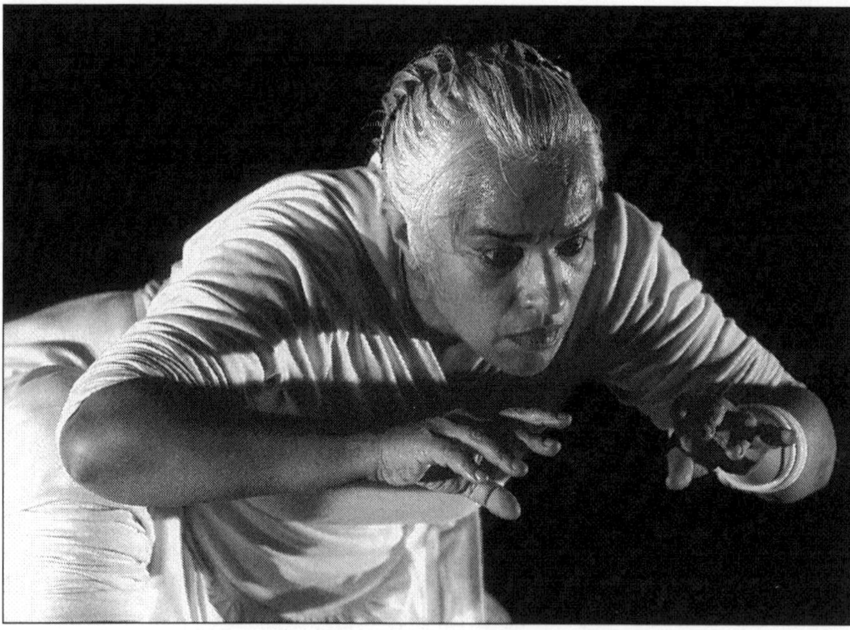

PLATE 12. 2: A Scene from *Khol Do*.
Source: Courtesy of S. Thyagarajan.

Ravanama

Of all my productions, *Ravanama* comes closest to a Kathakali-based performance. While doing the preparations for a presentation for a seminar on male impersonation, I was improvising on Lady Macbeth when it suddenly came to me that Lady Macbeth and Ravana are probably not very dissimilar people. They really have no idea of the circumstances they are in and how they get hurtled along despite themselves, in spite of themselves. They are doing ill; they are aware of doing wrong. And yet they carry on. I took Lady Macbeth's soliloquy, 'Come, thick night'. For me, through that single line Ravana becomes his mother and so for me through the line 'Come, thick night' I imagine a mother with her baby. The mother looks up at the skies and for a long time, for many cycles of beats, she just looks and looks deeper. Only after about three minutes or many cycles of beats later, suddenly the realization dawns on her that Ravana is her stepbrother. So for me this is Lady Macbeth looking out into the sky. I wore just bits of Kathakali costume, and even though I cannot stand it when dancers talk, because when the mouth opens the *abhinaya* is gone; I had to challenge myself to use some voice. At the same time I was being influenced by many bits and pieces of memories such as the Kathakali episode of Ravana and Mandodari.

The first sequence of *Ravanama* centres around a woman who opens her newspaper, turns the page and looks, and her gaze is fixed. I have never liked using the form of a play within a play—about the actor in the search of a form. But in case of *Ravanama*, I fell into all of that myself because I wanted to approach Kathakali and I didn't know how. I have loved the way Kathakali imagines Ravana. Paula Richman's writing and her book *Many Rāmāyaṇas* also fired my imagination.[4] The tension between Sita as Ravana's daughter and lover was for me the most energizing and generated a lot of the improvisations that I finally used in the performance. Everything about beauty came to reside right there. When I get these questions, 'So, is this about incest?' I can't bear it. It is as far away from that as can be. But it is about a shifting space between genders, between characters and human complexities.

Walk

I think I really am a creature of circumstance, and I am a very political person. Circumstance is, to a large extent, the main determinant of the form, because I never think about my next show and what form I shall take up. I only think through improvisation. There is also a large element that I know I'm going to improvise during the show. Otherwise, I'm lost, because I don't know any other ways to make shows. So, for me as an improviser, I need to be completely taken over, I need to be infected by and absorbed by and washed over by the circumstances in which the show gets made.

Walk got made after the heinous rape of Jyoti Pandey in Delhi on 16 December 2012. It shook my world, and of many others. Huge numbers of people, all ages, sexes, and walks of life gathered every day to protest. A large number of young people were among the protesters. Every day I would turn on the television and find out where the kids were and I would join them in Jantar Mantar and just walk with them. I was in a political group in my student days. But for many years I wasn't joining rallies because I was busy looking after my family and teaching. I couldn't sit at home at that time, when all these people were out there walking for justice. I would go with a camera and turn on my mic and just record people, because I didn't know what to do with myself. We were just walking with that storm in our belly and a lot of pain in our chests. So when I look at the making of *Walk*, first I don't see it as a performance; I see it as a state of being. It's just you being somewhere. Even when I say the first word *Walk*, I am actually in that place where they were all walking, which is very different from all the shows that I made, which come from another context. Before that you prepare yourself, you do your yoga, you get into a quiet zone, you choose some music to play, you set up your camera, you turn it on and then you start improvising. You are in this zone where the actor prepares and you wait for the imagination and you see yourself definitely as a person who is about to launch into a journey of creativity.

But *Walk* didn't happen like that. *Walk* happened because, while these protests were on, one day I was meant to be rehearsing for a comedy show, and when my rehearsal team arrived I told them I wouldn't be able to rehearse. I was supposed to prepare for the NSD's annual festival Bharat Rang Mahotsav. And this is twenty days before the show. No rehearsal had been done. I just could not rehearse, and told my rehearsal team that I could not rehearse the comedy. I told them we would just do it on stage somehow and for the moment we should focus on the technical part of the rehearsal. And one of people from the team happened to say—I thank that boy forever and ever—'If you are so overwhelmed by this rape, which we all are, why don't you just do something around the rape and put it into the comedy?' I said, 'Are you mad? How does one respond to that horrible circumstance of the rape and put it into a comedy show?' He said, 'Why not?' and just then the phone rang; it was a call from Jawaharlal Nehru University (JNU), asking: 'Will you please come tomorrow and express whatever you want, but not through a speech? It has to be a performance.' My head was buzzing because I was thinking, 'This boy has just suggested this and now I get a phone call. It's like a sign.' I actually wanted to say, 'No, sorry. For something as horrific as this I can't say tomorrow I'll be on stage.' Instead the word that came out was 'Yes'. After agreeing to perform at JNU, I put down the phone and looked at my team and said: 'What have I said? What have I done? What do we do?' So I went on to YouTube and listened to a tune but it did not move me. I told myself that the second tune is—whatever it is—use that. I thought, 'I am going to have to do something NOW, because tomorrow I'm going to be on stage.' So I just played the next tune that came, and while improvising on it the first word that I thought of was *Walk*. I usually use a camera to record my improvisations, but that was not on and I worried that if I stopped the improvisation to set up the camera, then I would get out of the creative zone. So I was keying in the words on the laptop and semi-improvising, which is really not the way I have ever made a show. Keying in words means I move out of the improvisation zone and am in a playwright zone and I hate being there because I can't script words. I can only create words when I'm improvising.

On the day of the performance, I continued improvising and was thankful that those boys were there because that meant that I had a ready-made audience. Then I downloaded the tune. I decided to go on stage without text and improvise whenever I forget the words that I had put down while improvising. For the first time it was a piece that had not come from within me, but from the world outside which had pulled something out of me, and I had felt duty-bound to live up to what was being expected of me. For the first in my life in theatre, during the JNU show, which happened in Munirka, near the site of the crime, I took these sheets with me and I was holding them in one hand. I did not want to miss a single word because it felt like I owed it to Jyoti Pandey and I owed it all these people. So that was a very different way of making a show. It was about Jyoti Pandey—about the girl who needed to walk, who needed to sit, who needed to lie in any place, in any part of the city, at any time of the day or night. And she could not. And they were two of them, Jyoti and her friend. A boy and a girl together. I kept thinking about that boy who is alive. For me, it's a bit like Sirajuddin of *Khol Do*. The father had to go on living after his daughter has been raped and killed. So while *Khol Do* was personalized, *Walk* was about the street. In making *Walk* I wasn't thinking about making a show, rather I was thinking about doing something (Plate 12.3).

The Audience

USM: What or who do you want your audience to see in your performance?

MKR: I never want to explain to anyone the meanings of what I am doing in a show, because if I have to explain it, then for me it is lost. But some memories remain precious. Once, when I did *Khol Do* in some auditorium somewhere in Delhi, a few days after the performance a man met me at the Shri Ram Centre and came forward to tell me, 'Madam, yours was the first time I saw a play in an auditorium.' He had never

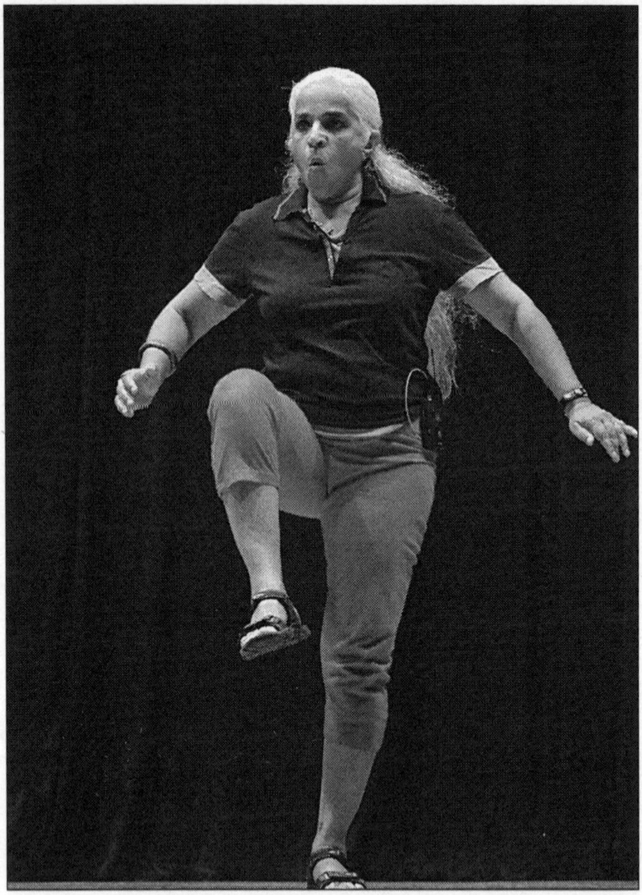

PLATE 12.3: *Walk*: A Performance Created after the 16 December 2012 Gang-Rape Incident in Delhi. *Source*: Courtesy of S. Thyagarajan.

before been in an auditorium. So we sat on the curve at that road outside Shri Ram Centre. And I asked him, 'What did you feel about it? What did it mean to you?' The interpretation that he came up with, this man from a neighbouring village of Delhi, gave me an interpretation of *Khol Do* that was so inspiring! He had got the idea of loss so clearly! It was exactly similar to the experience of my performance of *Khol Do* for an all-Palestinian audience once. They were all weeping in the audience. And I could hear the weeping and it changed the way I was performing *Khol Do*. These incidents continue to amaze me, and that's when I firmly tell myself that if I make my shows *here* in Delhi and if I trust that, there'll be plenty in the audience who'll respond from *there* (belonging to different cultures and social conditions) and I don't have to explain things to them.

Life, Art, and Pedagogy

USM: How does an artist bring art and life together?

MKR: What really excites me now that there are so many pathways of traversing those lines between life and art and if we've got our antenna nicely plugged in, we can be more aware or more open to shifting those lines and finding them or blurring them or walking in and out of the art space and something that is out there as part of life. People keep asking me: 'What audience do you keep in mind when you improvise?' I do not make a show for an audience. I have always said that I work around thoughts that take me from the personal to the political and back. I have mentioned in some of my earlier interviews that for me the performance must bring out the bigger picture through a personal narrative.

I have grown up watching my mother, a dancer herself, and at the same time being influenced by the Beatles and all that was typical of the 1960s. My mother made me learn the songs of the Beatles along with Carnatic music. Once I was 15, she was taking me to adult films. And yet she was the strictest of mothers. No making a noise while eating! But you must do all this. I don't know where it came from. So I grew up with this. In our first year in college we were influenced by Marxism and feminism. Both were such strong influences in my life, it was like breathing and living them all the time. So I did not have to work very hard to become Feminist. My activism was strongly grounded on these influences, especially feminism to begin with.

Rape has been a repeated theme in my plays. In 1979, we had done a number of street plays, and one of the plays was on rape. Once in the early 1980s, when we were doing the direct play on violence against women based on a real story, the mother of the victim happened to be in the audience one day. When we finished the show, this Punjabi lady just ran to me and put me on her lap and she went on thumping me like her daughter had come to life. And she thumped me and thumped me and it was hurting me and I was crying and she was putting her whole big body on me. That is the moment I realized the strength of the performance and felt really shaky about having blurred the boundary between art and life. Since then *Khol Do* has had a similar theme and then, finally, my work *Walk* has of course been made as a reaction to the shock of the 2012 Delhi gang rape.[5] Even when I made *Heads are Meant for Walking Into*, it was also a show that came out of a contemporary situation, and reaction to whatever was happening in Manipur after the rape of Manorama by the Indian Army, and the subsequent protest of the naked women outside the garrison gates of Kangla Fort in Imphal.[6]

In the new course we have started at the Shiv Nadar University, Uttar Pradesh, we have been getting students who are studying either engineering or computer science and they are undergraduate students, and every term you have to offer a new course. Many are boys who come with heavy heads. They don't even know they have a body, and they usually come to the class on the first day without any idea about what they are supposed to do. At NSD, everybody is very aware of their bodies. If you don't stump them on the very first day, you cannot get their attention. After all, they are about 19 years old and their hormones are running everywhere and they are just dying to be distracted and I want their attention. So my strategies are to stump and stun them and it is not because I had worked this out. It was a strategy born out of survival. So, one day, to get them into a zone of complete attention, I say, 'freeze'. And they are not freezing; and then you say, 'I want to you to freeze your eyes at wherever you are looking. Stop!' And that gets them to look at a particular spot and try freezing. 'Why is the foot shifting? Freeze!' The first few days go on like this, and all the other people can go to hell. So you do this for the first few days. It is like a liberal arts set-up. So then they are thinking, 'Wow! This is different from doing engineering.' For me that is already the beginning. The next phase consists of exercises where I say to them: 'Wherever you are, I want you to freeze and I'm going to count to ten. And you will all go into a sitting position within that time. And I don't want any stopping and I want you to all go in a flow.' And then they start flowing. They were thinking, 'What the hell does that mean?', and so then I say, 'flow'. So, what happens is, they start to gain a sense of body awareness. So then it goes on to a sit. And then from there I slowly build up.

In one class I took Brecht's 'The Job' as the text. I read the story. It's only two pages long. And all the students read it too. And they are very warm. I told them it's a true story. Then I would slowly put them in situations where they are Frau Hausmann, and this is a whole lot of boys. I had only three girls in that class. By the end of the term I had boys from Hyderabad, Visakhapatnam, and other places. There was one boy whose change was really evident by the end of the semester, when he was wrapping bandages around his chest to dress up as the woman in the play while looking at himself in the mirror. I was not thinking about the transgression of gender there. Instead, I was hoping that this sense of adventure would stay with him for life because this is probably the moment when he is as closest to being inside the skin of a woman, which only theatre can help one do. So I just keep making exercises and terrorizing my students. That's how I teach. I've also learnt an important lesson: one must try to hold their attention, put them into groups so that they learn to own their own stuff. For me the process starts with the exercise and the imagination and stretching it. Challenging dancers and actors to be creative by pulling them out of their comfort zones of gender constructs, social norms, and habits remains one of my favourite tools.

Notes and References

1. In her essay 'Pandita Ramabai', Maya Krishna Rao writes, 'Our folk forms—in song, dance, theatre, art—are rich with devices of "distancing", storytelling, play-making and participation, For me, the most exciting part of the journey begins now: to rediscover some of these forms, distil them and take them into workshops for teachers so that they can be equipped to use them for promoting learning with students.' This question is framed on precisely the same context. Maya Krishna Rao, 'Pandita Ramabai: The Making of a Participatory Theatre Programme around a Character from Indian History', in *Learning Through Theatre: The Changing Face of Theatre in Education*, ed. Anthony Jackson and Chris Vine, London and New York: Routledge, p. 206.
2. Anuradha Kapoor, a friend from college days.
3. The story of 'Khol Do'.
4. Paula Richman, *Many Rāmāyaṇas: The Diversity of a Narrative Tradition in South Asia*, Berkeley: University of California Press, 1991.
5. The first of what now has become one of Maya Krishna Rao's most significant performances is *Walk* which took shape as a protest/response after a woman was brutally gang raped in a moving bus in south Delhi. She and her male companion were brutally assaulted and thrown out of the vehicle without clothes on the streets after the ghastly crime. The victim succumbed to her injuries on 29 December 2012.
6. While talking about her creative process during the making of *Heads are For Walking Into*, Maya Krishna Rao referred to one specific event, when on 10 July 2004, the bullet-riddled body of 32-year-old Thangjam Manorama was found a little distance away from her home in Manipur. She had been raped, shot sixteen times in her genitals and murdered by Assam rifles after being picked up from her home on charges of having links with the separatist rebels. This sparked off large-scale protests in which hundreds of women also took to the street. On 15 July, about twelve women stormed and staged a naked protest in front of the Assam Rifles headquarters at Kangla Fort, Imphal, holding placards that read: 'Indian Army rape us' and 'We are all Manorama's mothers'.

13 Moving with a Purpose

Women Dancers in Dialogue with Empowerment, Rehabilitation and Therapy

AISHIKA CHAKRABORTY
URMIMALA SARKAR MUNSI

Flowing against the Stream (the Mainstream): Dancing Empowerment

SOHINI CHAKRABORTY

For her dance is not just entertainment nor is it a high aesthetic performance. Her dancers are neither objects of dollification nor figurines of beauty and spectacle. Working with the victims of sexual violence and survivors of human trafficking, Sohini Chakraborty, the founder-director of Kolkata Sanved (2004), uses dance as a therapeutic tool to heal the insulted and injured bodies of women who survived sexual abuse, violence and trafficking.

'Sanved' means 'that which responds to stimulus'. As a dance-sociologist and dance-activist, Sohini works through Sanved, which has developed over the last decades a multifaceted rehabilitation process, involving not merely therapy, self-expression, and healing but also advocacy, capacity building, and community development. Trained in contemporary dance and theatre movements, she is simultaneously engaged in breaking the barriers of traditional dance before transforming steps of dance movement into a unique counselling concept hitherto untried in South Asia, enabling the traffic victims to emerge as advocates of change, empowerment, and revolution. To Sohini, dance comes as a medium for mainstreaming victims and survivors of abuse by transforming them as free agents of life.

Sohini has received many awards including the prestigious Diane Von Furstenberg Award in 2011, an award recognizing those who transform the lives of other women. Her organization now works in partnership with other non-governmental organizations (NGOs) in rural and urban India, Bangladesh and Nepal, facilitating survivors of trafficking to fight against violence. Today Sohini is committed to harnessing and channelizing the power of dance among the underprivileged communities, and to building up the ecosystem for Dance Movement Therapy (DMT) across Asia by creating leaders and change-makers in the field from the victims of violence.

Sohini Chakraborty, interviewed by Aishika Chakraborty, 8 January 2015, Kolkata

> *My Body is used. My Dance is an escape.*
> *My Body is damaged. My Dance is my power.*
> *My Body has been restored . . .*
> *My Dance is a Revolution.*

Here are some random expressions written on chits of paper by participants of a DMT class organized by Kolkata Sanved. Inside Kolkata Sanved's studio, dance becomes something more than fun and amusement. The dance they 'do' is not always choreographed and staged for the sake of pleasing others, but is a tool to rehabilitate the survivors of sexual violence and other marginalized communities. It is a medium to transform marginalized, stigmatized, and silent bodies into proactive advocates who stand up and voice their concerns. Taking dance beyond the studio and stage, Sanved extends the 'power of dance' into uncharacteristic spaces, grounding it deep into bodies of survivors and fighters. Addressing the unique psychosocial challenges of individuals who have experienced the violation of the self, it takes dance as an alternative approach to empowering survivors of human trafficking and sexual violence. In a culture where a woman's body is seen as merely a tool for childbearing, sex, and labour, or as a signifier of tradition and culture, Sanved enables and transforms the body of a survivor (of sexual violence, rape, or trauma) as active citizens and change-makers by the sheer power of DMT.

Aishika Chakraborty (hereafter AC): Tell us about your journey with Sanved.

Sohini Chakraborty (hereafter SC): I want to describe myself first as an individual and, then, as a rebel. Ever since my childhood, I have been a rebellious person and I have always questioned social structures and the system. As a young girl I was admitted to a dance school but I left it as soon as I felt that the 'notion' of dance was too constricted to break the fetters, too rigid as a structural form. The school's authorities prevented me from being free to explore my dance and myself beyond their system.

I started to think beyond the box: perhaps I had the 'freedom' within myself. I have always thought that dance is more than entertainment and more than an elite art. I knew there was a space in between; I had to decide to whom I should turn to learn dance. From whom would I find the right direction?

When I experienced the dance and ideology of Manjusri Chaki-Sircar, my decision was clear: if I dance, it will be through the teachings of Manjusri di. Her dance imparted much more than mere technical skill; her feminist approach taught me an entirely new understanding of dance. As a performer I have also associated with Kolkata-based theatre artist Usha Ganguly. In their teachings I found I could combine my two passions.

Meanwhile I completed my master's degree in Sociology with 'criminology' as my special paper. My dissertation paper looked at violence against women. While I am a dancer, I am also a sociologist.

AC: Did you develop a training methodology of your own?

SC: From their training, I explored the potential of transforming dance into a medium to heal the bodies of survivors of sexual violence and trafficking. I also investigated the power of dance and the therapeutic use of dance and movement to heal, empower, and transform individuals. I strongly believe in the power of movement, which can break exploitative, patriarchal, and oppressive boundaries. As cycles of violence begin and end with the body, I wish, through movement, to engender freedom within these bodies, breaking the mental and emotional patterns of violence.

I involved myself with the Muslim girl students of Maulana Azad College in a dance programme. It was not just dance. Far more important was the cultural process in that shared space. It was beyond (anybody's) imagination to get involved in such a process where non-dancer, minority, and marginalized women came up to dance at Rabindra Sadan. The success boosted my confidence. In my next venture I chose to work with women domestic workers who had to struggle every day to support their families and got them to participate in another performance. These performances were all striking hits. In a sense they signified my moments of triumph and a winning moment for the disadvantaged women as well.

When women face violence, it immediately sparks a debate over the body: its control, mobility, and surveillance. All violence, I believe, is socially controlled, be it domestic violence or its many other forms. The highest form of gender-based violence is sex trafficking and this too is socially controlled. Here dance can be used as an immediate means of liberation. With dance, the body has an autonomous agency; dance has its control over one's self and one's body. This agency is inherent in dance, and therefore in DMT.

I increasingly felt that this was my calling. In 1996, I started working with survivors of trafficking. I was so young, still pursuing my master's degree. I did not consider myself a therapist at that time, but rather as a performer professing postmodern dance. However, I knew that I was doing something really new, something not tried by anyone before. Being a Sociologist, I believed my concepts of rehabilitation were clear. But when I started working practically, I understood that theory and application are entirely different. I decided I would have to unlearn a lot, especially what I had thought were my clear concepts about rehabilitation. Slowly, I changed my movements and the nuances. I started with storytelling sessions.

AC: How different is your therapeutic movement of dance from the existing model practised in the West?

SC: I came to know that in the West there is something called 'Dance Movement Therapy', which talks about the emotional, cognitive, physical and social integration of the individual, connecting the mind with the body. This is something akin to what I have been practising here in Kolkata for the last few years. So, I am in the right field. I did not teach DMT through this existing approach but the process I was exploring had many similarities. I started to contact people in the American Dance Movement Therapy Association. Instead of pursuing a typical degree, I attended various workshops and went through my own process to understand the field. During this time, I recognized that in Indian classical dance there are various healing elements which could be used to create an Eastern model of DMT. This became my new focus: to build something new. With this understanding, Kolkata Sanved was born in 2004. At the time, the concept of therapy remained very elitist in the Indian context. We needed to break this notion, to create therapy which was more individualistic and capable of impacting communities on a large scale. Our new form of therapy would bring a social transformation, speak about empowerment, and become a catalyst for agency. It would lift up survivors with the strength of transformation (Plate 13.1).

Today, DMT is an emerging sector across the globe, especially in India. Our DMT practitioners go into various institutions to approach various communities, including hospitals, railway platforms, and care homes. Encouraged by our success with survivors of trafficking, we expanded our base of work. In addition to communities plagued by

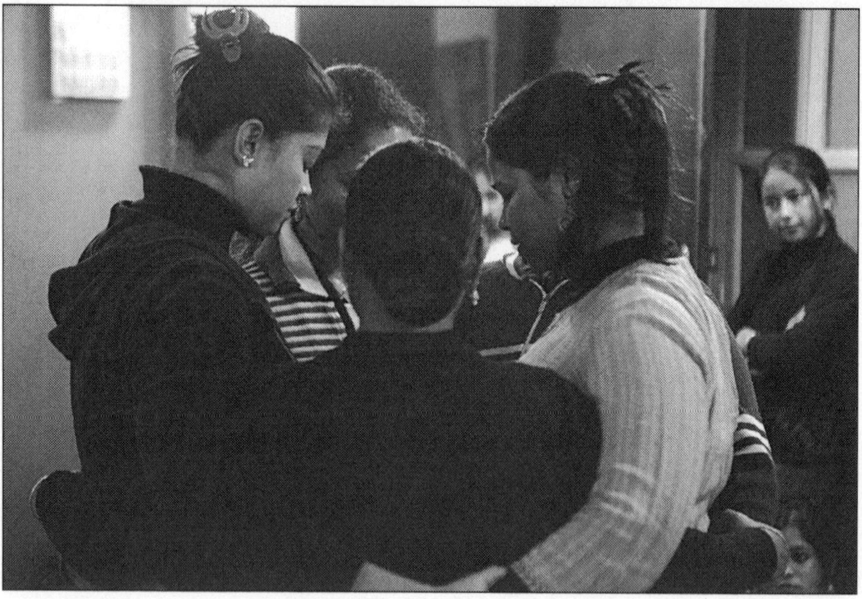

PLATE 13.1: A Dance Movement Therapy Workshop in Progress.
Source: Courtesy of Amy Parish.

violence, sexual abuse, exploitation, and sex trafficking, we have reached mental hospitals and schools. Sanved also provides institutional care to marginalized communities, especially to the children—both adolescent and youth—affected by gender-based-violence, sex-trafficking. We reach out to children living in the red-light areas, slum and villages, those living with HIV/AIDS and mental illness. As Sanved takes dance to the shelters and orphanages children await eagerly the much needed escape through their creative catharsis. The dance is designed to allow them to release their trauma of past experiences, to harness excess energies and to give the children ownership over their own bodies (Plate 13.2).

Kolkata Sanved's model is DMT for Change. We have four programmes within our model, with the two most important being Sampoornata (meaning completeness), which is the direct service of our unique DMT classes facilitated in various partner organizations and the Sanved Academy which trains and nurtures DMT practitioners hailing from both mainstream and underprivileged communities to offer rehabilitation and operate as advocates for change. The Sanved Academy offers Training of Trainers which is geared towards training individuals from underprivileged communities, and the Certificate Course which is accredited by the Tata Institute of Social Science (TISS), Mumbai and is held in both Kolkata and Mumbai. I believe

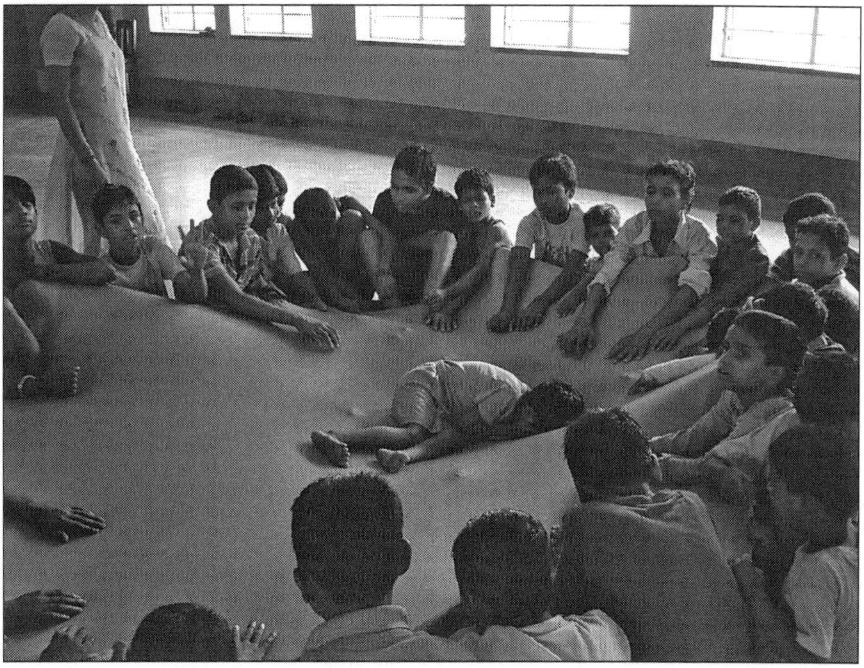

PLATE 13.2: Reaching out to the Children
Source: Courtesy of Urmimala Sarkar Munsi.

this is India's first certified course in DMT. While not yet a diploma or a degree, a certificate programme ensures the quality of our DMT practitioners who work through their own experiential transformation and learning to promote widespread change for both mainstream and marginalized populations.

AC: Why is this model different and called 'DMT for Change'?

SC: Western DMT historically divides the roles of therapist and client, therapy and performance, therapeutic space and outside community. Sampoornata reflects the global development trend of community-led development: participants become practitioners and performers responsible for both their own and community advocacy. This enables participants to continue their healing journey, through not only cognitive and emotional development in the therapeutic space, but also as DMT practitioners, performers and empowered community activists thinking, opining and directing their own lives actively. In India we have many healing elements in our culture as well as in our dance and these elements we have incorporated into our curriculum (Plate 13.3).

These elements include, first of all, a breathing exercise, leading to

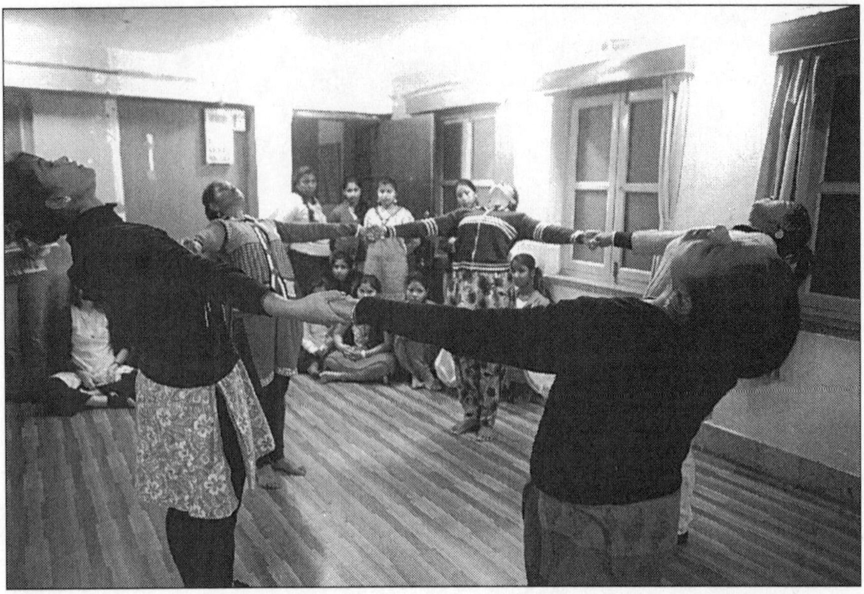

PLATE 13.3: A Class during the Dance Movement Therapy Certificate Course Conducted by Kolkata Sanved and Tata Institute of Social Sciences
Source: Courtesy of Amy Parish.

a coordination of body and mind. This is followed by a practice of *hastamudras*, or hand gestures, which is used as a tool to narrate a story, in this case one's life story, with an application of facial expressions which help face muscles to exude emotions using eye contact and eye–hand coordination. An exercise in *navaras*, exploration of nine emotions, works as a cathartic and emotional release. Sanved also imparts training both in Indian classical and folk and tribal dance practices acquainting students with the diverse rhythms and gestures. While the gentleness of Manipuri dance builds up inner peace, the formation of geometric lines and shapes of Bharatanatyam helps dancers to develop memory. The rhythmic footwork, piquet and pricking turns of Kathak are used as therapeutic means for anger release. Group dancing enables dancers to connect through bonding and connecting and releasing emotions as well as for fun or for a spiritual experience. Healing touch and meditation with guided imageries are also essential to our therapy. We use the healing power of dance on the body and mind adding legitimacy to the embodied approaches of rehabilitation, taking the power of movement to a wider audience.

This model goes beyond the clinical aspects of DMT; it also allows for artistic practice including performance which occurs with the consent of participants. The model imparts the importance of empowerment and individual rights while advocating for human rights. First, an individual transforms his/her own life and then brings social and structural change through the continuation of their work; this is our vision for change. In this way we have been able to provide a holistic approach to psychosocial rehabilitation as well as social transformation which is innovative across the fields of social development and DMT.

AC: You have already charted a long and unique journey making your mark in the global DMT movement. What are the future plans?

SC: Within the next ten years, I want to see Kolkata Sanved develop further as a centre of excellence focusing on DMT, working with creative processes of well-being with the help of dance as its main tool. The idea is to create a strong school of thought in DMT within the Indian context. We have already moved into the second decade of our work and along with this I would like to take a new leap in my own life. Within Kolkata Sanved there will be more holistic involvement. Beyond the practical application of DMT, Kolkata Sanved will undertake academic research, documentation and various other methods to not only improve our work in the field but to also encourage the acceptance and use of Sampoornata on a wider scale. To achieve this, mainstream individuals and underprivileged communities will walk the path of change together.

Thus our journey continues. Kolkata Sanved has pioneered the use of DMT as a therapeutic tool for those who are the most vulnerable and underprivileged, enabling young female survivors of trafficking to emerge as self-sufficient leaders and as DMT practitioners.

II

Prison Plays: Dancing Freedom inside the Jail

Dance emerged central to an exploration of discipline, rehabilitation, and recidivism or criminal justice when Alokananda Roy decided to train the male convicts of Kolkata's Presidency Correctional Home. Bringing a sense of normalcy to the outlaws, whom the larger society has given up, Roy has transformed the incarcerated prison into a transformative space, imparting a new meaning to the lives of the prisoners.

Once an acclaimed classical-creative dancer, Roy has ended up as a 'reformer of souls' by bringing rhythm to the life of the convicts. In the prison-based intervention, she uses dance in an artistic setting rather than as a therapeutic one, as the spurned and proscribed bodies experienced a soul transformation—connecting, expressing, and transforming their emotional experiences as a cathartic relief. The goal is to reduce recidivism and make sure these people are better citizens when they come out of jail. The positive intervention of dance within incarceration has, since then, continued as an enduring story of success in Calcutta's prisons. As a facilitator of dance-as-rehabilitation, Roy not merely enabled the convicts in incarceration to perform as artists on a public stage, forging a connection with the world outside, but also sensitized the mainstream society about the humaneness and creative potential of the jail inmates, by bringing the outlaws closer to the society at large—dance-wise, and also otherwise.

Under Roy's inspiring intervention, the disowned 'selves' of the outlaws take the risk by coming back to their 'body' before opening out in public to speak up and find expressions through dance. In healing the emotional wounds of the inmates, Roy invoked the spirit of human rights, where creative activity has had a direct relational effect on their behavioural patterns whose emotional discharge was slowly channelized into their creative liberations. Roy uses dance as a creative impulse rather than a therapeutic one. But the outcome was far-reaching, an aesthetic, psychological, and, more importantly, spiritual makeover. It was not 'dance therapy'. She called it 'love therapy'.

Alokananda Roy interviewed by Aishika Chakraborty, 4 October 2015, Kolkata

Aishika Chakraborty (hereafter AC): I remember you playing Shyama, the flawed court dancer in Tagore's dance drama back in the early 1980s. Swathed in blue, you glided across the stage, as I remember how deftly you manipulated and sacrificed your admirer (Uttiya), begging and imploring the royal guards (Kotal) to save the life of your 'imprisoned' lover (Vajrasena)! You love story began within a prison. After years, you made a 'comeback' as Goddess Saraswati in *Valmiki Pratibha*, in a real-life prison play. You activated the pioneering transformative dance therapy movement within Presidency Correctional Home, Kolkata. How has it all started?

Alokananda Roy (hereafter AR): If I want to talk about my journey, it spans a period of 60 years as a dancer. I will not call it a 'career'. I have never done it 'professionally', though I have been on the 'professional' stage for the last 60 years. But I have never danced for money and just did it for the sheer love of it! As a student of Children's Little Theatre (CLT), my first solo was *Gahana kusuma kunja majhe*, a Tagore song from *Bhanusinher Padavali*. I can still vividly remember the movements.

In fact, my journey with *Shyama* went through several stages of transformation. In 1967, when I was only fifteen, I made my debut as

Shyama. To be very honest, as a young dancer I reproduced whatever I was taught without realizing what I was doing. My emotions were all fixed, established in advance. I cried and laughed as I was told to do so. I cried when I was 'alluring' my admirer, Uttiya, though I was actually seducing him to sacrifice his life for another love interest. Later I realized the complexities. I tried to understand that Shyama is actually playing a foul game with Uttiya. Thereafter I stopped crying on stage. I discovered and reinterpreted Shyama at different stages of my life; it was not an unvarying journey. Each time I played a different Shyama—not only did I change the form, I also enacted different emotions each time.

I have broken a lot of norms; I enjoyed the freedom of the stage, where I can be of my own, not to be guided by somebody. My journey as a dancer is also about my own transformation, an inward journey that changed my realization of each character I played. Each experience helped me think differently.

AC: When did you decide to take dance out of the stage-space as a tool to change the lives of inmates of prison?

AR: *Jail* happened in 2007. It was 8 March—International Women's Day. I was invited as a guest of a programme at the female ward, organized by the women prisoners by the then Inspector General of Correctional Services, West Bengal Police, and head of all prisons of the state, B.D. Sharma. Sharma, who was in the process of ushering reforms in the jail, touching and transforming the lives of prisoners, invited me in the hope that I might be able to do something for the women prisoners. Sharma took charge as the Inspector General (and subsequently as the Additional Director General) of Correctional Services, West Bengal Police, on 7 November 2005, and indeed, kickstarted the entire process. Without his initiative to break barriers within the prison, the 'transformation' would not have taken off at all.[1] Sharma took the rehabilitative ethos of the new Act (West Bengal Correctional Services Act, 1992) as the benchmark. But he continued to improvise—most of which were the first of their kind in Indian prisons.

Jail was a very different experience—*it was so 'open' inside the 'jail'*. It was so tranquil and absolutely cut off from the world outside. Looking at the wide field and tall trees, I was reminded of the divine vision (*bhagawat darshan*) experienced by Rishi Aurobindo inside this (Alipore) jail. For me, it was, I think in hindsight, a spiritual beacon. Little did I know how the reality would hit my soul, and *hit* it did!

When I was walking out of the jail, I noticed some boys strolling aimlessly in the compound. It was then that I was 'hit'. They are convicts; some of them were sentenced to life imprisonment. The boys looked lost and cut off from the world. I was instantly moved. Any one of them could have been my child. The maternal instinct within me surfaced. I saw my son in each one of them in the sense that they are also somebody's son, somebody's father, somebody's husband—so that's how I saw them right from the beginning. No one is born criminal. It can be the influence of environment or poverty that makes them 'criminals'.

I asked Mr Sharma, 'Can I also teach the boys?' Sharma was surprised: 'Do you have the courage?' I nodded. I dared.

My Journey Begins

AC: So you took up the challenge, determined to go ahead!

AR: I returned to the jail and ended up with a programme that was much bigger than what Sharma had in mind. While the number of the women in the jail numbered 400, male convicts totalled around 2,000.

It was a slow and cautious start. Not everybody joined readily. Dance is still considered a feminine art, an emasculating exercise for men.[2]

I started with the movement of karate and martial arts of Kerala, Kalaripayattu, a powerful way of disciplining the body and mind. I slowly introduced them to soul-lifting dandiya and bhangra, the folk dances practised across the country. It worked. The inmates themselves started making dandiya sticks with much care and innovation. I wanted to train the inmates, both male and female, engaging them in myriad creative activities. I initially started with twenty boys and ten girls. Within no time the number doubled.

AC: What was the first performative venture within the jail?

AR: The first attempt at breaking the ice, frozen hard within, was 'Brotherhood beyond Boundaries'. It set the prelude. The adult male prisoners allowed themselves to get involved in this process through various phases of self-realization, confidence-building and also through spiritual awakening.

In 'Brotherhood beyond Boundaries', by weaving a collage of dance sequences I captured the diversities, the ethnic plurality, of India. As I said, not everyone joined dance instantly. Many would sit behind the performers, watching the rehearsals with extreme circumspection. But some joined immediately; many wrote songs for the production, while others made props, costumes, and accessories. I went to Burrabazar to buy metres and metres of cloth for sixty-odd participants. The prisoners made their costumes almost overnight! I asked one of the prisoners to compose a song of a wandering *baul* (a Bengali mystic mendicant singer) who travels all over India, from north to south and from east to west, to capture India's varied cultural traditions. The *baul* attains liberation in realizing that boundaries are senseless and that violence and evil serve no purpose. 'Brotherhood' was severally staged within the jail before officials, police persons, and bureaucrats, each time winning accolades from the audience.

I was approached by one among the audience to stage the performance outside the jail, at the Uday Shankar Dance Festival in Rabindra Sadan. That year (2007) the inmates got the first ever opportunity to travel outside the prison to perform outside. And it was the beginning of their journey. But it had to be a highly escorted performance. The programme went under strict vigilance. Each convict was attended by one police man, who guarded them everywhere—keeping vigilance at changing entries and exits from different wings.

AC: What was the reception among the audience?

AR: The performance was a huge success. The audience gave a standing ovation, which went on for several minutes. The performers never anticipated such a reception; they afforded and risked being non-violent and vulnerable by standing tall and confident on public stage. The work of the outlaws was appreciated, valued, and respected by the law-abiding civil society. Dance brought tears to their eyes. And, indeed, they did not realize what was happening to them. They never expected it, they had committed a crime for which they were punished, but now they were being applauded for their performance (Plate 13.4).

The Transformation

AC: You have been able to rehabilitate them in a space which so long banished them. The inmates changed themselves, repairing their ruptured selves by reconnecting their body with their minds. Did the old emotional wounds resurface?

AR: This is where the architects of the project saw the possibilities of 'reform'. The inmates of the state prison offered themselves to allow their 'self' to the process of an aesthetic, psychological and, more importantly, spiritual makeover. My initial aim was to place dance on an artistic-creative basis rather than on a therapeutic one. But ultimately it succeeded to open up a wider space for new possibilities, to encourage and empathize with the inmates to create something new to expend their raw energy. Dance offered the challenge to break the tedious routine of prison life, its hyper-vigilance, and to build trust among prisoners (Plate 13.5).[3]

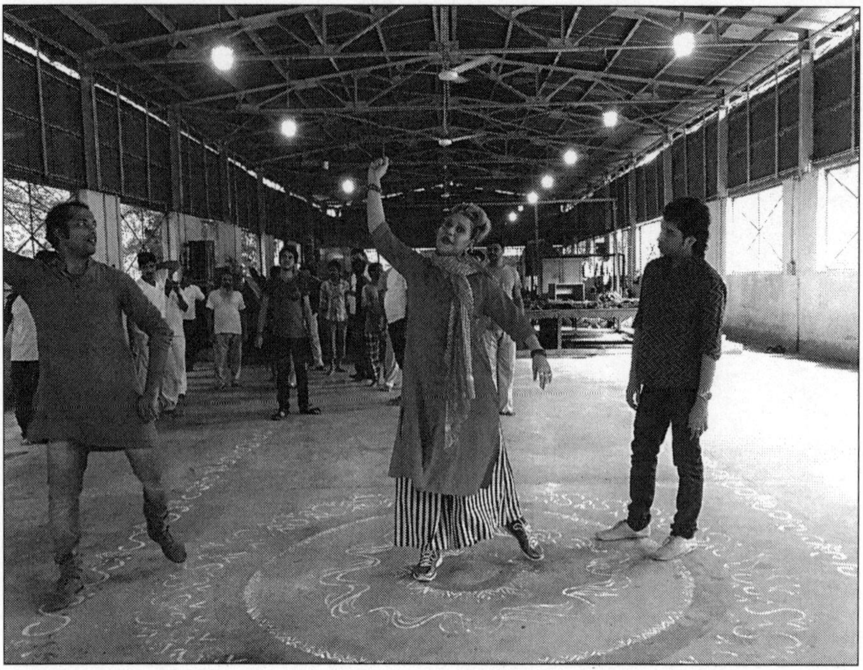

PLATE 13.4: Alokananda Roy, Assisted by Two Kolkata-based Choreographers, Conducting a Rehearsal at the Prison
Source: Courtesy of Alokananda Roy.

My lack of so-called formal training in dance therapy or experience to work with prisoners became my strong point. From the beginning it was an emotional involvement, free from prejudice. I have *never asked them about their past*. I have never enquired about the crimes they have committed[4]:

'Each One of Them is my Valmiki'

AC: To the public memory it was *Valmiki Pratibha* that comes as the real turning point. The dance-drama was in sync with the 'real' life stories of the prisoners for it shows the transformation of an erred soul into a consecrated one.

AR: *Valmiki Pratibha* happened after their realization of the transformed soul. I decided to take up the musical drama because it tells their story. The process of self-disclosure began in the most non-violent way. Through a lot of non-verbal negotiation and cooperation with one another, they reclaimed the 'space', by transforming themselves.

AC: Tell us something about the process.

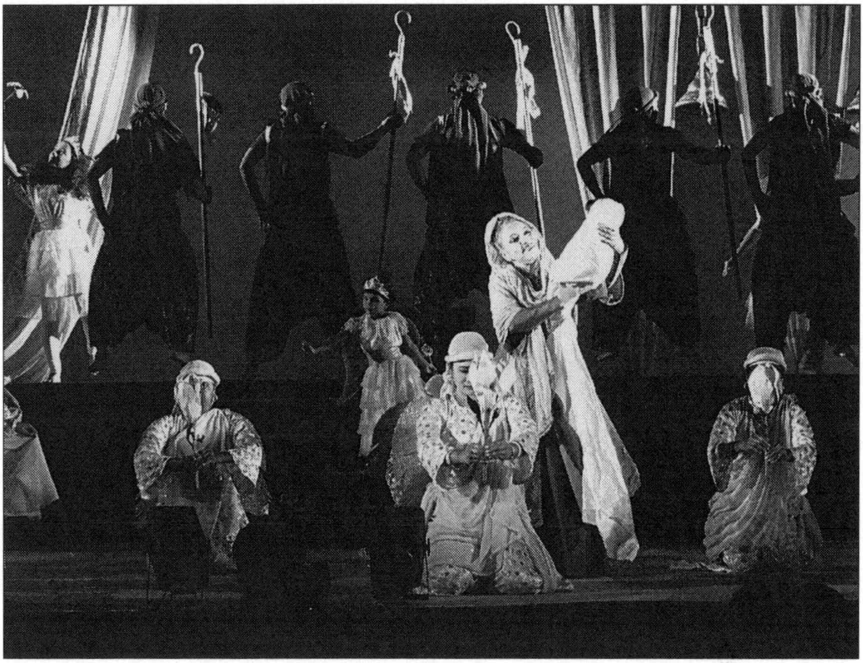

PLATE 13.5: A Group Choreography from the Prison Performance *Balmiki Pratibha*. *Source*: Photo courtesy of Alokananda Roy.

AR: Have I not set an example for society which resonates the transformation of Valmiki? It was not just 'dance' that I was teaching the prisoners. And I was not just 'teaching' them. I was connecting with them as human beings, something they had perhaps forgotten to be in the confines of the jail. I think I restored their faith in themselves. It was not dance therapy at work but love therapy.

Valmiki Pratibha instantly captured public imagination. The musical drama composed by Rabindranath Tagore in 1881 tells the story of the spiritual transformation of Ratnakar, the ferocious dacoit-turned-saint-poet Valmiki, the composer of the *Ramayana*. It explores the journey of a violent outlaw who converted and reformed himself to emerge as a pious soul.

Not one but many, in fact, each one of them is my Valmiki because each one has washed off their sins with tears of repentance. They realized the value of life through hard work and dedication. That, in a nutshell, is what 'correction' in the correctional homes is really all about. Many jailors and policemen participated in the programme. IG (Prison) Sharma himself rendered his voice to sing the songs of Valmiki.

Valmiki Pratibha went through several stages—from narrating the script (storyline) to the prisoners, to making them identify with the characters, orienting their bodies to the patterns of rhythm and movement, to training their voice for recorded and live vocal performance. The prisoners were trained in the nuances of theatre acting and facial expressions, timing, and stage entries. From procuring the textile woven by the inmates on the handloom of the jail, which the inmates stitched to make their own costumes, to making torches (*mashals*), bows and arrows, flowers out of paper and wire, spears, swords and shields, the entire paraphernalia for the stage act was made by them. Their raw energy churned out everything from out of the blue. What came out is sheer *pratibha* (creative genius). Now that's my Valmikis in action (Plate 13.6)!

My experiences over these years of social realignment and communication through dance and music has made me conclude that not just a theory but the practice of acceptance, love, forgiveness, humility, and peace can only make this world a better place to live. The therapeutic quality in recreational dance lies in the happiness that is felt when one dances to the music and its rhythm. Dance facilitates harmony

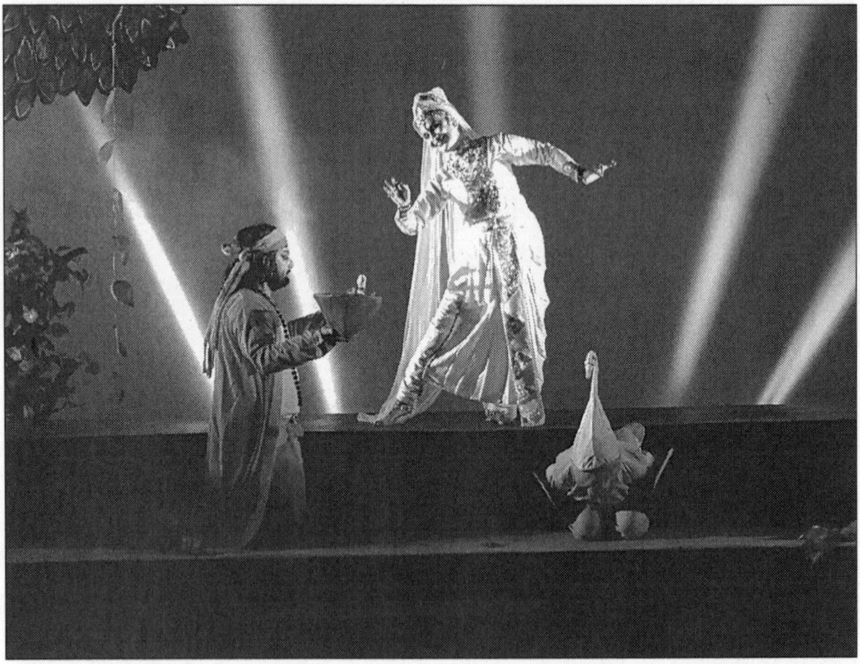

PLATE 13.6: Alokananda Roy as Saraswati and Nigel Akkara as Valmiki in *Valmiki Pratibha*. *Source*: Courtesy of Alokananda Roy.

within the body and cannot be compared with sport because sport is a very competitive activity devoid of empathy.

Valmiki Pratibha was staged on 15 November 2007 at 6.30 p.m. at Science City Auditorium and then after a month's break, on 15 December in Rabindra Sadan, Kolkata. It was considered by B.D. Sharma as the moment of truth.

> There was much excitement for the forty-five men and thirteen women inmates, who being accorded the treatment of performing artists, were visibly overwhelmed with the experience. At that moment, the anticipation and excitement of performing before a live audience transcended their sense of being prisoners. As they scurried around putting on make-up and costumes in the green room, they were like any other performing artist, just concentrated on the moment and the performance ahead of them. What ensued in the next two hours was something to witness. The audience was spellbound; first, by the sheer brilliance of the production. It was hard to imagine that the performers were . . . inmates who were lodged in jails.
>
> Second, the audience were witnessing history. For the first time perhaps in the history of prisons in the world, jail staff were performing along with prisoners in the same play. For the prisoners, who were performing, it was truly a journey from darkness to light. Many of them had tears in their eyes.[5]

Touchstone of Love

AC: What other work have you done with them?

AR: I did and am still doing a lot of work with them on and off stage. As far as the dance dramas are concerned I have been selective in my choice of theme. Each dance drama has a story to tell, with a latent potential to transform; there is a hint of a transformation. I have composed a piece on communal harmony (*Gahi Samyer Gaan*) on Kazi Nazrul Islam's songs and poetry, where Sufi song and dance are introduced. *Mokshagati*, which preaches forgiveness, is a message to civil society which was made along the lines of the life and philosophy of Emperor Ashoka's own transformation from Chandashoka to Dharmashoka. Aggression, offence, and crime cannot be negated or go unpunished. But forgiveness from the wronged can only incite repentance, catharsis, and redemption.

AC: What is Touch World?

AR: Touch World is a non-profit organization that I set up with the children of the inmates of the correctional homes. We look after the families of the inmates with the sole objective to integrate them into mainstream society in sustainable ways.

It is also part of my ongoing journey as a social activist. I have started with Inspiration Foundation with the underprivileged street children. The same journey continues with another expanded space.

I don't follow the treaded path. I always want to be different, to look different. I always wanted to challenge social extremes. Touch World, my jail project, is the outcome of my spiritual quest for inner freedom. I would prefer to call it a movement now!

Many convicts I worked with are now free. But I am working with a new group of prisoners. That's why the government and jail authority compares the correctional home to a dialysis machine. But here, impure blood comes in and pure blood gets out. I am part of the purification process.

I am always in touch with my children within and outside the prison. They are always in touch with me. They are my extended family. They call me 'Ma' (mother). They invite me on every occasion, big or small, and ring me up whenever they have something to share. If I fall ill, they all sit together and pray for me. During Durga Puja they composed a song for me:

There is Ma Durga; she comes every year.
Every time, she kills the demon with her mighty power!
And, here is our Ma (Alokananda)
She does not kill the demon,
She transforms the devil into a human.

Have I ever thought that I would attain my freedom, my salvation, within the prison?

III

Sensitizing through Performance: 'Shakti', a Feminist Dance Project

Lubna Marium is a dancer, researcher, and cultural activist based in Dhaka, Bangladesh. She is part of a Trust that manages 'Shadhona—A Center for Advancement of Southasian Culture', through which diverse activities to preserve and enhance cultural practices of Bangladesh are run. Shadhona creates and produces dance theatre—both traditional and contemporary; it works for the preservation and enhancement of 'intangible cultural heritage'; runs various 'dance outreach' programmes for children with special needs, people from marginalized communities, etc.; and it supports dancers through training programmes and scholarships. Though trained in traditional forms of South Asian dance, Lubna has always been fascinated by dance as a tool for change. Intrinsically an introvert, Lubna remembers how dance, and later performance, gave wings to her even as a child. This inspired her to delve deeper into the meaning and purpose of dance as a transformative cultural practice, through her studies in Indian aesthetics. Her area of interest is Tantra—Kashmiri Shaivism, and Buddhist Vajrayana—and how these kinaesthetic practices intersect with dance. She also runs Kolpotoru, a dance school she established in 2008. Lubna writes a regular column called 'Arts Gaze' on contemporary arts practice in Bangladesh. She was awarded the First Bishwaratna Bhupen Hazarika International Solidarity Award, 2013, by the Assam Sahitya Sabha on 28 March 2013 at Guwahati (Assam). Lubna is affiliated with the World Dance Alliance–Asia Pacific and is Vice-President for South Asia.

Lubna Marium interviewed by Urmimala Sarkar Munsi, 12 September 2015, Dhaka

Urmimala Sarkar Munsi (hereafter USM): How did 'Shakti' come about as a project that used the creative power of dance to change lives? What made you see Shadhona as the organization facilitating such an innovative process in Bangladesh?

Lubna Marium (hereafter LM): This project 'Shakti' is an attempt to create a space where dancers can question the meaning and purpose of their dance, analyse the narratives usually performed in their dances, discuss the necessity to contextualize age-old narratives and, finally, debate on the need to create new narratives by bringing present-day realities into their own performance. 'Shakti' is a work-in-progress.

There is an inherent interrogation of 'performance' as it is practised now. The implication is that there is a lack of 'sensitivity' towards present-day realities, but also a strong belief that it can be transformed.

USM: Could you describe Shadhona's initiatives and the work that it has been able to do?

LM: To examine and change this practice of dance, Shadhona[5] initiated 'Shakti', a unique initiative, to empower young dancers to include issues of social justice, viewed through the perspective of feminist ideology, into their work in mainstream performance, through a countrywide project. 'Shakti' aims to create a space for critical reflection, based on the conviction that the arts, and the artists who practise them, do not exist in a vacuum, but are active participants in the process of shaping our culture. It aims to direct young dancers and performers to believe that creativity and imagination are powerful instruments to change lives and build a better world (Plate 13.7). The first workshop came up with a powerful presentation entitled 'Are We Loud Enough?'

The Context

USM: How has the worked shaped up in the context of Bangladesh?

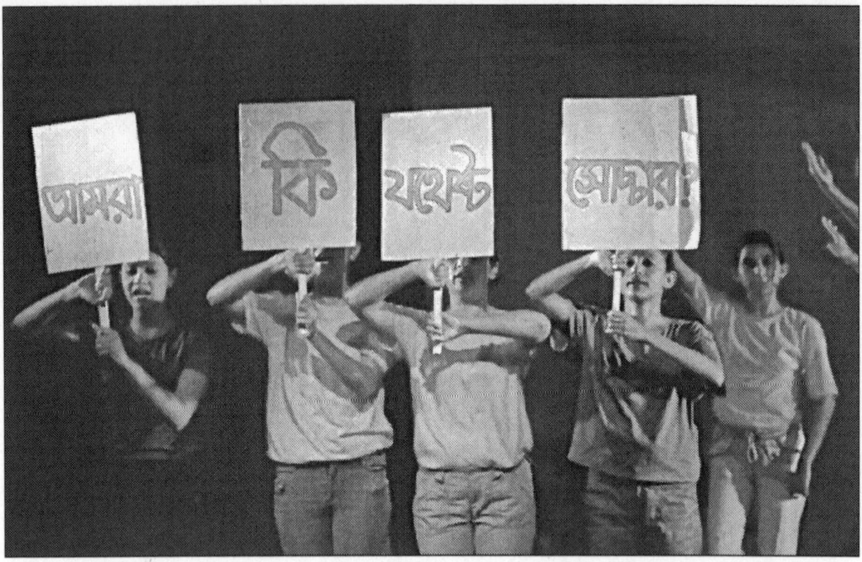

PLATE 13.7: 'Are We Loud Enough?': Shadhona Workshop on Dance as a Political Tool. *Source*: Courtesy of Lubna Marium.

LM: The practice of dance in Bangladesh is bound to conventions and traditions, both in the urban and rural space. In urban centres rules are set from the outset, because the *guru-shishya* (mentor-disciple) methodology of imparting knowledge is followed, based on the genuineness of the guru, and the respect, commitment, devotion, and strict obedience of the student. Here, very often the student is not encouraged to think independently, improvise or create. The emphasis is more on the reproduction of the teachings of the guru, rather than reinforcement of the creative ability of the *shishya*. Also, often performances are based on age-old narratives grounded on ancient myths. Outstanding in beauty and skill, they are handed down from one generation of dancers to another, in an unchanging repetition of repertoire. Meanwhile, in the rural centres many popular performances, though based on ritual and myth, and comparatively more open to improvisation. But they rarely address current issues from our day-to-day reality. At the end, that dance could be a political, performative tool for change remains almost unacknowledged.

Under these circumstances, a conscious decision was taken to break the boundaries of performance, and if necessary pedagogy too, to create a space which encouraged dancers to think anew.

The Intention

USM: You have told me before in many conversations that the intention of 'Shakti' was inspired by the work of great stalwarts of theatre and dramaturgy, both abroad and at home. Could you explain the process?

LM: One of the most inspiring examples of facilitating processes of empowering human beings as agents for social change is Paulo Freire, the Brazilian scholar in educational philosophy. In his book *Pedagogy of the Oppressed*,[7] Freire challenges cultural norms and puts forward path-breaking concepts. He writes:

> Man's ontological vocation is to be a Subject who acts upon and transforms his world, and in so doing moves towards ever-new possibilities of fuller and richer life, individually and collectively.
>
> Every human being, no matter how 'ignorant' or submerged in the *culture of silence* he or she may be, is capable of *looking critically at the world in a dialogical encounter with others.* Provided with the proper tools for this encounter, the individual can gradually perceive personal and social reality . . . become conscious of his or her own perception of that reality, and deal critically with it.[8]

Inherent in Friere's words is the belief that people can 'rehearse new forms of being together and working towards a more diverse world'.[9]

German playwright and dramaturgist Bertolt Brecht (1898–1956) proposed the genre of Epic Theatre, as opposed to conventional Dramatic Theatre, highlighting the constructed nature of the theatrical event to communicate that the audience's reality was equally constructed and, as such, was changeable. Brecht proposed that:

Epic Theatre turns the spectator into an observer, arouses his capacity for action and forces him to take decisions.

The observer is alterable and able to alter. Observers' eyes are on the course, rather than the finish.

Each scene stands for itself and the presentation is a montage.

Social being determines thought, in contrast to thought-determining being.[10]

On the other hand, Indian aesthetics proposes that theatre is an *alaukika*, or an extra-empirical, space, where the events are neither 'subjective' or 'objective'; and goes on to state that there is a willing suspension of purposivity which helps evoke, develop, and consolidate the emotional disposition of the spectator. Abhinavagupta (ninth century AD), a polymathic personality who exercised strong influences on Indian culture, states that theatre (*nātyam*) requires a reorganization of sensory knowledge and data through a conscious and consistent assimilation of new experiences (i.e. viewed on stage). Reception of theatre produces such reorganizatons of emotions already in the spectators' consciousness (*anuvyavasāyatmakam*). This needs to be acknowledged as another mode of cognition (*vikalpa-samvedanam*).[11]

Inherent in this statement is the recognition of theatre as a tool for changing perceptions.

'Shakti', therefore, is based on the concept of performance as a tool for change.

Understanding 'Shakti'

Here at Shadhona, we begin with a diverse group of dancers and aim to transform them into a 'community' working together with the aim of self-expression and political change (Plate 13.8). This involves basic exercises in defining both 'community' and 'performance' and trying to figure out how 'community performance' can analyse reality and impact it. The idea is to 'facilitate an exchange, bring people together, enable ways for the group to find its ways of working, and allow a group to value all its members'.[12] The first task is to build an atmosphere of consensus and collaboration, as most participants are unfamiliar with the idea of collectively determining the content and form of performance, as opposed to being given a predetermined framework. Here issues such as

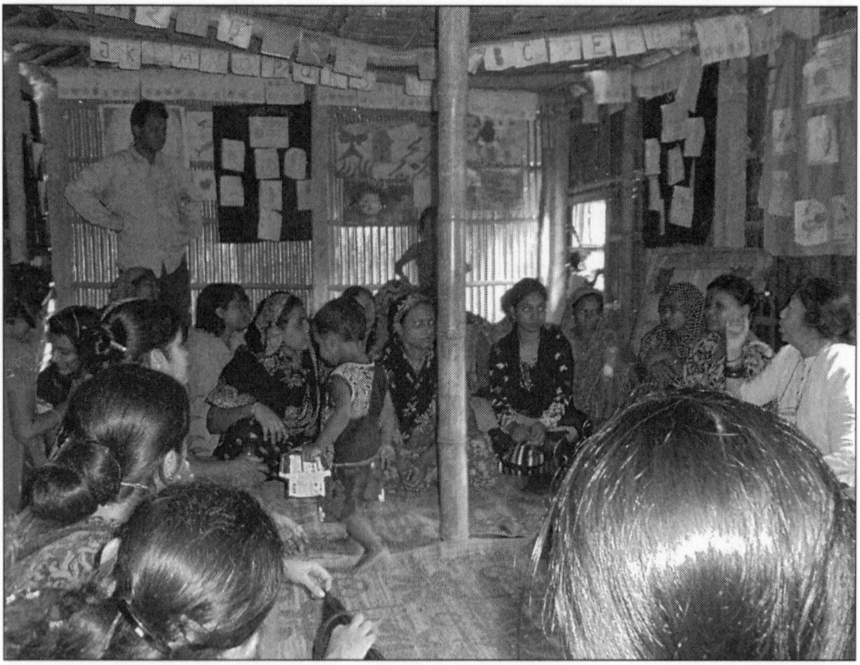

PLATE 13.8: Shadhona's Community Workshop with Women.
Source: Courtesy of Lubna Marium.

democratic decision making, allowing a space to vulnerable and minority voices, and cohabitation with alternative perspectives and lifestyles are raised and debated upon with the intention of finding common ground.

There is an added need to establish an 'ethics of accommodation' that needs to redefine who makes art, what art is, and the nature of beauty and pleasure, and appropriate ways of appreciating these. Second, the performance needs to be collectively created. The performance is not individually authored and predetermined by a dancer who directs the group towards the goal. This proves to be one of the most contested exercises, as dancers are comfortable with being 'directed', rather than being in the driving seat. This inherently implies a questioning of the decision-making process and the inherent submission to power.

Finally, and more importantly, 'Shakti' believes in an underlying politics of performance. 'The real politics of the performance space may well lie in the field of its external relations; in its actual or potential conflictual engagement with all the other shrines of power, and in particular, with the forces that hold the keys to those shrines.'[13] To confront the question of power, 'Shakti' adopts feminism as an ideology, which advocates 'equity' in all matters of social interaction.

Gradually, the project included participants from different target groups, i.e. female farmers, sex workers, children with special needs, street kids, etc., making it an inclusive performative interaction with society at large.

Why Feminism?

An important element of 'Shakti' is the evaluation and understanding of issues of social justice based on a liberal ideology of equity and fairness. Feminism being one of the most just philosophies of life, is addressed and studied intensively. All decisions are consciously measured and considered on the weighing scale of Feminism. Black feminist bell hooks defines Feminism thus: *feminism is a movement to end sexism, sexist exploitation and oppression.*[14] This clear and simple definition makes it totally clear that Feminism is not anti-men. It is against discrimination and sexism; it is against patriarchy. Feminism, like most other ideologies, is a discourse, an ideology, a way of looking at the world *and* it is a programme of action and activism. Feminism thus walks on two legs of theory and action. The actions are to challenge patriarchy and unequal power relations within families and societies; while the activism is the raising of the voice to implement actions that lead to an end of inequity.

Understanding the Process

'Shakti' is implemented through short, seven- to ten-day workshops. Though the workshops do consciously come up with a 'product', 'Shakti' is more about the process rather than the product. The focus is in the act of working together, by allowing different voices, bodies, and experiences to emerge.

Taking notes from Augusto Boal's Theatre of the Oppressed, 'Shakti' workshops comprise three kinds of activities.

The first is background information: getting to know each individual participant, discussing the raison d'être behind 'Shakti', and understanding feminism.

Second, since 'Shakti' is principally about dance, movement classes, games, and exercises take up a large part of the learning process. A difficult but necessary segment is unlearning. Martha Graham's important observation—'Whether it means to learn to dance by practicing dancing or live by practicing living, the principles are the same . . . Blood Memory is, after all, the memory that comes not from the mind or the intellect, but from the blood and bone'[15]—has remained significant to me in these works. This is akin to unlearning learnt usage of the body and devising new ways in which a trained body can tell different stories.

The third is a more structured activity, where genuine content is added to movements.

Practicalities

Script: Narratives are collected by going through current news, sharing personal experiences, re-reading epics, folk tales, popular literature, or simply by enacting concepts. Field trips are regularly undertaken to collect different narratives.

Genre of dance: A basic difficulty is the genre of dance to be utilized. Perforce, to accommodate dance and dancers from various backgrounds, there is an amalgamation of styles.

Music: This is a major area of concern—the soundtrack. To overcome this, 'Shakti' has, till date, always included singers and musicians in its workshops.

Having said that, the most positive outcome of each 'Shakti' workshop is the process which involves highly interactive imagining, group solving, physical involvement, trust and fun, all combining to create vigorous interpersonal dynamics through which a new world can be envisioned.

Managing Logistics

We can honestly state that the process is arduous and would have been almost impossible without outside support.

The project is funded by a non-governmental organization (NGO). This process too is fairly new to the world of dance. However, gradually 'Dance Outreach', which involves kinaesthetic activity, is being recognized as a tool for social communication to build bridges. 'Shakti' has done exemplary work with children with special needs and street kids.

Any framework for procuring and sustaining funding necessitates the need for documentation, evaluation, and reporting. This required us to start 'writing dance'—how dance evolves, how it builds bridges, and how it helps to create awareness about social issues.

'Shakti' also spurred us into regularly documenting the personal narratives and journeys of our participants. Initially, it was a process to assist us to report to our donors, but gradually it has in itself become a process, which helps enhance our work. Our documentation takes the form of: (1) videos of workshops/performances; (2) capturing the performance on tape; (3) reviews/questionnaires; (4) project notes; and (5) looking at target audiences to increase the reach of the work.

Furthermore, by sharing evaluations, outcomes, and achievements 'Shakti' has been able to further increase its reach.

Lastly, the entire process of documentation has enhanced our skill in writing proposals for development grants.

Looking Ahead

'Shakti' is now looking towards building sustainability by reaching out to a larger audience—student community, ethnic minority communities, etc.—by taking the project beyond the present target group; making 'feminist' performance a mainstream genre of dance productions; it also documents and records the process of transformation.

Notes and References

1. In 1992, the West Bengal State Legislative Assembly passed the West Bengal Correctional Services Act, which repealed the former colonial law based on retributive principles in West Bengal, India. The new Act promises, among many things,

> to give correctional treatment to the prisoners in custody so as to efface from their mind the evil influence of antisocial ways of life and rehabilitate them in the society as good and useful citizens; 2 (c) to adopt measures whereby a prisoner confined therein may not fall prey to the depriving mental attitude which may make him believe that he is lost to the society and it is his fate to pass the rest of his life as a social outcaste (pp. 494–5).

Cited in Nayanee Basu, 'Improvising Freedom inside Prison', *Critical Studies in Improvisation*, vol. 8, no. 2, 2012, http://www.criticalimprov.com/article/view/2143/2941, accessed 25 July 2016.

2. Nigel Akkara who rose to fame as the protagonist in *Valmiki Pratibha,* the first public success story of the dance therapy in the correctional home, was initially reluctant to join the dance class. He felt that his fellow inmates would mock at him by saying, *ghaghra choli pehnlo. Ghunghroo bandh kar naachna suru kar diya* . . . (You better wear a skirt and blouse. You have started dancing like a woman). Cited in Tumpa Mukherjee, 'Dance Therapy in Correctional Homes in West Bengal', paper presented at the national workshop titled 'Embodying Gender: Body and Dance in Social Context', organized by the School of Women's Studies, Jadavpur University, 29 March 2013.
3. This is what Sundarland describes as the unprocessed emotional material that has been banished to unconsciousness. 'Using body as a vehicle to connect with, express and transform emotional experiences offers cathartic relief, at the same time as transforming emotional discharge into creative, as opposed to neurotic action.' See Jennifer Brown, Sarah Houston, Lisa Lewis and Gerda Speller, 'Dancing Inside', a research evaluation conducted on behalf of Motionhouse Dance Theatre, Dance Studies Department, University of Surrey, November 2004, http://www.motionhouse.co.uk/documents/SurreyFinalreportnov04.pdf, accessed on 18 May 2016.
4. Brown observes just as aspects of the environment within the prison become rejected, aspects of the self are also rejected and disowned. The vocabulary of the identified self becomes verbal, and of the disowned self, kinaesthetic. The work of maintaining this split and keeping the disowned self out of our awareness is aided by the bodily nature of repression itself. . . . 'It is through movement that we express feeling, manipulate and shape the environment, relate and react to others, create and modulate boundaries, and defend our integrity . . .'. Brown et al., 'Dancing Inside', p. 7; James I. Kepner, *Body Process: A Gestalt Approach to Working with the Body in Psychotherapy*, Gestalt Press, 1999, p. 16.
5. Interview with IG (Prison) B.D. Sharma, in Basu, 'Improvising Freedom inside Prison'.
6. Shadhona is a cultural organization founded by Lubna Marium in Dhaka, Bangladesh, in 1992. Though Shadhona's scope of work encompasses many genres of art and the target group is diverse, the defining character of the organization is the hard-core, intensive work that it does with the arts and artistes, in the areas of: (a) research, documentation; (b) training; and (*c*) production and presentation.
7. Paulo Freire, 'Pedagogy of the Oppressed', New York, NY: Continuum, 1999.
8. Freire, *Pedagogy of the Oppressed*, in Petra Kuppers, *Community Performance: An Introduction*, London: Routledge, 2007, p. 6.
9. Kuppers, *Community Performance*, p. 6.

10. Bertolt Brecht, *Brecht on Theatre*, tr. John Willett, London: Methuen, 1964, quoted in Kuppers, *Community Performance*, p. 7.
11. 'Abhinavabharati'—Commentary on Sixth Chapter of *Natyashastra* by Acarya Abhinavagupta (tenth century AD). The translation has been collated from various sources, including Raniero Gnoli's *Aesthetic Experience according to Abhinavagupta*, Roma: Istituto Italiano per il Medio ed Estremo Oriente.
12. Kuppers, *Community Performance*, p. 10.
13. Ngũgĩ wa Thiong'o, *Penpoints, Gunpoints, and Dreams: Towards a Critical Theory of the Arts and the State in Africa*, Oxford: Clarendon Press, 1998, p. 40.
14. See Bell Hooks, *Feminism is for Everybody: Passionate Politics*, New York: Routledge, p. 117.
15. Martha Graham, Ninth Annual Virginia Arts Festival 2005, Martha Graham Dance Company, p. 4, http://marthagraham.org/wp-content/uploads/2012/02/MarthaGraham2005.pdf (accessed 7 September 2016). This quote refers to Martha Graham's autobiography, *Blood Memory*, New York: Doubleday, 1991.

Editors and Contributors

URMIMALA SARKAR MUNSI is Associate Professor, Theatre and Performance Studies, School of Arts and Aesthetics, Jawaharlal Nehru University, New Delhi. Her focus is on dance anthropology, living traditions, feminist studies, audio-visual documentation, and visual anthropology. She is a choreographer and a dancer, trained at the Uday Shankar India Culture Centre in Kolkata.

AISHIKA CHAKRABORTY is Associate Professor and Director of School of Women's Studies, Jadavpur University, Kolkata. She specializes in history, gender studies and dance studies with special focus on Bengal modern dance movement. A student of Manjusri Chaki-Sircar, she is currently engaged as a choreographer and researcher of Dancers' Guild, a contemporary dance institute set up by Chaki-Sircar.

SAMIK BANDYOPADHYAY is a theatre scholar and leading critic of theatre in India. He is currently affiliated to Jawaharlal Nehru University, New Delhi, as the Tagore Scholar, under a scheme of the Ministry of Culture, Government of India.

ANURIMA BANERJI is currently Assistant Professor, Department of World Arts and Cultures/Dance, University of California, Los Angeles. She is also an Odissi dancer and a poet, and teaches theories of performance, introduction to dance studies, histories of Odissi, and issues in Indian classical dance.

PRIYANKA BASU has recently been awarded a Ph.D. from School of Oriental and African Studies, University of London. Her research interests are popular folk traditions like *Kobigan* and contemporary global forms like Bollywood dance. She is an Odissi dancer and continues to perform in India and in the United Kingdom.

SOHINI CHAKRABORTY is a specialist in Dance and Movement Therapy and the Director, Kolkata Sanved, an NGO which provides a joint diploma on Dance and Movement Therapy with the Tata Institute of Social Sciences (TISS), Mumbai. A recipient of multiple international awards for her ground-breaking work with survivors of trafficking, she is a trained dancer, and is also currently pursuing her Ph.D. on Dance and Movement Therapy at TISS, Mumbai.

UMA CHAKRAVARTI taught history at Miranda House, University of Delhi, from 1966 to 2008. She is now an independent historian who writes on gender and caste in India.

PALLABI CHAKRAVORTY is Associate Professor and Director of the Dance Program, Department of Music and Dance, Swarthmore College. She teaches anthropology of dance, mapping culture and difference through dance, patterns of Asian dance and music, visual anthropology of performance, and Bombay film dance. She is a dancer and a choreographer, trained in Kathak under Guru Bandana Sen.

RATNABALI CHATTERJEE is former professor at the Department of Islamic History and Culture, University of Calcutta. She served as the Director of Women's Studies Research Centre University of Calcutta.

BISHNUPRIYA DUTT is currently Dean, School of Arts and Aesthetics, Jawaharlal Nehru University, New Delhi. She is also a Principle Investigator of the University Grants Commission (UGC) UK India Education Research Initiative (UKIERI) project. 'Gendered Citizenship: Manifestations and Performance', a multidisciplinary collaboration involving faculty and students from University of Warwick and Jawaharlal Nehru University, New Delhi. She is a scholar of theatre studies.

LUBNA MARIUM is General Secretary/Artistic Director of Shadhona, Dhaka. She is a dancer, choreographer, entrepreneur, and independent researcher, well-versed in Sanskrit and cultures in South Asia and is interested in dance and aesthetics and phenomenological perspectives of dance.

SADANAND MENON is an arts editor, journalist and cultural critic, photographer, and prolific speaker on politics, ecology and the arts. He is currently Adjunct Faculty, Asian College of Journalism, Chennai.

MAYA KRISHNA RAO is Professor at the Department of Education, School of Humanities and Social Sciences, Shiv Nadar University, Dadri, Uttar Pradesh. She is also a theatre practitioner trained in Kathakali, and has taught acting at the National School of Drama (NSD), Delhi. Her interests are in devising theatre, instant creations and the use of drama for community and children and actor training.

ALOKANANDA RAY is a classical dancer, dance educationist, choreographer, and social worker. She is the founder-director of Inspiration Foundation and is well-known for her work with the convicts of Presidency Correctional Home, Kolkata, as with other correctional homes of West Bengal where she uses dance for therapeutic purposes.

NIRMALA SESHADRI is a multidisciplinary artist, choreographer, movement educator, researcher, and writer. She is also the founder and artistic director of N Dance & Yoga. After twenty years of training and practice in Yoga, she also began devising a wellness and creativity-focused mind-body technique, Antarika, which she now imparts in the sphere of education.

Index

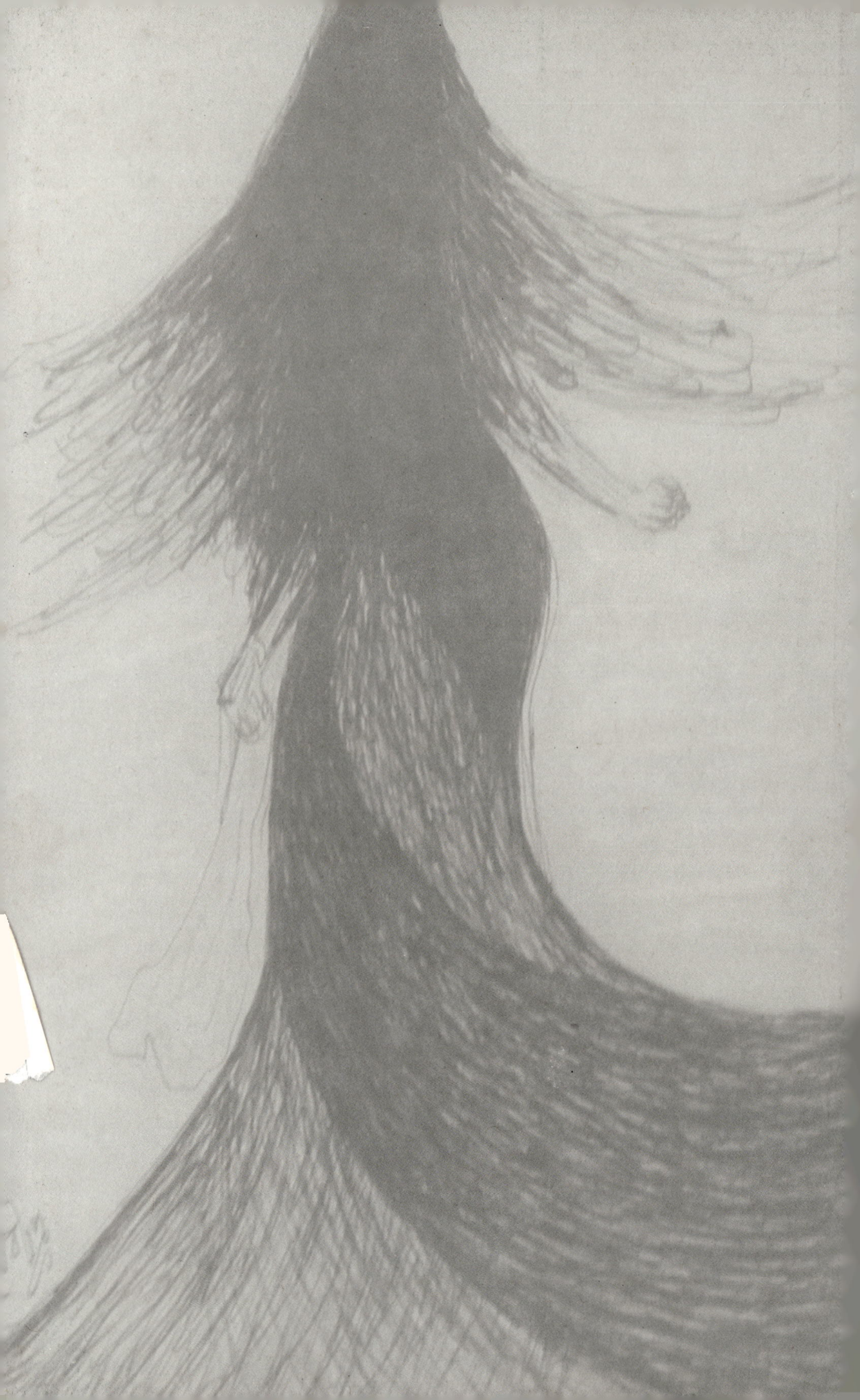